CHILDREN AT RISK

AN EVALUATION OF FACTORS CONTRIBUTING TO CHILD ABUSE AND NEGLECT

CHILDREN AT RISK

AN EVALUATION OF FACTORS CONTRIBUTING TO CHILD ABUSE AND NEGLECT

Edited by

ROBERT T. AMMERMAN

Western Pennsylvania School for Blind Children
Pittsburgh, Pennsylvania

and

MICHEL HERSEN

University of Pittsburgh
School of Medicine
Pittsburgh, Pennsylvania

PLENUM PRESS • NEW YORK AND LONDON

Library of Congress Cataloging-in-Publication Data

Children at risk : an evaluation of factors contributing to child
  abuse and neglect / edited by Robert T. Ammerman and Michel Hersen.
       p.   cm.
    Includes bibliographical references.
    Includes index.
    ISBN 0-306-43437-7
    1. Abused children--United States. 2. Child abuse--United States.
  3. Child abuse--United States--Prevention.   I. Ammerman, Robert T.
  II. Hersen, Michel.
    [DNLM: 1. Child Abuse--epidemiology. 2. Risk Factors.   WA 320
  C536517]
  HV741.C536135   1990
 _362.7'6'0973--dc20
  DNLM/DLC   72227
  for Library of Congress   90-7228
                                                               CIP

© 1990 Plenum Press, New York
A Division of Plenum Publishing Corporation
233 Spring Street, New York, N.Y. 10013

Printed in the United States of America

To Caroline and Helen

CONTRIBUTORS

ROBERT T. AMMERMAN, Western Pennsylvania School for Blind Children, Pittsburgh, Pennsylvania 15213

JAY BELSKY, Department of Individual and Family Studies, College of Health and Human Development, Pennsylvania State University, University Park, Pennsylvania 16802

BEVERLY A. BUSH, Department of Psychology, University of Maryland–Baltimore County, Catonsville, Maryland 21228

JUDITH A. COHEN, Department of Psychiatry, Western Psychiatric Institute and Clinic, University of Pittsburgh School of Medicine, Pittsburgh, Pennsylvania 15213

HOWARD DUBOWITZ, Department of Pediatrics, University of Maryland School of Medicine, Baltimore, Maryland 21201

DAVID C. FACTOR, TRE-ADD Program, Thistletown Regional Center for Children and Adolescents, Rexdale, Ontario, Canada M9V 4L8

JAMES GARBARINO, Erikson Institute for Advanced Study in Child Development, Chicago, Illinois 60610

ROY C. HERRENKOHL, Center for Social Research, Lehigh University, Bethlehem, Pennsylvania 18015

MICHEL HERSEN, Department of Psychiatry, Western Psychiatric Institute and Clinic, University of Pittsburgh School of Medicine, Pittsburgh, Pennsylvania 15213

JEFFREY A. KELLY, Division of Psychology, University of Mississippi Medical Center, Jackson, Mississippi 39216

JOHN R. LUTZKER, Department of Psychology, University of Judaism, Los Angeles, California 90077

ANTHONY P. MANNARINO, Department of Psychiatry, Western Psychiatric Institute and Clinic, University of Pittsburgh School of Medicine, Pittsburgh, Pennsylvania 15213

GARY B. MELTON, Department of Psychology, University of Nebraska–Lincoln, Lincoln, Nebraska 68588–0308

MAXINE R. NEWMAN, Department of Psychology, University of Judaism, Los Angeles, California 90077

RANDY K. OTTO, Department of Law and Mental Health, Florida Mental Health Institute, University of South Florida, Tampa, Florida 33612–3899

RAYMOND H. STARR, JR., Department of Psychology, University of Maryland–Baltimore County, Catonsville, Maryland 21228

JOAN I. VONDRA, Department of Psychology in Education, University of Pittsburgh, Pittsburgh, Pennsylvania 15260

DAVID A. WOLFE, Department of Psychology, University of Western Ontario, London, Ontario, Canada N6A 5B8

LISE M. YOUNGBLADE, Department of Individual and Family Studies, College of Health and Human Development, Pennsylvania State University, University Park, Pennsylvania 16802

PREFACE

During the past decade, a dramatic increase in research and clinical interest has risen in child abuse and neglect. This recent growth in awareness is due at least partly to the alarming statistics documenting the incidence of child maltreatment. Almost one million children are reported to be abused and neglected each year, and many experts believe that this figure underestimates the true incidence. Indeed, recent surveys suggest that almost 1.5 million children are the targets of domestic violence every year. A significant proportion of these children die as a function of this maltreatment, whereas the remainder suffer a variety of short- and long-term deleterious medical and psychosocial consequences. Child maltreatment is a universal problem that has precipitated a mobilization of effort from a variety of disciplines, including psychology, medicine, psychiatry, social work, sociology, and criminology.

Particular attention has been directed toward the prevention and treatment of child abuse and neglect. Such endeavors require the screening of large groups in order to identify families that are at high-risk for engaging in such behavior. Delineating those characteristics that differentiate high- from low-risk families and children is one of the obvious priorities for researchers and clinicians in the future. This book, therefore, carefully considers the status of research on risk factors of abuse and neglect in children. Adduced data undoubtedly will have practical value for subsequent intervention efforts. As research in child abuse and neglect approaches its fourth decade of modern investigation, it is especially timely to assess the progress made in this field and provide guidelines for future empirical work.

Children at Risk is divided into five parts. In Part I (Introduction), an overview of risk research is presented, and guidelines for continued empirical investigation are outlined. In Part II (General Issues), critical areas of child maltreatment are examined, including the epidemiology of abuse and neglect, legal issues, research practices and methodological approaches, and the psychosocial sequelae of maltreatment of child victims. Part III (Risk Factors Associated with Child Abuse and Neglect) includes evaluations of the three primary contributing factors to the etiology of maltreatment: sociological and ecological variables, parental characteristics, and child characteristics. Important new developments in the prevention and treatment of abuse and neglect are covered in Part IV (Prevention and Treatment). Finally, Part V (Conclusions) provides the agenda for future research and clinical endeavors in combatting child maltreatment.

A number of people devoted considerable time and effort in assisting us in the compilation of this volume, and their patience and dedication to the project are greatly appreciated. First, we thank the contributors who have graciously reviewed their respective areas of expertise. Second, we greatly appreciate the technical assistance provided by Mary Anne Frederick, Mary Jo Horgan, Jenifer McKelvey, Louise E. Moore, and Mary H. Newell. Third, we extend our gratitude to J. Lawrence Aber III for his helpful comments on our original outline for the book. Finally, we are indebted to the support and invaluable assistance provided by our editor, Eliot Werner, who proved himself a model of tolerance.

Robert T. Ammerman
Michel Hersen

Pittsburgh, Pennsylvania

CONTENTS

Chapter 3

Trends in Legislation and Case Law on Child Abuse
and Neglect 55

Randy K. Otto and Gary B. Melton

Chapter 4

Roy C. Herrenkohl

Chapter 5

Lise M. Youngblade and Jay Belsky

PART III. RISK FACTORS ASSOCIATED WITH CHILD ABUSE AND NEGLECT

Chapter 6

Joan I. Vondra

Chapter 7

David C. Factor and David A. Wolfe

Chapter 8

Robert T. Ammerman

PART IV. PREVENTION AND TREATMENT

Chapter 9

Maxine R. Newman and John R. Lutzker

Chapter 10

Anthony P. Mannarino and Judith A. Cohen

Chapter 11

Jeffrey A. Kelly

PART V. CONCLUSIONS

Chapter 12

James Garbarino

PART I

INTRODUCTION

CHAPTER 1

RESEARCH IN CHILD ABUSE AND NEGLECT

CURRENT STATUS AND AN AGENDA FOR THE FUTURE

ROBERT T. AMMERMAN AND MICHEL HERSEN

INTRODUCTION

It is common to decry the relative paucity of empirical research in newly emerging fields, and the area of child maltreatment is no exception. Yet, during the past decade, we have seen an explosion of investigative activity that has thrust research in child abuse and neglect to higher levels of understanding and sophistication. Indeed, the growth in knowledge has been so extensive that recent endeavors have brought the field to something of a watershed. Therefore, it is timely to assess the gains that have been achieved and review the changes in investigative practices and theoretical formulations that have thus far characterized the field. From a research perspective, a transition has occurred from unidimensional design approaches to multivariate strategies (e.g.,

ROBERT T. AMMERMAN • Western Pennsylvania School for Blind Children, Pittsburgh, Pennsylvania 15213. MICHEL HERSEN • Department of Psychiatry, Western Psychiatric Institute and Clinic, University of Pittsburgh School of Medicine, Pittsburgh, Pennsylvania 15213.

Gaines, Sandgrund, Green, & Power, 1978) that more adequately reflect the complex nature of child maltreatment. Similarly, current theoretical views reject single-factor explanations of maltreatment in favor of more intricate models describing the reciprocal interplay between causative variables in the development and maintenance of abuse and neglect (e.g., Starr, 1988; Wolfe, 1987). Although this shift in focus of attention from simplistic conceptualizations to complicated multicomponent models began in the late 1970s (Belsky, 1980) it is now almost universally acknowledged (Starr, 1988).

The dramatic growth in understanding the etiology and consequences of child abuse and neglect can be charted by the seminal articles and reviews that mark the progression of the field in its first 25 years (Belsky, 1980; Elmer & Gregg, 1967; Friedrich & Boriskin, 1976; Gelles, 1973; Kempe, Silverman, Steele, Droegemueller, & Silver, 1962; Parke & Collmer, 1975; Spinetta & Rigler, 1972). In fact, each of these contributions is as relevant today as when they were first published, because they highlight and underscore the critical methodological and conceptual issues faced by researchers of child maltreatment. Thus, although the field has advanced tremendously since the appearance of these works, their impact on current empirical efforts is considerable.

Kempe and coworkers (1962) were the first to describe the symptoms and characteristics of maltreated children and deserve credit for rekindling modern-day interest in this area. In addition to launching a field of scientific inquiry, they elucidated one of the most controversial problems in child abuse and neglect—how to define the phenomenon objectively—and relied primarily on physical evidence to identify abuse and neglect. The evidence included multiple fractures, bruises, scars, abrasions, and frequent accidents of suspicious origin. Since that time, however, a significant expansion has taken place in the definition of child maltreatment to comprise severe physical punishment without permanent injury, placing the child in dangerous situations, and emotional abuse (Brassard, Germain, & Hart, 1987). Although the broadening of criteria constituting child abuse and neglect has directed attention toward previously ignored maltreated populations, it also has led to methodological dilemmas and legal policy confusions (Besharov, 1982).

The pervasive deleterious consequences of maltreatment were first outlined by Elmer and Gregg (1967). Their short- and long-term evaluations of maltreatment (Elmer, 1977) documented the severe negative sequelae resulting from abuse and neglect in such areas of functioning as intelligence, academic achievement, social and cognitive development, and emotional adjustment. Although methodological limitations mitigate conclusions drawn from these studies, their efforts stimulated extensive research in the consequences of child abuse and neglect (see

Ammerman, Cassisi, Hersen, & Van Hasselt, 1986; Friedrich & Ein-bender, 1983).

The literature in the early and mid-1970s was dominated by the search for causative variables in maltreatment. Kempe *et al.* (1962) specu-lated that parental psychopathology was the most important determi-nant in the etiology of abuse and neglect. Subsequently, in their review, Spinetta and Rigler (1972) concluded that psychopathology and psychi-atric disorder in parents were crucial factors in the development of abuse and neglect. In turn, this review resulted in a burgeoning of more well-controlled empirical studies examining the characteristics of abusive par-ents. However, findings from these investigations failed to support Spinneta and Rigler's (1972) initial conclusions. Rather, although current data indicate that most abusive parents exhibit deficits in a variety of areas of functioning, they rarely suffer from severe psychiatric distur-bances (Wolfe, 1985).

On the other hand, Gelles (1973) proposed that societal factors are the primary causes of abuse and neglect. Within this framework, it is posited that maltreatment stems from stress engendered by poverty, educational disadvantage, and cultural sanctioning of physical punish-ment. Moreover, Gelles (1973) addressed the intergenerational transmis-sion of child abuse and outlined factors that led many abused children to grow up to become abusive parents. This model remains a major contri-bution to the understanding of the causes of child abuse and neglect, and has received compelling empirical support (e.g., Garbarino, 1976). However, it is clear that societal elements *alone* are neither necessary nor sufficient to bring about child maltreatment. Evidence for this derives from the fact that most families experiencing economic hardships do not engage in abuse and neglect. Similarly, child maltreatment occurs at all levels of socioeconomic status. Furthermore, the extent of intergenera-tional transmission of maltreatment does not appear to be as extensive as was previously posited (Kaufman & Zigler, 1987).

The next significant theoretical development in the field was Parke and Collmer's (1975) treatise hypothesizing that maltreatment was best understood within the context of the parent–child relationship. Specifi-cally, they contended that maltreatment was most likely to occur in particular situations (e.g., parent–child conflict) in which both parent (e.g., poor behavior management skills) and child (e.g., oppositionality) characteristics contribute to abuse. Thus, the interaction of parent, child, and situational variables combine and interact to result in domestic vio-lence. A large body of data has accrued supporting the social-situational approach (see Wolfe, 1987) and forming the basis of subsequent models of maltreatment.

Parke and Collmer's (1975) model suggests that the child can play a role in the development and maintenance of abuse. In their review of the literature up to that time, Friedrich and Boriskin (1976) speculated that certain child characteristics increased the risk of maltreatment. Contributing child risk factors consisted of prematurity, low birthweight, mental retardation, being unwanted, and the presence of a physical handicap. Other researchers (e.g., deLissovoy, 1979) broadened this supposition to include attributes that made the child more difficult to manage and, thus, "abuse-provoking." These factors include noncompliance, oppositionality, acting out, and hyperactivity. The importance of child variables in determining maltreatment risk has since become a matter of dispute. Although some authors suggest that certain selected child characteristics may contribute to the development of maltreatment (Ammerman, Van Hasselt, & Hersen, 1988), others reject this association (Starr, Dietrich, Fischhoff, Ceresnie, & Zweier, 1984).

Belsky (1980) provided one of the first integrations of causative factors into a multidimensional model. His ecological formulation describes the mutual influences of individual, situational, and societal variables in determining abuse and neglect. By identifying multiple elements of causative determination, he takes into account the finding that no single variable fully explains the development of maltreatment. Furthermore, this model reveals several levels of dysfunction that can be targeted for remedial intervention or prevention. Although subsequent formulations also use a multidimensional approach (e.g., Starr, 1988), Belsky's (1980) model can be credited with stimulating increased and more sophisticated theoretical and empirical efforts in this area.

The above articles do not constitute an exhaustive list of important contributions to the field of child abuse and neglect, but rather highlight salient progressions in the development of theory and research. Moreover, they underscore four critical issues that continue to challenge investigators: (1) the problem of objectively defining abuse and neglect, (2) determining the consequences and effects of maltreatment on children, (3) identifying causes and risk factors for abuse and neglect, and (4) using etiological models to develop effective treatments and prevention programs. The remainder of this chapter will review the current status of knowledge regarding these issues. In addition, future directions that empirical efforts might take in these areas will be presented.

THE PROBLEM OF DEFINITION

The study of child abuse and neglect has been impeded by the failure to establish a consensus regarding an objective operational definition of what constitutes maltreatment. Unfortunately, the diverse and, at times, competing needs of the fields involved in child abuse and neglect (e.g., criminology, public health, psychology, psychiatry, sociology) preclude reaching an agreement on acceptable criteria. Furthermore, by its very nature, child maltreatment is an ambiguous and elusive construct that defies precise explication.

Starr (1988) stated that there are four elements involved in defining child maltreatment: (1) the intentionality of the act, (2) the impact of the act on the child, (3) value judgments about the act, and (4) the cultural and societal standard upon which the act is evaluated. The fluctuating nature of these mediating factors differentially affects attempts to arrive at a universally acknowledged definition. Moreover, this task is further confounded by the private and socially undesirable nature of abuse and neglect. Information gathered typically derives from self-report or tangential evidence, both of which are susceptible to error, distortion, and confabulation.

Initially, the "battered child syndrome" (Kempe et al., 1962) was identified via objective evidence secondary to physical injury (i.e., burns, multiple fractures, bruises). Likewise, severe cases of neglect typically led to pervasive and observable negative consequences, such as poor hygiene, failure to thrive, and even death. Most instances of maltreatment, however, are not so severe as to result in such tangible consequences. In fact, 88% of reported cases of physical abuse involve minor physical injuries that usually do not result in permanent damage (American Humane Association, 1984). In addition, most instances of maltreatment consist of neglect which, in its less severe form, is largely dependent on the judgment of the professional involved. Thus, in the majority of cases, physical evidence will be sufficiently unclear or absent as to cast doubt upon the occurrence of abuse or neglect.

Psychological abuse also complicates efforts to define maltreatment clearly. Psychological or emotional maltreatment comprises repeated verbal assaults and manipulations that can lead to lowered self-esteem in the child (Garbarino & Vondra, 1987). Although victims of psychological abuse are often in need of therapeutic intervention, the construct has proven to be difficult to isolate and define succinctly.

Problems in defining child maltreatment affect researchers and service providers alike. Researchers select their samples based upon criteria that differ from study to study. The criteria used in these investigations include parents who have engaged in substantiated incidents of maltreatment, those who are referred to child protective service agencies because of suspicions regarding maltreatment, and those who are judged "at risk," based upon various standards determined by caseworkers and/or other clinicians. As a result, comparability across studies is limited. On the other hand, lawyers and criminal justice workers are more likely to emphasize physical evidence in determining the existence of maltreatment, as compared to the more vague definitions often used by social science researchers. These discrepancies have impacted upon attempts to reform legal guidelines regarding abuse and neglect (Mac-Murray & Carson, in press) as well as research efforts.

In summary, arriving at a universally accepted operational definition of maltreatment has proven to be a dilemma that is virtually insurmountable. The primary reasons for this finding include the private nature of abuse and neglect resulting in tangential and unclear indicators, and the reliance on fluctuating community-based standards and judgments regarding maltreatment. From a research perspective, however, all is not lost. Comparability and generalizability of studies is enhanced with clear descriptions of subject characteristics and recruitment methods. Although vague descriptions of methods have been the rule rather than the exception in child abuse and neglect research (Plotkin, Azar, Twentyman, & Perri, 1981), recent investigations provide more detailed information. Particularly noteworthy are the research efforts of Lutzker and his colleagues, whose subject descriptions are exemplary in their thoroughness and clarity (e.g., Barone, Green, & Lutzker, 1986; Lutzker, Megson, Webb, & Dachman, 1985).

CONSEQUENCES OF MALTREATMENT

Elmer and Gregg's (1967) seminal investigation suggested that the psychosocial effects of maltreatment on children are severe and pervasive. Since that time, extensive research has been conducted which has examined the sequelae of abuse and neglect. These studies have documented a variety of deficits and dysfunctions in maltreated children, including insecure attachment formation (Egeland & Sroufe, 1981), depression (Kazdin, Moser, Colbus, & Bell, 1985), anxiety (Green, 1978), conduct disturbance (McCord, 1983), poor peer relations (Bousha & Twentyman, 1984), academic underachievement (Morgan, 1979), and intellectual deficits (Hoffman-Plotkin, & Twentyman, 1984). In general, maltreated children are heterogeneous in terms of type and in severity of psychopathology. No syndrome has been identified that is specific to abused or neglected children, and no symptom is common to all victims of domestic assault (with the possible exception of insecure mother–infant attachment in maltreated infants). Although it is evident that the sequelae of maltreatment are deleterious, predicting their effects is impossible at this time (Ammerman *et al.*, 1986).

The varied clinical presentations of child victims of maltreatment are the result of several factors. First, the topographical characteristics of maltreatment differ from case to case; for example, some children only experience abuse or neglect, while others are abused *and* neglected. Other features of maltreatment that differentially mediate its effects consist of type of assault, severity of mistreatment, frequency of abuse, the situational context in which the assault takes place, the age of onset, and the length of maltreatment. Thus, it is possible that prolonged and frequent occurrences of relatively minor abuse are more highly associated with negative outcomes than a single-incident, severe assault. Although this is a widely held belief, there is little empirical research that examines the differential effects of varied forms of maltreatment.

A second determinant of the consequences of maltreatment is the biopsychological status of the child prior to abuse and/or neglect. Factors that enhance resiliency will mitigate negative sequelae and protect the child from long-term dysfunction. In similar fashion, increased vulnerability will maximize the likelihood that the maltreatment will have a detrimental effect. Resiliency and vulnerability, in turn, are determined by genetic factors, learning history, and ecological influences. The effects of maltreatment also are moderated by the developmental level of the child. Disruption and delay during critical developmental periods in mastering tasks involving social, affective, and cognitive skills and abilities will profoundly affect subsequent psychosocial growth. Indeed, recent findings confirm that children who are maltreated during infancy experience pervasive problems in a variety of developmental areas in later years (Egeland, Sroufe, & Erickson, 1983).

Although it is generally accepted that the features of maltreatment in combination with child characteristics will profoundly affect outcome, few investigations take such factors into account in evaluating the consequences of abuse and neglect. The reasons being (1) such data are extremely difficult to collect in *post hoc* studies, given their overreliance on error-prone parent reports, and (2) even when this information is available, it is very difficult to form homogeneous subgroups within subject samples for statistical comparison given recruitment limitations. However, researchers can address this problem in other ways. First, more detailed information about maltreatment characteristics should be collected and reported in the subject descriptions. Such instruments as the Child Abuse and Neglect Interview Schedule (CANIS) (Ammerman, Hersen, & Van Hasselt, 1987), a semistructured interview assessment of parents, can facilitate the gathering of detailed aspects of maltreatment. Second, broad distinctions between subgroups of maltreated samples can be made. For example, it was not until recently that researchers routinely differentiated abused from neglected children. Also, Kazdin and his colleagues (1985) contrasted abused children who had experienced past abuse, current abuse, and past *and* current abuse, whereas Kinard (1980, 1982) examined the effects of abuse characteristics on self-concept. Such studies as these are necessary if we are to isolate the relationship between types of maltreatment and their subsequent consequences.

Another problem in delineating the effects of abuse and neglect is the separation of maltreatment *per se* from other competing explanations of psychosocial dysfunction. Abuse and neglect rarely occur independently of other forms of family and individual psychopathology. Indeed, most theorists view maltreatment as a symptom of more global family dysfunction (Kelly, 1983; Starr, 1988; Wolfe, 1987). Therefore, identifying the effects of maltreatment independent of prolonged disturbances in family function is extremely difficult. A related concern is to determine cause and effect in maltreatment. Because much of the research in child abuse is retrospective, it is unclear to what extent psychopathology precedes or is caused by maltreatment. The most acceptable solution to these problems is the use of prospective longitudinal research designs. Such experimental strategies allow for the observation of the unfolding process of maltreatment and have yielded fruitful results when applied (Egeland & Brunnquell, 1979; Egeland *et al.*, 1983).

THE SEARCH FOR RISK FACTORS

From the early stages of research in child abuse and neglect, it was realized that delineating risk factors for maltreatment is of paramount importance. Identifying characteristics associated with risk is crucial in (1) the recognition and screening of maltreated children, and in (2) targeting populations in need of preventative intervention before abuse and neglect take place. In addition, the search for risk factors is intricately linked with the understanding of the etiology of child maltreatment.

As previously mentioned, initial formulations of risk focused on parental psychopathology. According to this approach, severe psychiatric disturbance (e.g., psychosis, antisocial personality) in perpetrators was thought to be the primary cause of maltreatment. Although recent evidence strongly disputes the role of severe parental psychopathology in maltreatment (see Wolfe, 1985), attention continues to be directed toward parental symptoms as risk factors. Indeed, a large proportion of research in child maltreatment has emphasized the study of parental characteristics. In general, these investigations have revealed a variety of features that distinguish maltreating from adequate care parents, including low-frustration tolerance, inappropriate expression of anger, social isolation, impaired parenting skills, unrealistic expectations of children, and a sense of incompetence in parenting (Wolfe, 1987). Research on parental contributions to maltreatment have produced useful results. Indeed, because maltreatment typically comprises the commission and/or omission of specific acts on the part of the parent or other adults, it is evident that parents should be the primary focus of attention in risk research.

However, several important limitations exist in the information gathered to date on this topic. First, although child abuse and neglect are committed by mothers, fathers, and non-parental figures, and occurs in all socioeconomic groups, research efforts have almost exclusively examined mothers from low SES backgrounds (Ammerman, 1989; Fantuzzo & Twentyman, 1986; Wolfe, 1987). This restricted range of investigation and sampling bias precludes a full understanding of the role of parental characteristics in child maltreatment. In particular, there is an urgent need to examine fathers implicated in maltreatment, given that they are involved in a significant proportion of substantiated reported cases and are more likely to inflict serious injury on maltreatment victims. A second concern is the relative paucity of prospective longitudinal research in the study of maltreatment. The bulk of empirical efforts in this area consist of *post hoc* comparisons of maltreating and non-maltreating parents. Thus, although it is clear that many abusive parents have poor parenting skills, it is not clear to what extent parents with these characteristics eventually become abusive and/or neglectful themselves. Such a distinction is critical for the development of prevention programs, because it is appropriate to target parents with poor parenting skills as a high-risk group *only* if a large percentage of them are likely to become maltreating. An important exception to this shortcoming in the literature is the work of Egeland and his colleagues (Egeland, Breitenbucher, & Rosenberg, 1980). Their prospective longitudinal research has done much to further our understanding of factors involved in the development of maltreatment. For example, Egeland *et al.* (1980) identified stress as an important determinant of maltreatment, especially in mothers who lack parenting skills and knowledge of children. Their empirical efforts, however, await replication and expansion.

Although child abuse and neglect occur at all socioeconomic levels, it has been noted for some time that a disproportionate percentage of maltreated children come from lower socioeconomic status (SES) families. Indeed, it seems logical that violence may emerge when individuals are confronted with severe and prolonged stress and hardship in the form of economic disadvantage, poverty, limited educational opportunity, and unemployment. The focus on societal risk factors has provided much insight into the antecedents of maltreatment. Indeed, Garbarino (1977) concludes from his research that such stressors in combination with social isolation lead to maltreatment. Despite the compelling evidence for the salience of social factors in maltreatment, such variables are of limited utility in determining risk status. As with parenting characteristics in abuse and neglect, the majority of economically disadvantaged families *do not* engage in maltreatment. Thus, viewing this population as being at high risk for abuse or neglect would result in a large number of inaccurately labeled families. Societal factors alone, therefore, are inadequate risk markers despite their prominent role in the origins of maltreatment.

The employment of child characteristics as risk factors has long been a source of speculation (Friedrich & Boriskin, 1976). In particular, samples of abused and neglected children contain a disproportionate amount of children with (1) prematurity, (2) low birthweight, (3) mental retardation, and (4) physical and/or sensory handicaps (see Ammerman et al., 1988). In addition, difficult to manage children (e.g., those with Attention Deficit Hyperactivity Disorder) have been posited to be at high risk for maltreatment. The processes through which children might play a role in the development of abuse is unclear, although disruptions in mother–infant attachment (Ainsworth, 1980), increased stress engendered by difficult to manage children (Ammerman et al., 1988), physiological arousal (Frodi, 1981), and heightened vulnerability to maltreatment (Morgan, 1987) have been proposed as possible explanations. Unfortunately, the majority of investigations of this topic utilize retrospective designs that have yielded unclear findings (see Starr et al., 1984). Moreover, the few prospective and longitudinal studies that have been conducted do not indicate that child characteristics are significantly involved in the development of abuse (Egeland & Brunnquell, 1979). There is convincing evidence, however, that oppositional and defiant children are involved in the exacerbation of parent–child conflict that can lead to an abusive incident (Loeber, Felton, & Reid, 1984). Also, some authors propose that certain populations of children (e.g., severely disabled, aggressive and oppositional) may be at heightened risk for abuse (Ammerman, Hersen, Van Hasselt, McGonigle, & Lubetsky, 1989), although such hypotheses await further empirical examination.

In summary, the search for risk factors in maltreatment have emphasized the contributions of parental, societal, and child characteristics. Although each of these provides a partial explanation of the etiology of maltreatment, and therefore suggests appropriate markers for risk, no one variable is sufficiently sensitive or specific to be used in the reliable identification of high-risk groups. Because of limited resources, it is virtually impossible to employ such broad criteria in accurately targeting populations for preventative interventions.

In response to the above problems in delineating risk factors for maltreatment, a number of authors have proposed multicomponent models of abuse and neglect (Belsky, 1980; Starr, 1988). These formulations acknowledge the varied causative paths that lead to the development of maltreatment. Although highlighting the importance of considering multiple levels of influence in etiology, these conceptualizations do not elucidate *how* contributing factors combine to bring about high risk of abuse and neglect. Understanding the processes involved in domestic violence, however, is crucial to the discovery of reliable risk markers.

Recent theoretical efforts have addressed issues of process in child maltreatment. Indeed, Burgess and Drapier (1988) view the interactional elements in family violence as critical in differentiating abusive from nonabusive problem families. In addition, of particular value is Wolfe's (1987) Transitional Model, in which abuse is conceptualized as growing out of three tiers of escalating conflict. Specifically, these are the three stages through which families pass in the development of violent domestic conflict: (1) Reduced Tolerance of Stress and Disinhibition of Aggression, (2) Poor Management of Acute Crises and Provocation, and (3) Habitual Patterns of Arousal and Aggression with Family Members. Within each stage there are destabilizing factors that increase the likelihood of aggression, and compensatory factors that mitigate the escalation of conflict. A variety of combinations of destabilizing and compensatory factors are possible that serve to promote or inhibit the probability of abuse. This model is the first to propose the specific elements that can contribute to an increase or lessening of risk for abuse. It also delineates how diverse interactions of variables can combine to form multiple pathways to maltreatment. Most importantly, the utility of the Transitional Model can be examined empirically. Future progress in the field will largely depend upon formulations such as this one, and their subsequent evaluation.

TREATMENT AND PREVENTION

One of the most significant developments to emerge in the past decade is a growing literature on the treatment and prevention of abuse and neglect. The need for remedial programs for maltreating families was recognized early, and a good deal of attention has since focused on perpetrators (see Ammerman, 1989). More recently, a number of authors have identified the implementation and evaluation of prevention programs as the single most important objective in the area of child abuse and neglect (Starr, 1988).

At this point, the primary form of intervention with maltreating families is medical and legal. As many children first come to the attention of medical professionals because of injuries stemming from maltreatment, physicians and nurses are called upon to provide emergency services and refer families to appropriate social agencies. Child protective services carry out preliminary legal interventions and determine the child's disposition based upon safety concerns. However, such medical and legal actions are predominantly reactive and crisis oriented. The long-term functioning of maltreated children and their families depends upon remedial programs designed to prevent the recurrence of maltreatment and enhance overall family adjustment.

Initial treatment efforts with perpetrators involved psychodynamic interventions based upon the premise that maltreating parents suffered from severe psychiatric disorders (see Kelly, 1983). Other programs, derived from findings implicating social factors and stress as causes of maltreatment, consisted of providing abusive and neglectful parents with in-home counselors to provide support and guidance in parenting. To a large degree, these approaches have received little empirical evaluation, although some evidence supports the use of in-home staff in preventing further maltreatment (see Rosenberg & Reppucci, 1985).

The greatest gains in the development of effective treatments have come from behavior therapy. These interventions grow out of the application of social learning theory to maltreatment and the expanding literature documenting a variety of psychosocial skills deficits in abusive and neglectful parents (see Ammerman, 1989). Behavioral interventions are competency-based and emphasize the acquisition of skills needed for effective parenting (Kelly, 1983). Typical treatment components include training in anger control, child management skills, stress reduction, and (in the case of neglect) home safety skills. Most importantly, these therapeutic approaches have been subjected to scientific scrutiny. On the whole, treatment outcome studies have demonstrated the short-term efficacy of these approaches to reduce recurrence of maltreatment and enhance overall family functioning. Several questions, however, need to be addressed in future clinical research investigations. First, it is unclear if treatment gains are maintained for longer than one year. Although recidivism data indicate a moderate decrease in maltreatment recurrence in treated relative to nontreated abusive and neglectful families (Lutzker & Rice, 1987), long-term follow-ups of more than 1 year for individual families have yet to be conducted. And second, research in this area has not evaluated if behavior therapy has broader beneficial effect beyond the specific areas targeted for change. Because maltreatment is acknowledged to be a reflection of more pervasive family dysfunction, it is imperative that future investigations conduct more comprehensive assessments in order to elucidate the full effects of behavioral interventions.

A relatively recent development is the treatment of child victims of abuse and maltreatment. This population has largely been ignored in the empirical literature, although anecdotal suggestions for treatment abound (Walker, Bonner, & Kaufman, 1988). Fantuzzo and his colleagues (Fantuzzo, Jurecic, Stovall, Hightower, Goins, & Schachtel, 1988), however, have demonstrated the usefulness of peer prompts to improve the social functioning of withdrawn abused children. Other areas of child dysfunction have not yet been investigated. Continued efforts in this direction are needed if we are to provide optimal care to maltreated children.

Finally, as previously mentioned, the creation and examination of preventative programs are critical for the next decade of child abuse research. Lutzker has led the way in this area with Project 12-Ways, a multicomponent secondary prevention program designed to help maltreating families and prevent recurrence of abuse and neglect (Lutzker, 1984). Short-term efficacy of Project 12-Ways has been documented (Lutzker, Campbell & Watson-Perczel, 1984), and long-term prevention appears to be quite promising (Lutzker & Rice, 1987). Moreover, his efforts, have stimulated similar programs with populations thought to be at high-risk for maltreatment (Ammerman, 1988).

Others have strongly advocated the use of primary prevention approaches to reach a larger population at risk for engaging in maltreatment (Starr, 1988). Even though such efforts are the major priorities for the future, empirical data regarding their efficacy are unavailable at this time. Moreover, as the debate continues over appropriate risk factors for maltreatment, it will be necessary to identify those populations that are most in need for preventative intervention. Wolfe (1987) suggests a multilevel prevention approach in which subpopulations at risk are recognized and given appropriate programs relevant to their specific areas of need. Thus, parents experiencing frequent and severe conflicts with their children may require group or individual training in behavior management skills. Socially isolated parents, on the other hand, may warrant community outreach or educational programs. According to this strategy, resources are allocated based upon level of risk and area of need. Given the heterogeneity of maltreating families, it is most likely that prevention programs emphasizing varied target populations and levels of intervention will have the greatest likelihood of success. Such efforts, however, await empirical investigation.

SUMMARY

It is encouraging that both the public and the research community have recently taken an active interest in child abuse and neglect. The past 25 years have seen tremendous growth in scientific investigation, and this has led to a complementary increase in our understanding of the antecedents and consequences of maltreatment. Although plagued by methodological impediments, research in child abuse and neglect has elucidated the contributing factors in etiology. In addition, promising developments in the treatment of perpetrators and child victims have emerged. The future holds promise, providing that researchers attend to the multivariate nature of maltreatment, and that they will direct their efforts toward the development, implementation, and empirical evaluation of comprehensive assessment, treatment, and prevention strategies.

ACKNOWLEDGMENTS

Preparation of this chapter was facilitated in part by grant No. G008720109 from the National Institute on Disabilities and Rehabilitation Research, U. S. Department of Education, and a grant from the Vira I. Heinz Endowment. However, the opinions reflected herein do not necessarily reflect the position of policy of the U. S. Department of Education or the Vira I. Heinz Endowment, and no official endorsement should be inferred. The authors wish to thank Mary Jo Horgan for her assistance in preparation of the manuscript.

REFERENCES

Ainsworth, M. D. (1980). Attachment and child abuse. In G. Gerber, C. Ross, & E. Zigler (Eds.), *Child abuse: An agenda for action* (pp. 35–47). New York: Oxford University Press.

American Humane Association. (1984). *Highlights of official child neglect and abuse reporting 1982.* Denver, CO: Author.

Ammerman, R. T. (1989). Child abuse and neglect. In M. Hersen (Ed.), *Innovations in child behavior therapy* (pp. 353–394). New York: Springer.

Ammerman, R. T. (1988). Prevention of mother-child problems in families with young multihandicapped children. *International Journal of Rehabilitation Research, 11,* 416–417.

Ammerman, R. T., Cassisi, J. E., Hersen, M., & Van Hasselt, V. B. (1986). Consequences of physical abuse and neglect in children. *Clinical Psychology Review, 6,* 291–310.

Ammerman, R. T., Hersen, M., & Van Hasselt, V. B. (1987). *The Child Abuse and Neglect Interview Schedule (CANIS).* Unpublished manuscript, Western Pennsylvania School for Blind Children, Pittsburgh, Pennsylvania.

Ammerman, R. T., Van Hasselt, V. B., & Hersen, M. (1988). Maltreatment in handicapped children: A critical review. *Journal of Family Violence, 3,* 53–72.

Ammerman, R. T., Hersen, M., Van Hasselt, V. B., McGonigle, J. J., & Lubetsky, M. (1989). Abuse and neglect in psychiatrically hospitalized multihandicapped children. *Child Abuse and Neglect, 13,* 335–343.

Barone, V. J., Green, B. V., & Lutzker, J. R. (1986). Home safety with families being treated for child abuse and neglect. *Behavior Modification, 10,* 93–114.

Belsky, J. (1980). Child maltreatment: An ecological integration. *American Psychologist, 35,* 320–335.

Besharov, D. J. (1982). Toward better research on child abuse and neglect: Making definitional issues an explicit methodological concern. *Child Abuse and Neglect, 5,* 383–390.

Bousha, D. M., & Twentyman, C. T. (1984). Mother-child interactional style in abuse, neglect, and control groups: Naturalistic observations in the home. *Child Development, 93,* 196–114.

Brassard, M. R., Germain, R., & Hart, S. N. (Eds.). (1987). *Psychological maltreatment of children and youth.* New York: Pergamon Press.

Burgess, R. L., & Draper, P. (1988). A biosocial theory of family violence: The role of natural selection, ecological instability, and coercive interpersonal contingencies. In L. Ohlin & M. H. Tonry (Eds.), *Crime and justice—an annual review of research: Family violence.* Chicago: University of Chicago Press.

deLissovoy, V. (1979). Toward the definition of "abuse provoking child." *Child Abuse and Neglect, 3,* 341–350.

Egeland, B., Breitenbucher, M., & Rosenberg, D. (1980). Prospective study of significance of etiology of child abuse. *Journal of Consulting and Clinical Psychology, 48,* 195–205.

Egeland, B., & Brunnquell, D. (1979). An at-risk approach to the study of child abuse. *Journal of the American Academy of Child Psychiatry, 18,* 219–236.

Egeland, B., & Sroufe, L. A. (1981). Attachment and early maltreatment. *Child Development, 52,* 44–52.

Egeland, B., Sroufe, L. A., & Erickson, M. (1983). The developmental consequences of different patterns of maltreatment. *Child Abuse and Neglect, 7,* 459–469.

Elmer, E. (1977). *Fragile families, troubled children: The aftermath of infant trauma.* Pittsburgh: University of Pittsburgh Press.

Elmer, E., & Gregg, G. S. (1967). Developmental characteristics of abused children. *Pediatrics, 40,* 596–602.

Fantuzzo, J. W., Jurecic, L., Stovall, A., Hightower, A. D., Goins, C., & Schachtel, D. (1988). Effects of adult and peer social initiations on the social behavior of withdrawn, maltreated preschool children. *Journal of Consulting and Clinical Psychology, 56,* 34–39.

Fantuzzo, J. W., & Twentyman, C. T. (1986). Child abuse and psychotherapy research:

Merging social concerns and empirical investigation. *Professional Psychology: Research and Practice, 17,* 375–380.

Friedrich, W. N., & Boriskin, J. A. (1976). The role of the child in abuse: A review of the literature. *American Journal of Orthopsychiatry, 46,* 580–590.

Friedrich, W. N., & Einbender, A. J. (1983). The abused child: A psychological review. *Journal of Clinical Child Psychology, 12,* 244–256.

Frodi, A. M. (1981). Contribution of infant characteristics to child abuse. *American Journal of Mental Deficiency, 85,* 341–349.

Gaines, R., Sandgrund, A., Green, A. H., & Power, E. (1978). Etiological factors in child maltreatment: A multivariate study of abusing, neglecting, and normal mothers. *Journal of Abnormal Psychology, 87,* 531–540.

Garbarino, J. (1976). A preliminary study of some ecological correlates of child abuse: The impact of socioeconomic stress on mothers. *Child Development, 47,* 178–185.

Garbarino, J. (1977). The human ecology of child maltreatment: A conceptual model for research. *Journal of Marriage and the Family, 39,* 721–735.

Garbarino, J., & Vondra, J. (1987). Psychological maltreatment: Issues and perspectives. In M. R. Brassard, R. Germain, & S. N. Hart (Eds.), *Psychological maltreatment of children and youth* (pp. 25–44). New York: Pergamon Press.

Gelles, R. J. (1973). Child abuse as psychopathology: A sociological critique and reformulation. *American Journal of Orthopsychiatry, 43,* 611–621.

Green, A. H. (1978). Psychopathology of abused children. *Journal of the American Academy of Child Psychiatry, 17,* 92–103.

Hoffman-Plotkin, D., & Twentyman, C. T. (1984). A multimodel assessment of behavioral and cognitive deficits in abused and neglected preschoolers. *Child Development, 55,* 794–802.

Kaufman, J., & Zigler, E. (1987). Do abusive children become abusive parents? *American Journal of Orthopsychiatry, 57,* 186–192.

Kazdin, A. E., Moser, J., Colbus, D., & Bell, R. (1985). Depressive symptoms among physically abused and psychiatrically disturbed children. *Journal of Consulting and Clinical Psychology, 94,* 298–307.

Kelly, J. A. (1983). *Treating child abusive families: Intervention based on skills-training principles.* New York: Plenum Press.

Kempe, C. H., Silverman, F. N., Steele, B. F., Droegemueller, W., & Silver, H. K. (1962). The battered child syndrome. *Journal of the American Medical Association, 181,* 105–112.

Kinard, E. M. (1980). Emotional development in physically abused children. *American Journal of Orthopsychiatry, 50,* 686–696.

Kinard, E. M. (1982). Experiencing child abuse. Effects on emotional adjustment. *American Journal of Orthopsychiatry, 52,* 82–91.

Loeber, R., Felton, D. K., & Reid, J. (1984). A social learning approach to the reduction of coercive processes in child abusive families: A molecular analysis. *Advances in Behavior Research and Therapy, 6,* 29–45.

Lutzker, J. R. (1984). Project 12-Ways: Treating child abuse and neglect from an eco-behavioral perspective. In R. F. Dangel & R. A. Polster (Eds.), *Parent training: Foundations of research and practice* (pp. 260–297). New York: Guilford Press.

Lutzker, J. R. Campbell, R. V., & Watson-Perczel, M. (1984). Using the case study method to treat several problems in a family indicated for child neglect. *Education and Treatment of Children, 7,* 315–333.

Lutzker, J. R., Megson, D. A., Webb, M. E., & Dachman, R. S. (1985). Validating and training adult-child interaction skills to professionals and to parents indicated for child abuse and neglect. *Journal of Child and Adolescent Psychotherapy, 2,* 91–104.

Lutzker, J. R., & Rice, J. M. (1987). Using recidivism data to evaluate Project 12-Ways: An ecobehavioral approach to the treatment and prevention of child abuse and neglect. *Journal of Family Violence, 2,* 283–290.

MacMurray, B. K., & Carson, B. A. (in press). Legal issues in violence toward children. In R. T. Ammerman & M. Hersen (Eds.), *Case studies in family violence.* New York: Plenum Press.

McCord, J. (1983). A 40-year perspective on effects of child abuse and neglect. *Child Abuse and Neglect, 7,* 265–270.

Morgan, S. R. (1979). Psycho-educational profile of emotionally disturbed abused children. *Journal of Clinical Child Psychology, 8,* 3–6.

Morgan, S. R. (1987). *Abuse and neglect of handicapped children.* Boston: Little, Brown.

Parke, R. D., & Collmer, C. W. (1975). Child abuse: An interdisciplinary analysis. In E. M. Hetherington (Ed.), *Review of child development research* (Vol. 5, pp. 509–590). Chicago: University of Chicago Press.

Plotkin, R. C., Azar, S., Twentyman, C. T., & Perri, M. G. (1981). A critical evaluation of the research methodology employed in the investigation of causative factors of child abuse and neglect. *Child Abuse and Neglect, 5,* 449–455.

Rosenberg, M. S., & Reppucci, N. D. (1985). Primary prevention of child abuse. *Journal of Consulting and Clinical Psychology, 53,* 576–585.

Spinetta, J. J., & Rigler, D. (1972). The child abusing parent: A psychological review. *Psychological Bulletin, 77,* 296–304.

Starr, R. H., Jr. (1988). Physical abuse of children. In V. B. Van Hasselt, R. L. Morrison, A. S. Bellack, & M. Hersen (Eds.), *Handbook of family violence* (pp. 119–155). New York: Plenum Press.

Starr, R. H., Dietrich, K. N., Fischhoff, J., Ceresnie, S., & Zweier, D. (1984). The contribution of handicapping conditions to child abuse. *Topics in Early Childhood Special Education, 4,* 55–69.

Walker, C. E., Bonner, B. L., & Kaufman, K. L. (1988). *The physically and sexually abused child: Evaluation and treatment.* New York: Pergamon Press.

Wolfe, D. A. (1985). Child abusive parents: An empirical review and analysis. *Psychological Bulletin, 97,* 462–482.

Wolfe, D. A. (1987). *Child abuse: Implications for child development and psychopathology.* Newbury Park, CA: Sage Publications.

PART II

GENERAL ISSUES

Chapter 2

THE EPIDEMIOLOGY OF CHILD MALTREATMENT

RAYMOND H. STARR, JR., HOWARD DUBOWITZ, AND BEVERLY A. BUSH

INTRODUCTION

Articles about child maltreatment appear daily in almost every metropolitan newspaper. It seems that children are being injured, molested, and even killed at an alarming rate. In an attempt to understand child maltreatment, the first question to ask is what do we really know about the extent of the problem? Answering that question is the purpose of this chapter.

The first part of this chapter deals with the critical need to define child maltreatment. Epidemiology cannot be considered independently of the definition of differing types of abuse and neglect. The next section of the chapter summarizes the results of three different types of study: (1) analyses of reported maltreatment cases, (2) examinations of both reported and unreported cases known to professionals, and (3) surveys of maltreatment among the general public. The implications of these data are discussed in the final section of the chapter.

RAYMOND H. STARR, JR. AND BEVERLY A. BUSH • Department of Psychology, University of Maryland–Baltimore County, Catonsville, Maryland 21228.   HOWARD DUBOWITZ • Department of Pediatrics, University of Maryland School of Medicine, Baltimore, Maryland 21201.

BASIC EPIDEMIOLOGICAL CONCEPTS

Epidemiology is "the study of the distribution and determinants of diseases and injuries in human populations" (Mausner & Kramer, 1985, p. 1). Thus, the field deals not only with issues of the incidence (the rate at which new cases occur in the population) and prevalence (the number of cases in a designated population at a given time or over a specific time period), but also with the risk factors that predispose particular persons or subgroups of the population to developing the condition of concern (Last, 1983). The purpose of epidemiological studies is to provide knowledge about disease and injury patterns that will aid in their treatment and prevention. This chapter focuses on current knowledge concerning the incidence and prevalence of maltreatment, problems in their determination, and what is known about broad, demographic risk factors. Discussion of more specific, individual risk factors will be limited because they are outlined in detail elsewhere in this volume.

THE DEFINITION OF CHILD MALTREATMENT

A fundamental starting point for examining the etiology of a problem is to define it. Unless a problem is defined, it will be impossible to determine its extent. Four factors are involved in defining maltreatment: (1) the intentionality of the act, (2) the effect of the act on the child, (3) the value judgment society makes about the act, and (4) the standard used to make the judgment (Garbarino & Gilliam, 1980).

A lack of definitional clarity in maltreatment research complicates the task of understanding its epidemiology. The most common definitions of different types of maltreatment are those specified in the Child Abuse Prevention and Treatment Act (National Center on Child Abuse and Neglect [NCCAN], 1988). Although most states have adopted these definitions, some modify them, making the direct comparison of reported cases from state to state difficult. Thus, there are many competing definitions of child maltreatment, none of which is universally accepted.

This is so because child abuse, in its various manifestations, resists easy definition. For example, Swedish law bans "all forms of physical punishment and other injurious or humiliating treatment of children" (Radda Barnen, 1980, p. 7) by parents. Most American parents would find such a law unduly restrictive while Swedish parents would see many routine acts of U.S. parents as abusive. Definitional differences occur not only between but within cultures (Korbin, 1987), further complicating the issue.

Not only are there different definitions of child maltreatment, but these often vary across professions, researchers, states, and agencies (Giovannoni & Becerra, 1979). Some of these differences were examined by Gelles (1982) and by Giovannoni and Becerra (1979) in studies in which members of various professional disciplines involved in child protection were asked to designate whether a number of acts were or were not maltreatment. The studies concluded that professionals do not use a consistent set of criteria in defining and reporting child maltreatment. However, Gelles concluded that judgments of intentionality were particularly important, because intentional acts are more likely to be reported. In spite of this finding, it must be remembered that intent is particularly difficult to determine. For example, how can intention be evaluated when significant parental psychopathology is a factor in a case of abuse?

Legal definitions of maltreatment typically are vague. Thus, the specific behaviors that constitute maltreatment often are not clearly stated; and such undefined terms as *mental suffering* and *unfit* abound (Giovannoni & Becerra, 1979). Some experts believe that definitional vagueness is desirable because it allows social service workers to consider specific, individual details of a particular case. Others think vagueness can lead to inconsistent case handling and due process violations (Valentine, Acuff, Freeman, & Andreas, 1984). At best, a definition can never be more than a guide. Each case of maltreatment is complex and, regardless of comprehensiveness, a definition cannot provide a simple answer to every case.

Because of the primacy of definitional issues, the remainder of this section consists of a brief presentation of specific issues. Rather than propose a uniform set of definitions, specific definitional criteria will be included in the discussion of individual studies of the epidemiology of maltreatment.

Child maltreatment is usually categorized into three types of abuse and two types of neglect: physical, psychological, and sexual abuse; and physical and psychological neglect. The major distinction between abuse and neglect is that the former typically involves an act of commission whereas neglect is the result of an omission.

Physical Abuse

Physical abuse occurs when a child is injured by a parent or other caregiver. Beyond this criterion other aspects of definitions are typically vague. Additional factors that may play a role in defining physical abuse include parental approaches to discipline, intent to injure, the effect of an act on the child, and the vulnerability of the child. Some of these variables, such as intent, are difficult—if not impossible—to assess. This increases the vagueness of definitions in which intent is a factor. A key variable that must be examined is whether the intent was to cause pain, in which case an act may not be considered physically abusive, or to physically injure, in which case abuse is more likely. In addition, in cases of repeated injury where parental psychopathology is likely to be present, it also is difficult to infer intent because of the psychopathology. Thus, the criterion of intent to injure, combined with other family circumstances, makes the definition of physical abuse complex.

As was indicated earlier, definitions of abuse vary between different professions. For example, a pediatrician may see spanking an infant as undesirable and possibly abusive and will talk with the parents about the negative effects of corporal punishment; a protective services worker might have more stringent criteria requiring bruises or other injuries to validate a report of physical abuse; and a prosecutor might work only with even narrower criteria. In addition to varying between the professions, working definitions also differ considerably within members of the same profession. It is just this sort of definitional variability that complicates the study of the epidemiology of child maltreatment.

PHYSICAL NEGLECT

Physical neglect is more difficult to define than physical abuse. Specific, child-centered criteria for diagnosing a case of neglect usually are missing. However, the more inadequate a parent's caregiving is, the more likely it is that parents and professionals will agree that it is physically neglectful (Polansky & Williams, 1978). For example, there is likely to be agreement that a child who has not been fed and whose diaper has not been changed for a day has indeed been neglected. In other, more ambiguous cases professionals have difficulty deciding if the injury to a child is the result of an act of omission or commission. For example, do we classify as physically abused or as physically neglected those children who are born with fetal alcohol syndrome or addicted to narcotics? Furthermore, homeless children represent still another gray area (Dubowitz, 1987).

PSYCHOLOGICAL ABUSE AND PSYCHOLOGICAL NEGLECT

Psychological maltreatment is a more abstract concept than physical maltreatment. Evidence often is intangible and more difficult to attribute to a specific parental behavior. Definitional variability is common. Some investigators think that any distinction between psychological abuse and psychological neglect is artificial (Garbarino, Guttman, & Seeley,

1986). Garbarino *et al.* believe that there is significant damage to a child's psyche in both cases and, therefore, argue for the primacy of the psyche in all types of maltreatment. However, the physical and not the psychological consequences of a parental action or inaction usually cause society to label the act as abusive or neglectful. Although the psychological damage typically lasts longer than the physical injury, all the varying effects of maltreatment must be considered. In contrast to Garbarino and coworkers, Whiting (1976) distinguished between psychological abuse and neglect. For Whiting, psychological abuse is present when parents cause a child to become emotionally disturbed; psychological neglect occurs when they refuse to allow their emotionally disturbed child to receive treatment.

Protective service agencies typically become involved in only the most severe cases of psychological maltreatment because of the difficulty in proving that parental acts cause a child to develop patterns of disturbed behavior (Dubowitz, 1987). Typically, psychological maltreatment is classified as abuse or neglect only when it is extreme, or when other forms of maltreatment are also present.

SEXUAL ABUSE

Sexual abuse is also difficult to define. This difficulty is partly the result of societal attitudes concerning sexuality and partly due to the fact that sexual abuse can involve family members or extrafamilial contacts. Additionally, there is a lack of consensus on what acts are sexually abusive. There need not be obvious physical injury, physical contact, or psychological harm for some definitions to classify a child as sexually abused. One study evaluated the role of various factors as determinants of sexual abuse and concluded that, in declining order, the most important factors leading those surveyed to see an act as sexual abuse were (1) the perpetrator's age, (2) the nature of the act, (3) whether the child consented to the act, (4) the age of the victim, (5) the sex and relatedness of victim and perpetrator, and (6) the consequences of the act for the child (Finkelhor, 1979).

SUMMARY

It can be concluded that "a myth of shared meaning surrounds the general area of child maltreatment and the specific area of child sexual abuse" (Haugaard & Reppucci, 1988, p. 29). Different professions use various definitions. Also, there is no consistency in the working definitions used within professions. For example, researchers use definitions in their studies that vary from those used in legal jurisdictions. These and other aforementioned problems impede the task of accurately determining the epidemiology of child maltreatment.

THE INCIDENCE AND PREVALENCE
OF CHILD MALTREATMENT

The epidemiology of child maltreatment has been examined in a number of ways. At the broadest level there are studies and surveys tabulating reported cases (American Humane Association, 1984; American Association for Protecting Children [AAPC], 1985, 1986, 1987, 1988; National Center on Child Abuse and Neglect [NCCAN], 1981, 1988; A. Russell & Trainor, 1984). More narrowly, there are numerous studies indicating the incidence of specific types of abuse (Gelles, 1978; Gil, 1973; Kinsey, Pomeroy, Martin, & Gebhard, 1953; Straus & Gelles, 1986; D. E. H. Russell, 1983, 1984).

It is helpful to consider the samples included in epidemiological studies as falling on a five-point continuum (NCCAN, 1988). At the first level there are cases reported to child protective services (CPS). At a second level there are maltreated children who have been detected by or referred to other agencies with investigative powers (e.g., police, public health departments) but who are not officially classified as abused or neglected. Cases of maltreatment known to noninvestigatory agencies (e.g., hospitals, mental health centers, schools) and not officially reported constitute the third level. Although these children are maltreated, professionals often do not file a report for a number of reasons—such as a belief that they are better able to help the family than CPS workers. At the next level are cases in which a lay person recognizes maltreatment but does not report it. Finally, at the fifth level, there are maltreated children who are not recognized as abused or neglected by anyone.

Analyses of Reported Maltreatment

Reported cases of child maltreatment,* those at the first level of the NCCAN (1988) categorization, are an important measure of incidence.

---

*Strictly speaking, we cannot discuss incidence and prevalence with regard to reported cases. Incidence figures may be inflated by reports of maltreatment of children already known to child protective services personnel who do not represent *new* cases. Similarly, prevalence cannot be determined based on reports, only on the total number of cases currently considered maltreated. For consistency, we use the terms rate and incidence in analyzing reporting practices in this chapter.

The American Association for Protect   ᴧnd its parent agency, the American Humane Ass   ɾunded since
1974 to prepare annual summaries of ch   ᴧ reports submitted to child protection agencies. The d   ᴧ to the AAPC include the total number of reports, the   ᴧᴄe, and the characteristics of the reporting system. In aᴧ   ᴧ, many state and local
agencies provide case level data.

The use of reported cases to examine child maltreatment incidence
has inherent problems. Foremost among these is reporting bias. For
example, poor and minority families are more likely to be reported as
maltreating (Hampton & Newberger, 1985; O'Toole, Turbett, & Nalepka,
1983; Pelton, 1977) due, in part, to their increased contact with social
service providers. Further evidence suggests that only about 40% of
maltreatment cases are reported to CPS (NCCAN, 1988). Other studies
have examined reporting practices in more detail (e.g., Adams, Barone,
& Tooman, 1982; Gelles, 1982; Knudsen, 1988; Morris, Johnson, &
Clasen, 1985; Newberger, 1983).

Results of the most recent AAPC data—for 1986—indicate that over
two million children (2,086,000) were reported as maltreated to protective services agencies, a rate of 33 per 1,000 children (AAPC, 1988).
Reports were filed on 1,335,000 families with a mean of 1.6 children per
family reported. These data indicate an 8% increase in reported cases
from 1985 and a 212% increase in the past decade, an average increase of
13% per year. However, these AAPC data need to be interpreted with
caution, because the figures may be overestimates due to the inclusion
of duplicate cases if more than one maltreatment report was filed for a
child in a given calendar year. Alternatively, they may be underestimates because reports on Native Americans are not included by some
states. Regardless of the accuracy of these data, most investigators do
agree that reported cases are only the "tip of the child abuse iceberg."

The AAPC (1988) has also analyzed available data by type of maltreatment in those cases in which an investigation indicated that maltreatment did indeed occur (J. Fluke, personal communication, November 22, 1988) (see Table 1). Most, but not all, of these indicated cases are
substantiated. The AAPC differentiates between indicated and substantiated cases with the former representing a slightly larger class. However, only some states differentiate between indicated and substantiated
cases.

The AAPC data are based on extrapolations from those states that
provide computerized records of maltreatment reports and that used
similar definitional criteria for the various forms of maltreatment. Physical neglect (deprivation of necessities) comprised a majority of cases.

TABLE 1. Summary Profiles for Indicated Maltreatment (1986)[a]

	Maltreatment type					
	All maltreatment	Physical abuse	Fatalities	Sexual abuse	Neglect	Psychological maltreatment
Percentage of all cases	—	27.6%	—	15.7%	54.9%	8.3%
Rate/1,000	12.4	3.5	—	2.9	6.8	1.1
Child						
Age (years)	7.3	8.0	2.8	9.2	6.2	7.9
Sex (male)	46%	51%	54%	23%	52%	48%
Race (white)	67%	68%	53%	77%	63%	77%
Perpetrator						
Parent	81%	82%	76%	42%	92%	90%
Other relative	7%	6%	4%	23%	3%	3%
Age (years)	32	32	27	32	31	33
Sex (male)	47%	50%	44%	82%	30%	42%
Caretaker						
Single female	25%	25%	24%	24%	51%	34%
Unemployed	35%	29%	—	26%	42%	33%

[a]Adapted from AAPC (1988). Indicated cases are those where abuse is deemed to have occurred as a result of investigation. Most, but not all, indicated cases are substantiated (J. Fluke, personal communication, November 22, 1988).

Slightly more than a quarter of indicated cases were due to physical injury, with major injury (e.g., poisoning, fracture, or brain damage) comprising 3% of cases, minor injury (e.g., bruises, cuts, or shaking) in 14%, and unspecified injuries 11%. According to the data, about one in six maltreated children was sexually abused. Less than one in ten (8%) was psychologically maltreated or experienced some other form of maltreatment. Some children were classified as having more than one form of maltreatment. Compared to the years from 1976 through 1982 (Russell & Trainor, 1984), the current data indicate increases in reports of physical injury and sexual abuse and a decline in reports of physical neglect and psychological maltreatment.

Data on the victims of maltre.   .nt and their families have also been examined. The figures differ by type of maltreatment (see Table 1). Mean child age is youngest for fatalities, where a blow of a certain intensity is likely to lead to greater physical injury, and oldest for sexual abuse. In general, there was a tendency for boys to be more maltreated for all maltreatment types except for sexual abuse where girls predominated. Black children were relatively more likely to be fatally injured and less likely to be sexually abused. Parents were most likely to perpetrate neglect and least likely to sexually abuse their child. However, other relatives were involved in almost a quarter of the cases of child sexual abuse. Males were typically the perpetrator of sexual abuse. Females were more likely to neglect, psychologically maltreat or murder a child due to, at least in part, their greater contact with children. Single females particularly tended to be more neglectful and psychologically maltreating. Unemployed, single females were at the highest risk for neglect. This latter finding is not surprising. Such women are at risk for increased reporting because of greater stress, poverty, and depression; not to mention the bias introduced by negative professional stereotypes and greater monitoring by social services agencies.

Other reporting trends were also found. Young children from black families were disproportionately more likely to be reported as abused or neglected (AAPC, 1988). Overall, 43% of reports in 1986 were for children less than 6 years old, with a mean child age of 7.2 years, compared to a national mean of 8.6 years for all children. Whites were underrepresented in reported cases. They constituted 81% of all U.S. children but only 66% of maltreatment reports. These reporting trends have existed since the first analyses of reports in 1976 (AAPC, 1988).

There are still more significant trends in the AAPC (1988) report. With the increase in recent years in the reporting of sexual abuse there has been a corresponding decrease in the percentage of all maltreatment reports involving boys. In 1986, 48% of all reports were for boys, a decline from 50% ten years earlier. Males were increasingly less likely to be the caretaker of the reported child (39%) but were disproportionately more likely to be the perpetrator of maltreatment (44%). The decline in male caregivers is positively correlated with changes in the percentage of reports for single-parent, female-headed families (32% in 1986). Almost half of all reports (49%) in 1986 were for families who received public assistance, although they comprise only 12% of families in the United States. A more detailed analysis of confirmed maltreatment reports from one state's central maltreatment registry supports these findings (Rosenthal, 1988).

Relying on reported, rather than substantiated or indicated, cases to examine the incidence of child abuse is questionable because allegations frequently are not substantiated upon CPS investigation. Data for 26 states showed that between 40% and 42% of reports were held to be valid by the reporting CPS agencies (AAPC, 1988). Using the 40% substantiation rate and applying it to the 1986 reporting rate of 33/1,000, a substantiated maltreatment rate of approximately 13/1,000 results, which is similar to the rate of indicated cases of 12/1,000 (see Table 1).

Substantiation rates varied from state to state in 1986 with a range of

23% to 64%, suggesting not only wide variability in definitions but also a relationship between case validation and number of reports. Nationally, 74% of states have substantiation policies. As might be surmised, these differ from state to state. Moreover, policies are used in a uniform way in only one half of the states that have them (Trainor, cited in Russell & Trainor, 1984). Other factors further influence substantiation rates. For example, overburdened caseworkers are less likely to classify a given case as one of maltreatment than are workers with lighter caseloads (NCCAN, 1981).

Secondary analyses of the American Humane Association and the AAPC data bases for 1980 and 1983 have also been performed (Maximus, Inc., 1986a,b,c). These support the above conclusion that between 40% and 45% of child abuse and neglect cases are substantiated (Maximus, Inc., 1986a). If the assumption is made that about 42% of abuse and neglect cases are substantiated, then slightly more than 737,000 children were classified as maltreated in 1986.

Another type of reported case concerns children who are fatally abused or neglected. Because fatalities are more likely to be officially reported, data concerning their incidence has been used to analyze temporal changes in child maltreatment. Results of one recent survey indicate that the number of fatalities increased from a projected 899 in 1985 to 1,181 the next year. There was a slight decline to 1,132 in the following year, 1987 (Daro & Mitchel, 1988). National data were extrapolated from reports of fatalities from between 34 and 39 states, the number varying each year.

Again, the counting of fatalities is not so simple as it may seem at first glance (Mitchel, 1987), because many fatalities due to physical abuse are misclassified as accidental deaths or sudden infant death syndrome. The actual incidence of fatalities may therefore be much higher than the suggested estimates of up to 5,000 a year (Christoffel, Liu, & Stamler, 1981; Mitchel, 1987). In general, studies have found few demographic or case differences between families in which a child is maltreated but not fatally injured and those in which the maltreatment is deadly (Mitchell, 1987). Fatalities that are due to maltreatment are a serious, and in all likelihood an increasing, social problem. It is hoped that better procedures for securing accurate fatality data will be developed in the near future so that the exact magnitude can be determined more accurately.

Research also has focused on reporting among more specific samples. Results of such studies complement the findings of larger, more comprehensive investigations (Pelton, 1981). In one such study, reporting patterns for a single Indiana county over a 20 year period (1965–1984) were examined (Knudsen, 1988). Demographic characteristics were not significantly different from national data for poverty level, education, occupational status, median age, and sex ratio. The overall rate of reporting and the percentage of substantiated reports increased over time and was greater for children less than six years of age. Knudsen considers this increase to be the result of a broadening of the definition of and to an increase in the actual incidence of maltreatment, and not just the result of increased reporting. The rate of maltreatment substantiation also increased over time, which would be the case if less severe forms of maltreatment were being reported. Reports of less severe maltreatment were seen as less likely to be substantiated. In 1984, the incidence rate for substantiation on a first report of suspected maltreatment was more than 10 per 1,000 children. In the last year of his study, 38% of all reports were for abuse and 62% for neglect. Most reports were for lack of supervision (38%), followed by physical abuse (20%), physical neglect and sexual abuse (14% each), other forms of neglect (10%), and psychological abuse (4%).

A detailed analysis of reported cases in one state, over an 8-year period, provides further information (Rosenthal, 1988). Although confirming other evidence showing that girls were more likely to be sexually abused than boys, Rosenthal also concluded that boys were more likely to be severely injured than girls. However, some age differences were present. For example, when the age of the child was considered, girls from 13 to 17 years old were more likely to be maltreated, even when sexual abuse was removed from the analyzed data. In addition, males were more likely to be the perpetrator with older children, and females the perpetrator with younger children. This latter finding is interpreted as evidence that male teens, who are likely to fight back when struck, are less likely to be abused and that, when abuse does occur, it is probably perpetrated by a relatively stronger adult male.

Still other analyses have examined what have been termed the "ecological correlates" of maltreatment (see a review by Zuravin, 1989). Ecological studies, based on the theoretical views of Bronfenbrenner (1977) and Bronfenbrenner, Moen, and Garbarino (1984), emphasize the relation of community and environmental characteristics to maltreatment. In one study, Zuravin (1989) examined the ecology of child maltreatment in an urban area using reported cases of abuse and neglect as the dependent variable and neighborhood characteristics for individual census tracts as the independent variable. Eliminating duplicate reports on families, she found that the average abuse incidence for 1983 and 1984 was 23/1,000 families with children. The corresponding figure for neglect was 26/1,000. The strongest correlates of both abuse and neglect were low income and the rate of vacant housing in the neighborhood. Although this correlation does not imply a cause and effect relationship, it does seem likely that poverty and maltreatment are related (Pelton, 1977). The work of Zuravin and others (e.g., Garbarino & Crouter, 1978; Spearly & Lauderdale, 1983) suggests that adopting an ecological perspective should provide information of value in understanding the epidemiology of child maltreatment.

In summary, relying on analyses of reported cases to provide reliable and valid information on the incidence of maltreatment presents problems—and foremost, the securing of accurate reports. Unfortunately, at present it is safe to conclude that relying on substantiated reports yields an underestimate of the true incidence of abuse and neglect. Investigators are currently evaluating other approaches to examining the incidence and prevalence of child maltreatment.

THE NATIONAL INCIDENCE SURVEYS

Two national incidence surveys of professionals and their reporting practices have been done to clarify incidence issues (NCCAN, 1981, 1988) at reporting Levels 1 (cases known to protective services) through 3 (cases known to professionals in major, noninvestigatory agencies). The first study involved a probability sample in 26 counties in 10 states of "community professionals" (NCCAN, 1981). The sample included CPS staff, and school, hospital, police, and juvenile services personnel who would be likely to have contact with maltreating families (NCCAN, 1981). Data were collected during 1979 and 1980. The second study, using a similar sample from 29 counties, was done in 1986 (NCCAN, 1988).

Both studies evaluated the occurrence of six major types and a number of subcategories of maltreatment: physical abuse (two subtypes), sexual abuse (six subtypes), and psychological abuse (eight subtypes); and physical neglect (seven subtypes), psychological neglect (five subtypes), and educational neglect (three subtypes). Each type of maltreatment was clearly defined in both studies. The second study used both the original and a revised, expanded definition (NCCAN, 1988). This allowed for the direct comparison of the 1979–1980 and the 1986 data, using the original definition of demonstrable harm to the child. The use of the revised definition with the 1986 data allowed for the inclusion in the incidence data of children who were both endangered and harmed, and for a wider variety of potential perpetrators for some forms of maltreatment. The revised 1986 definition thus yielded higher incidence and prevalence figures than did the original 1979–1980 definition.

Study data analyses consisted of (1) an assessment of countability, (2) unduplication, and (3) the weighting and estimation of incidence figures. All case reports were evaluated as to whether they were countable as cases of maltreatment according to study definitions. Intercoder reliability for countability was 86% for both sets of definitional criteria. Data were also reviewed for duplications because of the possibility that the same case might be known to more than one reporting source. In the case of duplication, a case was assigned to the highest appropriate level on the five-level model discussed earlier. Estimates of national incidence were obtained for each type of maltreatment using a complex weighting procedure. The results of the two studies are summarized in Table 2.

The National Incidence Studies are not without problems, as is the case with all incidence studies that have been done to date. Data concerning the incidence of sexual abuse present the major difficulty (Finkelhor 1984; Finkelhor & Hotaling, 1984). Finkelhor and Hotaling question the results of the first National Incidence Study indicating that a disproportionately high percentage of sexual abuse cases had been officially reported. Fewer cases were listed by individuals who knew about a case of sexual abuse, but did not file a report. Finkelhor and Hotaling (1984) cite additional evidence suggesting a low percentage of officially reported cases and conclude that definitional difficulties are also present. For example, a mother who allowed a child to be sexually abused but who did not play an active role in the actual abuse was still counted as a perpetrator. But, if each parent perpetrated a different type of maltreatment, both were listed as perpetrators of maltreatment. These issues complicate the task of determining what parental charac-

TABLE 2. Summary Results from the 1979–1980 and 1986
National Incidence Studies[a]

Maltreatment category	Original definitions		Percentage of change 1979–1980 to 1986	1986 Definition
	1979–1980	1986		
Total abuse	336,600 (5.3)	580,400 (9.2)	+72 (+74)	675,000 (10.7)
Physical	199,100 (3.1)	311,200 (4.9)	+56 (+58)	358,300 (5.7)
Sexual	42,900 (0.7)	138,000 (2.2)	+222 (+214)	155,900 (2.5)
Psychological	132,700 (2.1)	174,400 (2.8)	+31 (+33)	211,100 (3.4)
Total neglect	315,400 (4.9)	498,000 (7.9)	+58 (+61)	1,003,600 (15.9)
Physical	103,600 (1.6)	182,100 (2.9)	+76 (+81)	571,600 (9.1)
Psychological	56,900 (0.9)	52,200 (0.8)	−8 (−11)	223,100 (3.5)
Educational	174,000 (2.7)	291,100 (4.6)	+67 (+70)	292,100 (4.6)

[a]Adapted from NCCAN (1988). Numbers in parentheses are for incidence (rate/1,000 children) and for change in incidence.

teristics are associated with different forms of abuse or neglect. Finally, only intrafamilial sexual abuse was considered, resulting in a definition that differs considerably from that used in other studies which examine extrafamilial sexual abuse as well.

Overall, the maltreatment incidence in 1986 was approximately 16/1,000 (NCCAN, 1988), which represents slightly more than 1 million children. When the revised definition of maltreatment is examined these figures increase to 25/1,000 or in excess of 1.5 million children. Using the original definition, slightly more than half of all reported children were abused (56%) and slightly less than half were neglected (48%). However, the revised definition indicated relatively more neglect (63%) than abuse (43%). When the 1986 data are compared with 1979–1980 data, the results suggest that recognized maltreatment increased significantly, due largely to a 74% increase in the incidence of abuse. Neglect rates did not change significantly over the 6-year period. Hence, most of the overall increase in incidence was due to increased physical and sexual abuse and not to increased neglect. The greatest part of this increase was for those cases involving moderate injury, which increased 89%.

It is important to remember that these data do not represent the actual number of maltreated children and probably are underestimates. First, only 40% of the 1986 cases had been referred to CPS (46% using the revised definition). Second, abuse cases at Level 4 (cases known to other agencies and individuals) and Level 5 (undetected cases) of the five-part model are not included in the data from either survey. Thus, there is no estimate of the number of cases known only to such personnel as private physicians and mental health workers.

Three factors may account for the increase in physical and sexual abuse between 1979–1980 and 1986. First, the actual incidence could have increased with more children being maltreated. Second, professionals may be more likely to report abuse or neglect cases they see. Third, the results may be due to methodological differences in the two surveys. The authors propose that the second explanation is the more likely (NCCAN, 1988). Thus, much of the increase in reported cases in 1986 was due to children who had moderate injuries (72% of the total) followed by serious injuries (15%), probable injuries (12%), and fatalities (0.1%). The incidence of severe injuries did not increase significantly. If the actual incidence of maltreatment had increased, there should have been a significant rather than a nonsignificant increase in these cases. It is assumed that cases of severe injury were equally likely to have been reported at both survey times, given the importance of intervention when such injuries are present. However, moderate rather than severe cases are the ones that professionals, who are increasingly attuned to the detection of maltreatment, would be more likely to note, regardless of whether an official report of maltreatment was or was not filed. The second explanation also is supported by the finding of a more than 200% increase in the incidence of sexual abuse. Sexual abuse became a major child welfare issue during the period between the two surveys. It is unlikely that there was a threefold increase in the actual number of sexual assaults on children over a 6-year period.

A detailed examination of the six methodological changes introduced in the 1986 survey suggests that they account for, at most, a small portion of the increased incidence of abuse. It is more likely that professionals' greater awareness of and ability to identify maltreatment account for the increasing incidence of maltreatment. Also, it is plausible, but somewhat less likely, that the actual incidence of abuse has increased. Regardless of the interplay of all these factors, it is unlikely that the incidence of maltreatment declined across the 6-year period of the two studies, a finding that is important in clarifying the results of surveys by Straus and Gelles (e.g., Gelles, 1978; Gelles & Straus, 1987, 1988; Straus & Gelles, 1986; Straus, Gelles, & Steinmetz, 1980) discussed below.

National Incidence Study data also provide information about the types of children who were maltreated (NCCAN, 1988). The major findings revealed in this study were that

- Females were more likely to be abused (13/1,000 compared to 8/1,000 for males), mostly because of their increased susceptibility to sexual abuse (4/1,000 vs. 1/1,000)
- The incidence of child abuse increased with child age, particularly for physical abuse
- Impoverished children were much more likely to be maltreated or injured—children from families earning less than $15,000 a year were more than five times as likely to be maltreated and more than seven times as likely to be seriously injured or impaired
- Family size was unrelated to maltreatment using original definitions; with the revised definition family size was positively associated with abuse and neglect
- Race, ethnicity, and county metropolitan status were not related to the incidence of maltreatment

More detailed analyses of the first survey data have been done. One such analysis examined the national incidence data for hospitals, institutions at Level 3 of the five-level maltreatment awareness model (Hampton & Newberger, 1985). The subset of cases identified as maltreated by the hospitals surveyed showed several detection trends that differed from those found for the incidence study as a whole. The children detected by hospitals, compared with cases reported by other agencies, were more likely to: (1) live in urban areas (66% vs. 42%), (2) be younger, (3) have younger parents, (4) be black (25% vs. 16%), and (5) have been physically abused. Multivariate analyses of the data for cases that were and were not reported to CPS indicated four variables that were the key predictors of hospital-based reporting: (1) type of maltreatment, (2) family income, (3) maternal role in maltreatment, and (4) race or ethnicity. Psychologically abused children from white families with above average incomes, in which the mother was deemed responsible for the maltreatment, were least likely to be reported. Physically abused children from lower income, minority families, in which the alleged perpetrator was not the mother, were more likely to be reported. These results support the argument that a report is more likely to be made when there is a demographic difference between the reporter and the maltreating family (O'Toole *et al.*, 1983).

Study results also clarify some of the issues involved in interpreting the analyses of CPS reports discussed above (AAPC, 1985, 1986, 1987, 1988; American Humane Association, 1984; Russell & Trainor, 1984). Of particular importance is the elimination of the counting of duplicate reports in the NCCAN incidence studies. National Incidence Study data suggest that the increased recognition of maltreatment cases by sources other than CPS workers has not been reflected in an increased incidence of confirmed CPS cases. There are two likely explanations for this finding. First, the surveyed professionals may fail to report cases to CPS. Second, CPS may fail to confirm as legitimate maltreatment those cases that are reported. If the former is correct, efforts need to be made to increase the recognition of maltreatment and to convince professionals of the value of reporting it. If the latter view is correct, efforts need to be made to secure more investigative resources for CPS agencies. In reality, it is likely that both explanations contribute to this discrepancy.

SURVEYS OF THE GENERAL PUBLIC

Many studies have examined the epidemiology of child maltreatment by surveying either a random sample of the general public or special, at-risk populations. These studies provide data concerning Level 4 of the five-level model of maltreatment awareness. They represent the broadest base for formulating estimates of maltreatment incidence and prevalence. These studies have typically examined only one type of maltreatment rather than being comprehensive, as was the case for the studies in the earlier subsections of this chapter (AAPC, 1985,

1986, 1987; American Humane Association, 1984; NCCAN, 1981, 1988; Russell & Trainor, 1984).

Physical Abuse

Some of the earliest estimates of the incidence of physical abuse were based on surveys of nationally representative samples. Gil (1973) conducted a survey in 1965 in which 1,520 adults were asked about their personal knowledge of families who had injured "a child, not by accident, but in anger or deliberately" (p. 49). The results showed that 3% of the sample knew of at least one such incident. Allowing for error variance, between 2.5 and 4.1 million children were injured in the year prior to the survey—a figure that seems high even today. However, Gil's methodology has been criticized (Light, 1973). When Light controlled for errors in the Gil analysis, the incidence of physical abuse decreased to 500,000 children a year.

Straus, Gelles, and their colleagues conducted national surveys of the incidence of physical abuse in the general population in 1975 and in 1985 (Gelles, 1978; Gelles & Straus, 1987, 1988; Straus et al., 1980; Straus & Gelles, 1986). Physical abuse was defined as the parental use of certain violent acts toward a child as measured using the Conflict Tactics Scale (Straus, 1979). This questionnaire asks family members about how they resolve conflicts. There were slight differences in the scales used in the two surveys. The original, 1975 scale asked about throwing objects; pushing, grabbing, or shoving; slapping or spanking; kicking, biting, or hitting with a fist; hitting or trying to hit with an object; "beating up"; and threatening with or using a knife or gun (Straus & Gelles, 1986). Questions concerning scalding or burning were added in 1985.

Child abuse was defined as kicking, biting, punching, "beating up," and threatening with or using a knife or a gun (Gelles & Straus, 1987). Other violent acts—including hitting with an object and threatening with a weapon—were excluded. They were considered as variations of normal discipline, rather than abusive, or were deemed unlikely to lead to actual injury.

For the 1985 study, telephone interviews were conducted with a nationally representative sample of 1,428 families containing a male–female couple or one adult over 18 years old where there was at least one child from 3 to 17 years old. Overall, 84% of contacted families agreed to participate in the survey. Data are available for only two-parent families. The 1975 study was conducted using a different method (Gelles, 1978; Straus & Gelles, 1986). First, in-person rather than telephone surveys were conducted. Second, families were given the alternative of answering "never" with regard to the frequency with which a given act occurred in their home. In 1985, they were not directly told they could answer "never." Third, only two-parent families were interviewed. In 1975, 65% of approached families agreed to be interviewed, yielding a final sample of 1,146 families with a 3- to 17-year-old in the home.

The results of the surveys indicate that there was a significant decline in the rate with which parents reported using three forms of violence between 1975 and 1985: throwing something declined from 54 per 1,000 children to 27/1,000; kicking, biting, and hitting with a fist declined from 32/1,000 to 13/1,000; and hitting or trying to hit with an object declined from 134/1,000 to 97/1,000. The rate of acts that could be considered potentially abusive also declined significantly from 36/1,000 to 19/1,000 (Gelles & Straus, 1987).

The key question is whether these data indicate a real decline in the incidence of child abuse. Straus and Gelles (1986) consider several possible explanations for the disparate findings, including (1) differences in methodology, (2) an increasing reluctance to report family violence to an outsider, and (3) a real decline in family violence. With regard to methodology, Straus and Gelles cite several references for studies of the differences between in-person and telephone interviews, all of which note no significant differences in the results obtained using the two methods. Alternatively, as public knowledge about child abuse and recognition of its seriousness increases, people may be more reluctant to admit to experiencing family violence. The authors argue that, if this were the case, more families would have refused to participate in 1985 than did in 1975. However, it is difficult to evaluate this possibility because of the different survey techniques used in the two studies.

Factors cited that support an actual decline in the incidence of child abuse include structural changes in families, improved economic conditions, and the availability of prevention and treatment programs (Gelles & Straus, 1987, 1988). First, changes in family structure, including an increasing age at the time of first parenthood and declining family size, lead to less stress and, potentially result in decreased violence. Second, intact families were less likely to experience economic stressors in 1985 than they were ten years earlier. Finally, the increased availability of and publicity about treatment programs may mean that parents try to get help with childrearing problems before resorting to abusive violence.

It is important to recognize that the true incidence of physical abuse is probably higher than that reported by the surveys. First, many individuals are unlikely to admit to being violent. Second, the range of violent acts included in the survey was quite limited. Many other acts, such as burning and poisoning, result in physical abuse. For example, 5 in 1,000 families in the 1985 survey reported burning or scalding their child (Gelles & Straus, 1987). This finding suggests that the rate of child abuse is probably higher than the reported 19/1,000. Third, the surveys included only children over 2 years of age despite the fact that younger children were more likely to be physically abused than older ones (approximately 7% for 3- to 4-year-olds, and 4% for older children) (Gelles, 1978). The presence of an inverse relationship between child age and physical abuse is supported by other studies. For example, 79% of physical abuse reports in Arizona and 85% in Louisiana were for children less than four years old (Maximus, 1986b). The latter figures, in turn, are probably overestimates. Young children are more subject to scrutiny by professionals and are more likely to represent unconfirmed cases of physical abuse (Jason, Andereck, Marks, & Tyler, 1982). A fourth reason the Gelles and Straus findings are likely to be underestimates of physical abuse is that results are available for intact families even though only single-parent families are under greater stress and, as such, are more likely to be violent. In a reanalysis of National Incidence Study data, Miller (1984) found that teenage mothers, who are likely to be single parents, also were more likely to physically abuse their children than were older mothers. Furthermore, retrospective evidence suggests that single parents are more punitive toward their children (Sack, Mason, & Higgins, 1985). Thus, the Gelles and Straus data only suggest the incidence of physical abuse in the general population.

The Gelles and Straus (1987) data indicate that approximately 1.5 million children were subjected to potentially abusive violence in 1975 compared to about 750,000 children in 1985. Moreover, they suggest that the decline in incidence is most probably because of some combination of attitudinal and behavioral change rather than differences in survey methodology. Only further research can yield a conclusive answer about the validity of these alternative explanations.

The results of the 1975 survey do reveal something about the types of families that direct high levels of violence toward children. Examining the Conflict Tactics Scale variables that were used to determine child abuse (Straus & Gelles, 1986), approximately 4% of fathers and 6% of mothers were abusive (Gelles, 1978). This heightened level of maternal abuse may be due to the greater amount of time mothers spend with their children, to the greater degree to which children interfere with maternal daily activities (Straus et al., 1980), or to other factors related to family functioning. Boys were more likely to be subjected to physical abuse than were girls (approximately 6% vs. 3%) (Gelles, 1978). Although the exact reason for this difference is debatable, it does confirm the findings of the AAPC survey (1988) discussed earlier.

It is unfortunate that the data analyses of the Gelles and Straus family surveys did not focus more specifically on acts that they label physically abusive. Instead, most of their analyses are for total violent acts (including, for example, throwing objects, spanking, slapping, and hitting) rather than just abusive ones. Thus, when total violence toward children, including abusive violence, is considered, a number of demographic differences were found (Straus et al., 1980). For example, there was more overall violence in the midwest and west; in large cities; among non-Jews, younger parents, and parents with either some high school or who graduated from high school; in lower income and blue collar occupations, and in families where the husband worked part-time or was unemployed. No differences were found between black and white families.

Sexual Abuse

The preceding sections have noted the dramatic increase in public awareness concerning sexual abuse over the past decade. Given this recognition, it is not surprising that many studies have revealed its prevalence, including general population surveys and studies of special populations that are believed to have a high likelihood of sexual abuse (e.g., Gruber & Jones, 1983; Silbert & Pines, 1981).

It is important to remember that all the data in this section are for the prevalence of sexual abuse during childhood as measured retrospectively in adult samples. These data indicate how many adults were sexually abused during childhood. The rates reported are thus considerably higher than would be the case if the incidence per 1,000 cases per year (the measure used for all other data in this chapter) were used as a measure of problem magnitude.

There is considerable variation in study methodologies. Studies use dissimilar definitions, consider childhood to end at various ages, have different criteria about the inclusion of cases where there was consent to the maltreatment, use diverse question framing techniques, and interview samples with different characteristics using a variety of interview techniques.

As was indicated earlier, definitions are a major factor influencing the outcome of incidence and prevalence studies. Key variables are whether physical contact was involved, the age of the victim, the age differential between the victim and the perpetrator, and whether the perpetrator was a family member. These definitional factors make comparisons across studies particularly difficult because prevalence figures typically are lower when narrower definitions are used (Haugaard & Reppucci, 1988). In one study of the relationship between definitional restrictiveness and prevalence, the recalculation of data from a survey of black and white urban-area women (Wyatt, 1985), using a more restrictive definition, led to a 14% drop in the prevalence of sexual abuse (Wyatt & Peters, 1986a).

Given the current interest in sexual abuse it is surprising that only two national, representative sample surveys have been conducted in the United States (Kinsey et al., 1953; "22% in Survey," 1985). Kinsey and his colleagues found that 22% of women had experienced some sexual activity during childhood, with contact occurring in less than half of these cases (9%). The Los Angeles Times survey interviewed a national, random sample of 2,627 adults and asked 100 questions concerning sexual abuse ("22% in Survey," 1985). The results were that 27% of women and 16% of men reported sexual abuse as a child, with 55% of all victims experiencing sexual intercourse. Less than a quarter (23%) of abusers were relatives, and the modal age at the time of the abuse was 10 years. Unfortunately, specific details concerning aspects of the survey, such as the maximum victim and minimum perpetrator age and the frequency of contact versus noncontact abuse, have not been published, limiting the comparability of these data with those from other studies.

The only other national incidence data come from Canada (Committee on Sexual Offenses Against Children and Youth, 1984, cited in Haugaard & Reppucci, 1988) where 2,135 men and women over 17 years old were surveyed. Overall, 28% of the women and 10% of the men had experienced some form of sexual abuse as children. These results include cases in which the abuse was perpetrated by a peer (40% of cases) and in which no contact was involved (half of all cases). Thus, contact abuse had occurred for, at the most, 14% of women and 5% of men—a prevalence not very different from the Kinsey et al. (1953) findings for women.

Other estimates of prevalence at the fourth level of maltreatment recognition are provided by the results of a number of more limited surveys of varying groups including college students (Finkelhor, 1979; Fritz, Stoll, & Wagner, 1981; Fromuth, 1986; Haugaard, cited in Haugaard & Reppucci, 1988; Risin & Koss, 1987; Sedney & Brooks, 1984), and random sample surveys in specific geographic areas (Finkelhor, 1984; Kercher & McShane, 1984; D. E. H. Russell, 1983, 1984; Wyatt, 1985). These studies are summarized in Table 3.

The use of differing methodologies complicates comparisons among

TABLE 3. Summary Studies of Sexual Abuse Prevalence

	Geographic surveys			
	Finkelhor (1984)	Kercher & McShane (1984)	Russell (1983, 1984)	Wyatt (1985)
Sample size	700	2,000	930	248
Location	Urban Boston	Texas	San Francisco	Los Angeles
Response rate	74%	53%	64%	73%[a]
Male/female	Both	Both	Female	Female
Method	Questionnaire	Questionnaire	Interview	Interview
Maximum victim age	15	?	17	17
Minimum perpetrator age	None	None	None	None
Age differential required	Yes	No	No	No
Contact required	No	No	No	No
Abuse wanted/unwanted	Unwanted	?	Either	Either
Women abused as child	15%	11%	54%	62%
Men abused as child	6%	3%	—	—

	College and university student surveys					
	Finkelhor (1979)	Fritz et al. (1981)	Fromuth (1986)	Haugaard (1987)	Risin & Koss (1987)	Sedney & Brooks (1984)
Sample size	796	952	482	1,089	2,972	301
Response rate	92%	Unknown	Unknown	61%	98%	Unknown
Male/female	Both	Both	Female	Both	Male	Female
Maximum victim age	16	Prepuberty	16	16	13	Unknown
Minimum perpetrator age	None	Postadolescent	16	16	None	Unknown
Age differential required	Yes	Yes	Yes	Yes	Yes	No
Contact required	No	Yes	No	Yes	No	No
Abuse wanted/unwanted	Either	Either	Either	Unwanted	Either	Either
Women abused as child	19%	8%	22%	12%	—	16%
Men abused as child	9%	5%	—	5%	7%	—

[a]This figure may be 55% depending on how response rate is measured (Haugaard & Reppucci, 1988).

these studies. Thus, as indicated in Table 3, some studies examined only incidents involving contact, whereas others did not. In addition, the maximum age of the victim, minimum perpetrator age and whether the perpetrator had to be older than the victim or could be a peer also differed from study to study. Further complexities are introduced when the issue of whether the sexual contact was wanted or unwanted is added. Some studies (e.g., Finkelhor, 1979; Fritz et al., 1981; Fromuth, 1986) count both types of act as abuse; other studies analyze only unwanted contact (e.g., Committee on Sexual Offenses Against Children and Youth, 1984, cited in Haugaard & Reppucci, 1988); and still others vary for intrafamilial and extrafamilial abuse (D. E. H. Russell, 1983, 1984) or for children of varying ages (Wyatt, 1985).

These studies also have examined other key aspects of the prevalence of sexual abuse, including (1) abuse involving direct contact between victim and abuser, and (2) intrafamilial versus extrafamilial abuse. D. E. H. Russell (1983) found that 38% of her sample reported contact abuse before they were 18 years old. For less than 5% of the women surveyed, the perpetrator was a parent, was a family member for 16%, and was unrelated for 31% of her sample. If a more restrictive definition is used and only abuse in girls 13 years old or younger is considered, these prevalence figures decline to 28% of her sample experiencing abuse before 14 years of age, with 12% experiencing intrafamilial and 20% extrafamilial abuse. These data also indicated that, for intrafamilial abuse, stepfathers were much more likely to abuse (17% of her sample who had a stepfather present) than were biological fathers (2%); and that stepfathers, when they did abuse, perpetrated more severe forms of abuse (D. E. H. Russell, 1984).

Wyatt's (1985) reported prevalence of sexual abuse that involved contact was higher than Russell's—45% prior to age 18. Wyatt found that 76% of all sexual abuse (both contact and noncontact) was committed by nonrelatives, less than 2% by fathers, about 6% by nonrelated males in a father role, and 14% by other male relatives. Finkelhor (1984) reported that 80% of the abuse experienced by the subjects in his random survey involved contact, resulting in a female contact abuse prevalence of 12% and a male rate of 5%. A relative was the perpetrator in 32% of all the cases. In addition, it should be noted that he used a somewhat narrower definition of sexual abuse than Russell or Wyatt—an act was counted as abusive only if the person self-defined it as sexual abuse.

Data for college students come mainly from middle-class adolescents and young adults—a less representative sample than is the case for general population surveys. When the results of student surveys, all of which used questionnaires, are compared with those from the two more general questionnaire studies (Finkelhor, 1984; Kercher & Mc-Shane, 1984), there is considerable overlap in results for the various sample types. The prevalence range for general population surveys is 11% to 15% for women and 3% to 6% for men. Comparable data for college students are 8% to 22% for women and 5% to 9% for men (see Table 3). This variability is not surprising considering the different definitions and methodologies used in the various studies. Indeed, one study of male college students evaluated the effects of different definitions and found that the prevalence rate ranged from 4% to 24% depending on the definition of sexual abuse used (Fromuth & Burkhart, 1987).

There is even greater variation in the prevalence of sexual abuse when the data for both questionnaire and interview studies are considered. The range for women is from 62% (Wyatt, 1985) to 8% (Fritz *et al.*, 1981), while it is 9% (Finkelhor, 1979) to 3% (Kercher & McShane, 1984) for men. A number of factors account for these differences. In addition to the effects of differing definitions discussed by Fromuth and Burkhart (1987), methodological differences are also important. In an analysis of four representative studies (Finkelhor, 1979, 1984; D. E. H. Russell, 1983, 1984; Wyatt, 1985), Wyatt and Peters (1986b) examined the role of different data collection procedures. The prevalence rate was much higher in the two interview studies (D. E. H. Russell, 1983, 1984; Wyatt, 1985) and lower in the questionnaire studies (Finkelhor, 1979, 1984). Indeed, the results of the two interview studies in Table 3 are quite similar and those of the eight questionnaire studies are relatively similar, particularly for those including a male sample.

A second important methodological variable discussed by Wyatt and Peters (1986a,b) was the way in which information was gathered, particularly how questions about prior sexual abuse were framed. They propose that studies that asked more detailed questions about a variety of forms of sexual abuse yielded greater reporting of such maltreatment. The confounding of these two variables limits our ability to determine which is more important. In addition, published information concerning four of the other six studies summarized in Table 3 (Fritz *et al.*, 1981; Fromuth, 1986; Haugaard, 1987, cited in Haugaard & Reppucci, 1988; Sedney & Brooks, 1984) is not sufficient to determine the question framing procedure used. The remaining studies (Kercher & McShane, 1984; Risin & Koss, 1987) used a narrow framing procedure and the results are close to those of the Finkelhor (1984) geographic survey.

Other factors appear to be unrelated to the prevalence of sexual abuse (Wyatt & Peters, 1986b). These include whether random sampling or subject self-selection was used, the geographic area of the study, and the subject's race and education level. Taking all of this into consideration, Wyatt and Peters (1986b) conclude that not only is more research needed to clarify the exact extent of sexual abuse but that future studies should use in-person interviews so that the issue of sexual abuse can be embedded within a study described as having a broader purpose. They also suggest (1) matching subject and interviewer race, (2) using carefully trained project personnel, (3) ensuring interview confidentiality, and (4) paying subjects for the time and expense incurred.

What do these studies tell us about the prevalence of sexual abuse in addition to the fact that study design plays an important role in determining study outcome? A major conclusion, unfortunately, is that the prevalence of child sexual victimization is much higher than would have been predicted a decade ago. Although we cannot cite one prevalence figure as giving a single, valid indicator of the extent of child sexual abuse, we can state with certainty that females are at significantly greater risk. However, it is important to remember that, relying on the high prevalence figures cited by D. E. H. Russell (1983) and Wyatt (1985), less than 5% of women have been sexually abused by a parent or parent-figure. Since these studies examined prevalence rates and did not include males, the actual annual incidence of sexual abuse for the overall child population will be significantly lower. In spite of this caveat, sexual abuse is a major problem and most cases never reach the attention of authorities.

Psychological Maltreatment and Physical Neglect

It is surprising that there is so little information about what probably are the most common forms of child maltreatment. No research has been done studying psychological maltreatment or physical neglect at Level 4 of maltreatment. Although it is true that surveys at this level would be difficult to conduct, they would yield valuable information about how children are being cared for by their parents.

SUMMARY AND IMPLICATIONS

What is the answer to the question with which this chapter began: "What do we really know about the extent of the child maltreatment problem?" One obvious answer is that the determination of the "exact" incidence and prevalence of child abuse is a very complex process. We have discussed a number of studies that use different samples, definitions, and research methodologies. The best that can be done at present is to compare the incidence and prevalence data from studies of the first four levels of maltreatment: (1) cases known to protective services, (2) those that have been reported to other investigative agencies, (3) maltreated children who have been detected by other professionals and agencies, and (4) cases in which other individuals, including perpetrators and victims, know of the maltreatment.

A second answer to the above question is that much is known about the epidemiology of child maltreatment. Indeed, there is much data, much more than we have been able to discuss in this chapter. The problem is how to interpret and systematize the available findings. Table 4 summarizes data for the different maltreatment levels by the type of maltreatment.

The data in Table 4 indicate a wide variation in estimates of the incidence and prevalence of child maltreatment. The two data sets that are most similar are those for reported cases (AAPC, 1988) and for the National Incidence Study of cases that have either been reported or are known to agencies or professionals (NCCAN, 1988). Although it would be expected that the National Incidence Study data would show a higher incidence of maltreatment—because a broader sample of cases were included—this is not consistently the case. Thus, the data for the National Incidence Study indicate a lower incidence of sexual abuse than the AAPC data suggest. But the AAPC data are inflated because of the

TABLE 4. Summary of Incidence Data

	Total maltreatment	Physical abuse	Sexual abuse	Neglect	Psychological maltreatment[a]
Reported cases (AAPC, 1988)	12.4[b]	3.5	2.9	6.8	1.1
National incidence study (NCCAN, 1988)	16.3 (25.2)[c]	4.9 (5.7)	2.2 (2.5)	7.5 (13.7)[d]	3.6 (6.9)[e]
Cases known to individuals		19[f]	10%–58%[g]	No data	No data

[a]Includes both psychological abuse and psychological neglect.
[b]Rate/1000.
[c]The first figure is incidence using the original (NCCAN, 1981) maltreatment definitions; data in parentheses are for the revised definition (NCCAN, 1988).
[d]Data are for the sum of the incidence of physical and educational neglect. Figures include an unknown amount of duplicate cases where both were present.
[e]Data are for the sum of the incidence of psychological abuse and neglect. Figures include an unknown amount of duplicate cases where both were present.
[f]Data from Gelles and Straus (1987, 1988) and Straus and Gelles (1986).
[g]Lower figure is mean percentage for surveys of men and women reported in Table 3. Higher figure is mean for women only from detailed interview studies (Russell, 1983, 1984; Wyatt, 1985).

counting of duplicate cases (AAPC, 1988). Other differences in the reported incidence figures for the two studies may be due to the broader sample used in the National Incidence Study or to methodological differences (AAPC, 1988). It is likely that to at least some unknown extent the data from these two studies indicate a real discrepancy between the rate of indicated reported cases evaluated by the AAPC studies (1988) and both the reported and the known, but not reported cases assessed in the National Incidence Study (NCCAN, 1988).

The data presented in this chapter also suggest that the vast majority of cases of child maltreatment are never officially recognized. Incidence and prevalence rates for the two areas in which studies have been done (physical and sexual abuse) are much higher when surveys of the general public are conducted than when they are reported and/or when professionally known cases are considered. Many of the acts included in the Straus and Gelles study (Gelles & Straus, 1987, 1988; Straus & Gelles, 1986) have only the potential to injure. In addition, if injury does occur, the damage to the child may not be severe enough to require medical attention, or the case may not be considered physical abuse even if care is needed. Similarly, most incidents of sexual abuse are never brought to official attention. The *Los Angeles Times* survey concluded that sexual abuse victims report abuse to the police in only 3% of cases ("22% in Survey," 1985). Indeed, less than half of victims (42%) told *anyone* about the abuse and, of these, only 30% said their telling resulted in "any effective action" (p. 34). Data on police reporting are similar to those Russell (1983) found in her survey, 2% of cases of intrafamilial and 6% of extrafamilial abuse were reported to the police.

There are important factors that should be considered in interpreting the data presented in this chapter and in planning future research efforts. First, it is important to remember that epidemiology is the study not only of the incidence and prevalence of a problem, but also of the risk factors involved. With the exception of some discussion of demographic risk factors, this chapter has focused on the incidence and prevalence of maltreatment. Other risk variables are considered in Chapters 1, 6, 7, and 8.

Second, it is necessary to reiterate the key role that definitional issues play in determining the incidence and prevalence of child maltreatment. The studies reviewed in this chapter consider a wide spectrum of acts as abusive, ranging from fatalities at one extreme to indecent exposure at another. Reviewing and sorting out all of the important definitional variables is a difficult and complex task and is beyond the scope of this chapter. Child maltreatment is a complex phenomenon that is defined in many different ways. Each definition has implications not only for determining incidence and prevalence, but also for case finding, treatment, and prevention.

Third, progress has been made since 1975 when Cohen and Sussman stated "the only conclusion which can be made fairly is that information indicating the incidence of child abuse in the United States simply does not exist" (cited in Gelles, 1978, p. 582). But, much still remains to be done. For example, research groups could come together to agree on standardized definitions to be used in epidemiological studies. If a group liked a given definition better than the standard, agreed upon one, they could incorporate both definitions in their study. This was done in the most recent National Incidence Study to allow comparability of the 1979–1980 and 1986 data (NCCAN, 1988). Furthermore, better information is needed about the prevalence of neglect and psychological maltreatment at Level 4 of the National Incidence Study categorization of level of awareness (NCCAN, 1988). Ideally, a study could be conducted using a national interview sample in which the presence of all types of maltreatment is evaluated. Although planning and conducting such a study would be difficult, it would be a major step forward in obtaining a better idea of the actual dimension of the problem of child maltreatment in all its forms.

Another way to increase knowledge about the epidemiology of child maltreatment is to improve analyses of reported case data. The American Association for Protecting Children receives annual funding sufficient for only partial analysis of state report data. Annual data analyses are not needed. It would be a better investment to have detailed analysis of data every 5 years in order to obtain a fuller examination of reporting and case substantiation trends—the very data policy makers need to make informed decisions. It is unfortunate that existing data do not permit making a firm conclusion about the magnitude of child maltreatment and whether our prevention and treatment efforts are having a meaningful impact in reducing the extent of the problem. Perhaps future research and analyses of reporting trends will provide the answers to these as yet unanswered questions.

REFERENCES

Adams, W., Barone, N., & Tooman, P. (1982). The dilemma of anonymous reporting in child protective services. *Child Welfare, 61,* 3–14.
American Association for Protecting Children. (1985). *Highlights of official child neglect and abuse reporting 1983.* Denver: American Humane Association.

American Association for Protecting Children. (1986). *Highlights of official child neglect and abuse reporting 1984*. Denver: American Humane Association.

American Association for Protecting Children. (1987). *Highlights of official child neglect and abuse reporting 1985*. Denver: American Humane Association.

American Association for Protecting Children. (1988). *Highlights of official child neglect and abuse reporting 1986*. Denver: American Humane Association.

American Humane Association. (1984). *Highlights of official child neglect and abuse reporting 1982*. Denver: Author.

Bronfenbrenner, U. (1977). Toward an experimental ecology of human development. *American Psychologist, 32*, 513–531.

Bronfenbrenner, U., Moen, P., & Garbarino, J. (1984). Child, family, and community. In R. Parke (Ed.), *Review of child development research* (pp. 283–328). Chicago: University of Chicago Press.

Christoffel, K. K., Liu, K., & Stamler, J. (1981). Epidemiology of fatal child abuse: International mortality data. *Journal of Chronic Diseases, 34*, 57–64.

Daro, D., & Mitchel, L. (1988). *Child abuse fatalities remain high: The results of the 1987 annual fifty state survey* (Working Paper No. 8). Chicago: National Committee for Prevention of Child Abuse.

Dubowitz, H. (1987). *Child maltreatment in the United States: Etiology, impact, and prevention*. Washington, DC: Office of Technology Assessment.

Finkelhor, D. (1979). *Sexually victimized children*. New York: Free Press.

Finkelhor, D. (1984). *Child sexual abuse: New theory and research*. New York: Free Press.

Finkelhor, D., & Hotaling, G. T. (1984). Sexual abuse in the National Incidence Study of Child Abuse and Neglect: An appraisal. *Child Abuse and Neglect, 8*, 23–33.

Fritz, G. S., Stoll, K., & Wagner, N. N. (1981). A comparison of males and females who were sexually molested as children. *Journal of Sex and Marital Therapy, 7*, 54–59.

Fromuth, M. E. (1986). The relationship of childhood sexual abuse with later psychological and sexual adjustment in a sample of college women. *Child Abuse and Neglect, 10*, 5–15.

Fromuth, M. E., & Burkhart, B. R. (1987). Childhood sexual victimization among college men: Definitional and methodological issues. *Violence and Victims, 2*, 241–253.

Garbarino, J., & Crouter, A. (1978). Defining the community context for parent-child relations: The correlates of child maltreatment. *Child Development, 49*, 604–616.

Garbarino, J., & Gilliam, G. (1980). *Understanding abusive families*. Lexington, MA: Lexington Books.

Garbarino, J., Guttman, E., & Seeley, J. W. (1986). *The psychologically battered child: Strategies for identification, assessment, and intervention*. San Francisco: Jossey-Bass.

Gelles, R. J. (1978). Violence toward children in the United States. *American Journal of Orthopsychiatry, 48*, 580–592.

Gelles, R. J. (1982). Problems in defining and labeling child abuse. In R. H. Starr, Jr. (Ed.), *Child abuse prediction: Policy implications* (pp. 1–30). Cambridge, MA: Ballinger.

Gelles, R. J., & Straus, M. A. (1987). Is violence toward children increasing? A comparison of 1975 and 1985 national survey rates. *Journal of Interpersonal Violence, 2*, 212–222.

Gelles, R. J., & Straus, M. A. (1988). *Intimate violence*. New York: Simon & Schuster.

Gil, D. G. (1973). *Violence against children: Physical child abuse in the United States*. Cambridge: Harvard University Press.

Giovannoni, J. M., & Becerra, R. M. (1979). *Defining child abuse*. New York: Free Press.

Gruber, K. J., & Jones, R. J. (1983). Identifying determinants of risk of sexual victimization of youth: A multivariate approach. *Child Abuse and Neglect, 7*, 17–24.

Hampton, R. L., & Newberger, E. H. (1985). Child abuse incidence and reporting by hospitals: Significance of severity, class, and race. *American Journal of Public Health, 75,* 56–60.

Haugaard, J. J., & Reppucci, N. D. (1988). *The sexual abuse of children: A comprehensive guide to current knowledge and intervention strategies.* San Francisco: Jossey-Bass.

Jason, J., Andereck, N. D., Marks, S., & Tyler, C. W., Jr. (1982). Child abuse in Georgia: A method to evaluate risk factors and reporting bias. *American Journal of Public Health, 72,* 1353–1358.

Kercher, G. A., & McShane, M. (1984). The prevalence of child sexual abuse victimization in an adult sample of Texas residents. *Child Abuse and Neglect, 8,* 495–501.

Kinsey, A. C., Pomeroy, W. B., Martin, C. E., & Gebhard, P. H. (1953). *Sexual behavior in the human female.* Philadelphia: W. B. Saunders.

Knudsen, D. D. (1988). Child maltreatment over two decades: Change or continuity? *Violence and Victims, 3,* 129–144.

Korbin, J. E. (1987). Child abuse and neglect: The cultural context. In R. E. Helfer & R. S. Kempe (Eds.), *The battered child* (4th ed., pp. 23–41). Chicago: University of Chicago Press.

Last, J. (1983). *A dictionary of epidemiology.* New York: Oxford University Press.

Light, R. (1973). Abused and neglected children in America: A study of alternative policies. *Harvard Educational Review, 43,* 556–598.

Mausner, J. S., & Kramer, S. (1985). *Epidemiology: An introductory text.* Philadelphia: W. B. Saunders.

Maximus, Inc. (1986a). *Child maltreatment: A secondary analysis of the American Humane Association data base.* Washington, DC: Author.

Maximus, Inc. (1986b). *Child maltreatment: A secondary analysis of the American Humane Association data base: Exhibits.* Washington, DC: Author.

Maximus, Inc. (1986c). *Assessing alternative statistical estimation procedures for determining the incidence of child maltreatment: Appendix A: Reporting, substantiation, and confirmation rates, 1980 and 1983* (Final report, Task Order U, BOA 105-84-8103, prepared for the Office of Program Development, Office of Human Development Services). Washington, DC: Author.

Miller, S. H. (1984). The relationship between adolescent childbearing and child maltreatment. *Child Welfare, 63,* 553–557.

Mitchel, L. (1987). *Child abuse and neglect fatalities: A review of the problem and strategies for reform* (Working Paper No. 838). Chicago: National Committee for Prevention of Child Abuse.

Morris, J. L., Johnson, C. F., & Clasen, R. W. (1985). To report or not report: Physician's attitudes toward discipline and child abuse. *American Journal of Diseases of Children, 139,* 194–197.

National Center on Child Abuse and Neglect. (1981). *Study findings: National study of the incidence and severity of child abuse and neglect* (DHHS Publication No. OHDS 81-30325). Washington, DC: U. S. Government Printing Office.

National Center on Child Abuse and Neglect. (1988). *Study findings: Study of national incidence and prevalence of child abuse and neglect: 1988.* Washington, DC: U. S. Department of Health and Human Services.

Newberger, E. H. (1983). The helping hand strikes again: Unintended consequences of child abuse reporting. *Journal of Clinical Child Psychology, 12,* 307–311.

O'Toole, R., Turbett, P., & Nalepka, C. (1983). Theories, professional knowledge, and diagnosis of child abuse. In D. Finkelhor, R. J. Gelles, G. T. Hotaling, & M. A. Straus (Eds.), *The dark side of families: Current family violence research* (pp. 349–362). Beverly Hills, CA: Sage.

Pelton, L. H. (1977). Child abuse and neglect: The myth of classlessness. *American Journal of Orthopsychiatry, 48,* 608–617.

Pelton, L. H. (1981). Introduction. In L. H. Pelton (Ed.), *The social context of child abuse and neglect* (pp. 11–21). New York: Human Sciences Press.

Polansky, N., & Williams, D. (1978). Class orientations to child neglect. *Social Work, 23,* 397–401.

Radda Barnen. (1980). *The ombudsman and child maltreatment.* Stockholm, Sweden: Radda Barnen.

Risin, L. I., & Koss, M. P. (1987). The sexual abuse of boys: Prevalence and descriptive characteristics of childhood victimizations. *Journal of Interpersonal Violence, 2,* 309–323.

Rosenthal, J. A. (1988). Patterns of reported child abuse and neglect. *Child Abuse and Neglect, 12,* 263–271.

Russell, A., & Trainor, C. M. (1984). *Trends in child abuse and neglect: A national perspective.* Denver: American Humane Association.

Russell, D. E. H. (1983). The incidence and prevalence of intrafamilial and extrafamilial sexual abuse of female children. *Child Abuse and Neglect, 1987,* 133–146.

Russell, D. E. H. (1984). The prevalence and seriousness of incestuous abuse: Stepfathers vs. biological fathers. *Child Abuse and Neglect, 8,* 15–22.

Sack, W. H., Mason, R., & Higgins, J. E. (1985). The single-parent family and abusive child punishment. *American Journal of Orthopsychiatry, 55,* 252–259.

Sedney, M. A., & Brooks, B. (1984). Factors associated with a history of childhood sexual experience in a non-clinical female population. *Journal of the American Academy of Child Psychiatry, 23,* 215–218.

Silbert, M. H., & Pines, A. M. (1981). Sexual child abuse as an antecedent to prostitution. *Child Abuse and Neglect, 5,* 407–411.

Spearly, J. L., & Lauderdale, M. (1983). Community characteristics and ethnicity in the prediction of child maltreatment rates. *Child Abuse and Neglect, 7,* 91–105.

Starr, R. H., Jr. (1988). Physical abuse of children. In V. B. Van Hasselt, R. L. Morrison, A. S. Bellack, & M. Hersen (Eds.), *Handbook of family violence* (pp. 119–155). New York: Plenum Press.

Straus, M. A. (1979). Measuring intrafamily conflict and violence: The Conflict Tactics (CT) Scale. *Journal of Marriage and the Family, 41,* 75–88.

Straus, M. A., & Gelles, R. J. (1986). Societal change and change in family violence from 1975 to 1985 as revealed by two national surveys. *Journal of Marriage and the Family, 48,* 465–479.

Straus, M. A., Gelles, R. J., & Steinmetz, S. K. (1980). *Behind closed doors: Violence in the American Family.* Garden City, NY: Anchor Books.

Valentine, D. P., Acuff, D. S., Freeman, M. L., & Andreas, T. (1984). Defining child maltreatment: A multidisciplinary overview. *Child Welfare, 63,* 497–509.

Whiting, L. (1976). Defining emotional neglect. *Children Today, 5,* 2–5.

Wyatt, G. E. (1985). The sexual abuse of Afro-American and white-American women in childhood. *Child Abuse and Neglect, 9,* 507–519.

Wyatt, G. E., & Peters, S. D. (1986a). Issues in the definition of child sexual abuse in prevalence research. *Child Abuse and Neglect, 10,* 231–240.

Wyatt, G. E., & Peters, S. D. (1986b). Methodological considerations in research on the prevalence of child sexual abuse. *Child Abuse and Neglect, 10,* 241–251.

Zuravin, S. J. (1989). The ecology of child abuse and neglect: Review of the literature and presentation of data. *Violence and Victims, 4,* 101–120.

CHAPTER 3

TRENDS IN LEGISLATION AND CASE LAW ON CHILD ABUSE AND NEGLECT

RANDY K. OTTO AND GARY B. MELTON

INTRODUCTION

The recognition of child abuse and neglect as a significant social problem in the United States is a relatively recent development. Although most states had passed specific child maltreatment laws by the early 1920s, it was not until publication of a 1962 article describing the "battered-child syndrome" (Kempe, Silverman, Steele, Droegenmuller, & Silverman, 1962) that legislators and health care professionals paid considerable attention to the problem of child abuse and neglect. Since then, there have been several waves of legislation and judicial activity that have been nearly universal in American jurisdictions but that seldom have had unequivocally positive effects.

RANDY K. OTTO • Department of Law and Mental Health, Florida Mental Health Institute, University of South Florida, Tampa, Florida 33612-3899.   GARY B. MELTON • Department of Psychology, University of Nebraska–Lincoln, Lincoln, Nebraska 68588-0308.

JUSTIFICATION FOR STATE INTERVENTION

PARENS PATRIAE POWER

To evaluate the trends in law on child maltreatment, a useful starting place is consideration of the broad philosophical and empirical foundation of such policies. Without question, the state has a legitimate interest in the welfare of its citizens. Accordingly, under its *parens patriae* (sovereign as parent) power, the state may take actions to protect those individuals who are considered unable to protect or care for themselves (e.g., minors, the mentally disabled). In some cases, the state's interest as *parens patriae* is so compelling that it overrides even fundamental rights, such as the right to family privacy (see, e.g., *Prince v. Massachusetts*, 1944; cf. *Roe v. Wade*, 1973). Serious child maltreatment presents just such a situation.

Although the state's parens patriae power is expansive, it is not without boundaries (see, e.g., *Pierce v. Society of Sisters*, 1925; *Wisconsin v. Yoder*, 1972). For example, an involuntary intervention to protect child welfare can be justified only if no action less intrusive on family privacy would accommodate the state's compelling interest in the healthy socialization of dependent children. Indeed, family privacy is so fundamental that it must be considered even after children have been removed from the custody of their biological parents because of a demonstrated lack of safety in the home (Melton & Thompson, 1987). In *Santosky v. Kramer* (1982), the Supreme Court concluded that

> [t]he fundamental liberty interest of natural parents in the care, custody, and management of their child does not evaporate simply because they have not been model parents or have lost temporary custody of their child to the state. Even when blood relationships are strained, parents retain a vital interest in preventing the irretrievable destruction of their family life. (p. 753)

ORIENTATION AND SCOPE OF INTERVENTION

In the face of a need to balance critical needs to protect both child welfare and family privacy, no consistent orientation exists among child advocates about the nature of child maltreatment, the value of parental autonomy, and the merits of various interventions to prevent harm to children (Bourne & Newberger, 1977; Gelles, 1982; Melton, 1987a; Melton, Petrila, Poythress, & Slobogin, 1987). Accordingly, there is little agreement about either the specific circumstances that justify child protective jurisdiction or the level of coercive intervention that is desirable.

One school of commentators, emphasizing the deleterious effects of abuse and neglect, argues that the fundamental value placed on family privacy undermines the state's ability to protect children from abuse and neglect at the hands of their caretakers (e.g., Bourne & Newberger, 1977; Feshbach & Feshbach, 1976; Garbarino, 1977, 1982; Garbarino, Gaboury, Long, Grandjean, & Asp, 1982). This group perceives children as particularly vulnerable and in need of special protection by the state. "Family privacy" is considered merely to shield abusive families from public scrutiny, rather than protect them from unnecessary or unjustified state intervention. Accordingly, this group advocates minimal restrictions on the state in its attempts to identify and intervene in cases of suspected abuse. Such "child savers" support adoption of low standards for invoking state intervention and aggressive, high levels of intervention in cases of suspected abuse or neglect.

By contrast, two other schools of thought share the belief that state intrusion into family life is rarely advisable, even though they disagree why families should be better insulated against state intervention in cases of suspected abuse and neglect. One particularly influential family law scholar, Michael Wald (1975, 1976, 1982; Wald, Carlsmith, & Leiberman, 1988) has relied primarily on utilitarian arguments to support family integrity and privacy. Given the potential harm and lack of clear benefit frequently associated with state intervention in cases of alleged abuse (see, e.g., Children's Defense Fund, 1987; Clark Foundation, 1985; Mnookin, 1973), Wald has advocated clearly defined, strictly limited bases for state intervention. In short, he has concluded that more harm usually will be done by intervention than would have occurred if the state had ignored possible child maltreatment. Accordingly, Wald contends that coercive intervention should occur only when there is clear evidence that serious harm will result from inaction or a relatively unintrusive intervention.

An important step toward adoption of Wald's view came with the publication of the Juvenile Justice Standards Relating to Child Abuse and Neglect (Institute of Judicial Administration/American Bar Association [IJA/ABA], 1981). The Standards generally would limit state intervention to "situations in which there are findings that a child has suffered, or is at substantial risk of suffering, serious harm, and . . . intervention is necessary to protect the child from being endangered in the future" (Melton et al., 1987, p. 311). Although the Standards Relating to Abuse and Neglect, unlike most of the other volumes of the Juvenile Justice Standards, have not been adopted by the ABA as its official policy, the Standards remain an important reference for critics of the child welfare system.

A second school argues for family privacy and greater protection from state intrusion on the grounds that such intervention, insofar as it threatens children's perceptions of their "psychological parents," can have extremely deleterious effects (Goldstein, Freud, & Solnit, 1973, 1979). Like Wald (1975, 1982), these commentators would set a high threshold before state intervention could take place (indeed even higher than Wald advocates), but they differ from Wald in that they support aggressive intervention (even immediate termination of parental rights) once *serious* abuse or neglect is substantiated. Goldstein *et al.* believe that the best interests of the child (or, to use their term, the "least detrimental alternative") are best ensured by minimization of uncertainty and unpredictability and promotion of children's belief in the omnipotence of their parents. Their approach involves forceful, immediate measures, but only when it is clear that serious abuse or neglect has occurred. Otherwise, Goldstein *et al.* advocate virtually unfettered deference to parental autonomy.

With such a difference of opinion among experts in the fields of child mental health and family law, it is not surprising that the approach that states should adopt in cases of suspected abuse and neglect is controversial. Unfortunately, there is no reason to believe that this lack of consensus will be remedied in the immediate future.

Even if a consensus about the nature of child maltreatment and the appropriate policy responses to it is lacking, it is clear that the general direction since the 1960s has been toward more expansive concepts of abuse and neglect, accompanied by correspondingly increased intervention, despite the paradoxical evolution of constitutional law on family privacy during the same period (Melton, 1987c). The impression held by legislators and the public alike is that there is a need for broad standards for state intervention. For example, the scope of maltreatment for legal purposes has expanded to include emotional abuse and neglect, even though application of such concepts in a manner that is not arbitrary or discriminatory may be impossible (Melton & Thompson, 1987). Accompanying expanded definitions have been calls for greater use of criminal sanctions, especially in regard to sexual abuse. In that respect, in recent years, legislatures in every American jurisdiction have adopted procedural and evidentiary reforms designed to make prosecution easier (Bulkley, 1985), despite questions of the efficacy of a "get-tough" strategy generally (Melton, 1987a) or of utility of the specific reforms, many of which are of dubious constitutionality (Melton, 1987b; see *Coy v. Iowa,* 1988).

CRIMINAL AND CIVIL ADJUDICATION OF CHILD ABUSE AND NEGLECT

Criminal Adjudication

Although criminal prosecution has been rare until recent years, remedies for child abuse and neglect have been available in both the civil and criminal arenas for a considerable period of time (Davidson & Horowitz, 1984). All 50 states provide potential criminal sanctions for child maltreatment. As a matter of practice, though, criminal prosecution is generally reserved for sexual and the most serious cases of physical abuse. Data gathered by Midonick (1972) are illustrative, although somewhat out of date. Examining New York records, Midonick found that fewer than 10% of all reports of child abuse found their way to family court, and fewer than 10% of those cases adjudicated were referred to criminal court.

A philosophical argument can be made that child abuse and neglect should be adjudicated criminally because to do otherwise minimizes the seriousness of the behavior. "Decriminalizing" what is otherwise criminal behavior is considered to send a subtle message to the public. And as with other crimes, criminal adjudication is considered by some to promote specific and general deterrence (Chisolm, 1978; Davidson, Horowitz, Marvell, & Ketcham, 1981).

Advocates of criminal adjudication argue that it best ensures the safety of children in serious cases by incapacitating the abuser when necessary (Davidson, 1981). Even with the use of restraining orders, civil adjudication cannot guarantee that the abuser will not have further contact with the abused child (or other children).

Additionally, use of criminal prosecution is advocated because it is considered to better ensure compliance with sanctions that may be imposed by the judge. Compliance with criminal court-ordered treatment is thought by some to be more likely than compliance with civil court-ordered treatment (Urzi, 1981).

Criminal adjudication is also advocated on the grounds that law-enforcement officials will investigate allegations more aggressively if they believe that a criminal prosecution will result (Urzi, 1981). Criminal prosecution, because of the greater due process requirements and burden of proof, is also more protective of families' privacy rights than civil adjudication.

Finally, recent work suggests that criminal adjudication may be able to reduce recidivism in criminal behaviors traditionally considered to be psychosocial problems. Like child abuse, spouse abuse has traditionally been managed through noncriminal interventions (Costa, 1983). More recently, however, states have begun to respond to spouse abuse using the criminal justice system. This approach has met with some success and may have implications for the management of child abuse.

In a demonstration project conducted in Minneapolis, Sherman and Berk (1984) found that individuals arrested for assaulting their spouse showed a somewhat lower recidivism rate than those who were either counseled by, or simply separated from their spouse by the responding police officer. Certainly, these preliminary findings are open to interpretation but they do suggest that criminal adjudication may be indicated with some types of behavior traditionally considered to be psychosocial problems and amenable to treatment.

The parallel to child abuse and neglect is clear. Criminal sanctions may be effective in reducing child abuse and neglect, at least with a segment of the population. However, research comparing recidivism rates among abusive and neglectful parents who have been processed through the criminal justice and civil systems needs to be conducted.

It appears then that there are specific advantages associated with criminal adjudication. These include the provision of considerable procedural protections to families accused of abuse, ability to manage and control individuals who present a continuing, serious threat to their victims and other children, and the potential impact of general and specific deterrence by way of threatened imposition of criminal sanctions.

Civil Adjudication

Although criminal prosecution has become more common in child maltreatment, civil intervention long has predominated in such cases. The first child protective agency was established in New York in 1875, and by the mid-1920s all states had laws prohibiting child maltreatment (Besharov, 1983).

Perhaps foremost, civil adjudication of abuse and neglect has been based on the belief that these behaviors are psychosocial problems that can be differentiated from criminal behavior (Fontana & Besharov, 1979; Rosenberg, 1975; Urzi, 1981). Abusing one's child often is considered to be a mental health problem in itself, or at least indicative of underlying mental health problems. Such a belief predominates among the public even for sexual abuse (Finkelhor, 1984), the form of maltreatment by far most likely to generate a criminal complaint. Therefore, it is argued, intervention should be treatment-oriented, rather than punitive in nature. A collateral argument is that rehabilitation and treatment may not be accomplished, or are at least are compromised, when conducted under the auspices of the criminal justice system (Dickens, 1978).

Also supporting civil intervention in cases of child abuse and neglect is the belief that abusive and neglectful behaviors are particularly responsive to treatment (Midonick, 1972). This argument is appealing if maltreatment is indeed a product of parental pathology, inadequacy, or skills deficits remediable by therapeutic intervention. Court-ordered treatment or other coercive interventions pursuant to civil jurisdiction could be used to promote the family court's goals of maintenance of family integrity and prevention of further abuse.

In the same vein, civil intervention often is favored because it accords greater dispositional flexibility than do criminal sanctions. In civil adjudication, no one caretaker need be labeled as the problem. Rather, when appropriate, the family system or multiple caretakers may be identified as dysfunctional and interventions instituted accordingly. Critics of criminal sanctions argue that their usefulness as a means of family change is severely compromised by their focus on single individuals.

Such utilitarian arguments cannot be considered in isolation. If civil intervention is to be justified on the grounds that it facilitates appropriate treatment, then the efficacy of treatments available to the family court is relevant. Unfortunately, interventions aimed at decreasing abusive and neglectful behaviors have not met with much success. Recidivism rates in model demonstration projects for the treatment of abusive and neglectful parents approach 33%, with the best estimate being that approximately one third of treated clients show improvement during treatment (Cohn, 1979; Melton et al., 1987; Rosenberg & Hunt, 1984; Wald, Carlsmith, & Leiberman, 1988). Such findings call into question the justification of civil intervention on the ground that further abuse and neglect may be prevented through treatment.

Civil intervention in the case of abusive and neglectful caretakers also has been justified on the grounds that it is less likely to traumatize the child than criminal adjudication. Criminal adjudication may create further stress for a family already in crisis, thereby placing the child at greater risk for abuse or neglect (Dickens, 1978; IJA/ABA, 1981). Although there is little empirical support for such a claim (Melton, 1987b), many commentators believe that children may be revictimized if they are required to testify in a criminal court in which the defendant's rights to a public trial, a jury trial, and confrontation of witnesses are preserved (DeConey, 1975).

It is also claimed that interventions should be nonpunitive in order to encourage self-reporting (Dickens, 1978). Knowing that they are subject to criminal penalties (including prison sentences and resulting separation from their family), parents may be less likely to come forward and admit to abuse or neglect (Fontana & Besharov, 1979). Such an argument ignores the fact that even in noncriminal dispositions the potential sanctions are severe and may serve to deter self-reporting. In civil adjudication, the possibility remains that the abusive caretaker or abused child will be separated from the family. Thus, even under the current system, whereby abuse cases are frequently adjudicated by civil courts, the large majority of cases are not reported by the abusive caretaker or his or her spouse.

Critics also argue against criminal prosecution, because it requires a more rigorous standard of proof and accordingly may result in more false negative errors and, therefore, less protection of children (Midonick, 1972). Because of the need for stronger evidence in criminal than in civil cases, criminal prosecutors also may be more likely to seek the testimony of child victims, who correspondingly may be especially leery of testifying because of the combination of procedural protections of the rights of criminal defendants and because of the penalties that they ultimately may endure (DeConey, 1975).

In summary, as compared to the criminal system, civil adjudication increases the likelihood that intervention can be ordered (as a result of lower burdens and less procedural rigor), provides the decisionmaker with more latitude in identifying those who are responsible for the abuse and are in need of treatment, and often offers a greater range of possible interventions. It does so, however, at the cost of increasing the likelihood of incorrect adjudications and unnecessary or overly intrusive interventions.

Discussion

The debate about the relative merits of criminal and civil intervention does not result in a clear answer. Each form of intervention has advantages and disadvantages of varying importance in particular cases, and both civil and criminal sanctions may be sought in some instances. Some (e.g., Chisolm, 1978) have argued that the courts and child protective workers should choose the judicial intervention accordingly, with the child's best interest being of paramount concern. Such a principle may be attractive to legal decision makers because of its consistency with the historic individualized approach to children's cases. However, such an approach is not without problems. As a practical matter, courts (and the experts advising them) may be unable to differentiate "dangerous" and "non-dangerous" caretakers (as suggested by Chisolm, 1978). Moreover, a policy of individualized justice increases the probability of discrimination on the basis of ethnicity, social class, or other suspect classifications. Perhaps most fundamentally, case-by-case decisions about the path that adjudication will take beg the question of whether maltreating parents deserve punishment, as a matter of justice.

Although the political climate has changed sufficiently that an unequivocal "model" answer no longer would be likely to emerge, the Juvenile Justice Standards (IJA/ABA, 1981) provide a clear preference for civil action because of the paramount interests of the child and the presumed adverse effects of the criminal process on the victim:

> Criminal prosecution for conduct that is the subject of a petition for court jurisdiction filed pursuant to these standards should be authorized only if the court in which such petition has been filed certifies that such prosecution will not unduly harm the interests of the child named in the petition. (IJA/ABA, 1981, p. 180)

Whatever the preferred balance between treatment and punishment and between the interests of the victim in a rapid return to normalcy and of society in seeking retribution, concepts of the nature of children, abusers, and maltreatment itself have had an ongoing effect on legal policy. As each new social construct has been "discovered," a wave of legislation has followed.

LEGISLATIVE RESPONSES

The First Wave of Legislation: Child Abuse Reporting Statutes

The first such wave followed publication of the seminal article on the "battered child syndrome" by Kempe and his colleagues (Kempe, Silverman, Steele, Droegenmueller, & Silver, 1962). With the discovery of a purported medical syndrome, case-finding was the logical public health response. Accordingly, between 1963 and 1967, all 50 states and the District of Columbia passed statutes requiring that health professionals report cases of suspected abuse (Brown, 1974).

Current child abuse statutes typically identify different types of behavior defined as constituting abuse or neglect, specify the agencies that are responsible for abuse investigation, name those individuals required to report abuse, and list penalties for failure to report. Additionally, these statutes generally contain clauses overriding professional privileges (with the general exception of the attorney–client privilege) and granting immunity from civil liability for good faith reporting.

Initially, only physicians were statutorily mandated to report cases of suspected abuse, presumably because they were considered to be in a unique position to identify such cases (Isaacson, 1975; Paulsen, 1967). Gradually, however, legislators expanded reporting statutes to the point that most child professionals and many laypersons are required to report suspected abuse (see Myers, 1986, for a review of the 50 state reporting statutes).

This first wave of legislation had a considerable impact on the number of suspected abuse cases reported to child welfare and law-enforcement authorities. Besharov (1983) noted that there was an eightfold increase in the number of cases of suspected abuse reported between 1966 (150,000) and 1980 (1.1 million).

Reporting statutes have certainly not been the panacea that some might have hoped. The most common criticism of these statutes is that they are vague and overbroad (Besharov, 1983, 1984; Davidson & Horowitz, 1984; Flicker, 1977; Melton, 1987a; Melton & Thompson, 1987). Representative of states' abuse laws is New York's reporting statute, which mandates that health care and law-enforcement professionals report abuse when "they have reasonable cause to suspect" abuse (New York Social Services Law Sec. 413, McKinney, 1988). Exactly what the professional needs to see or believe in order to report abuse and thereby comply with the reporting statute is not made clear in most statutes.

There may also be difficulty reaching a consensus about the behavior that falls within the scope of child maltreatment. Research has shown that there is considerable disagreement between professionals regarding what constitutes sexually abusive behavior on the part of caretakers (Atteberry-Bennett, 1987; Atteberry-Bennett & Reppucci, 1986). It can even be difficult to reach agreement about the boundaries of physical abuse (Giovannoni & Becerra, 1979). There is considerable disagreement about the circumstances under which spanking and other, less severe forms of corporal punishment should be viewed as abusive (Alvy, 1975).

The matter becomes still more complicated when neglect or "failure to provide" is considered. All states consider parents' failure to provide their children with basic care and necessities to be neglectful (Davidson & Horowitz, 1984). Nonetheless, the scope of "basic care and necessities" is not self-evident. Although some state statutes requiring parents to provide adequate shelter, food, and care have been struck down as unconstitutionally vague, others have withstood judicial scrutiny. In the latter cases, the courts have generally held that such broad language is necessary to ensure the protection of children (Davidson & Horowitz, 1984).

Further complicating matters is the issue of intent. Should impoverished parents who are unable to provide basic necessities (e.g., food, clothing, a safe physical environment, and medical care) be treated differently from parents who are financially able, but who decide not to provide such necessities? Although there may be general agreement that the latter case constitutes neglect and some form of coercive intervention is indicated, whether and what type of state intervention is required in the former case is less clear. Because the civil child protective system is supposed to be nonpunitive, intervention is premised on consequences of behavior rather than blameworthiness, but intrusion into the family nonetheless seems unfair when the harm is not the parents' fault.

Perhaps most difficult to define are the concepts of emotional or psychological abuse and neglect, which are included in the majority of state reporting statutes. Not surprisingly, sections describing emotional abuse and neglect lack specificity. Most statutes refer to infliction of "mental injury," without a more precise definition (Melton & Corson, 1987). The nature of the triggering behavior by a parent or response by a child is unclear. For example, should the state intervene when the parent engages in an admittedly abusive behavior when there is no apparent injury to the child, or is it the child's emotional adjustment that should serve as the triggering mechanism? The analogue to the problem of blameworthiness is even more acute in emotional maltreatment than it is in physical neglect, because some intentional parental behavior (e.g., divorce) that is known often to have harmful psychological effects on children seems intuitively to lie outside the boundaries of abuse (Melton & Thompson, 1987). Other behaviors that may have predictable consequences often viewed as negative for children are strongly linked to social class. A purely outcome-based definition thus risks class-based intrusions into family life.

Given these difficulties, allegations of emotional abuse are usually joined with allegations of physical maltreatment or sexual abuse, and they are rarely filed alone. Because of the difficulty drawing a causal nexus between the parent's allegedly abusive behavior and the child's psychological state, many argue that the child's mental injuries should be both substantial and observable, and be clearly linked to parental behavior (Besharov, 1984; Melton & Thompson, 1987).

Data regarding the proportion of abuse reports that are later substantiated support the conclusion that the reporting standards are, at a minimum, unclear and possibly overbroad. Currently, between 40% and 43% of abuse and neglect reports are substantiated, and approximately 25% of these require some type of court action (National Center for State Courts, 1988). Thus, less than one half of current child abuse and neglect reports are substantiated. The high rate of unsubstantiation probably results from a number of factors, including defensive practice by professionals fearing repercussions for failure to report (but see Maney & Wells, 1988, on underreporting by professionals), inadequate investigatory resources in child protective services (CPS), and the intrinsic difficulty of proving some forms of maltreatment of young children. Failure to substantiate maltreatment may also result from professionals' confusion because of vague and possibly overbroad standards.

One of the criticisms of such vague and apparently value-laden standards is that they open the door to arbitrary, discriminatory application of state power. Mandated reporters effectively can pick and choose standards to apply, and thus may impose their own values on individuals of different cultural backgrounds and socioeconomic status (Davidson & Horowitz, 1984; Dickens, 1978; Melton, 1987a; Melton et al., 1987).

Attempts to prevent and manage child abuse and neglect through state legislation clearly have not met with complete success. Although some gains have been made (e.g., the number of abused children coming to the attention of authorities), there have been associated costs (e.g., a considerable number of unsubstantiated reports; interventions that sometimes may be more disruptive than helpful). Moreover, professionals are confused about their roles and responsibilities. The mixed picture probably has resulted in part from the often quick and essentially unplanned manner in which state legislatures often have approached the difficult policy problems related to child maltreatment (Lucht, 1975; Nelson, 1984).

CHILD ABUSE PREVENTION AND TREATMENT ACT OF 1974

The picture at the federal level is a little rosier. The federal government has been a late and ambivalent participant in policy on child maltreatment. Until 1974, virtually all government activity on child maltreatment was at the state level. With passage of the federal Child Abuse Prevention and Treatment Act (CAPTA) of 1974 (Public Law 93-247), the federal government began to set the agenda for child abuse prevention and treatment. Prior to enactment of CAPTA, federal support for abuse and neglect programs was limited largely to Title IV-B of the Social Security Act, which authorized general child welfare services. However, in 1973, the year before passage of Public Law 93-247, only $507,000 of Title IV-B monies went toward child abuse activities nationally (House of Representatives Report No. 685, 1974).

Noting that state efforts largely went toward reporting and that there was inadequate follow-up, the Child Abuse Prevention and Treatment Act attempted to establish a research agenda and prevention and treatment programming to be coordinated through the newly established National Center on Child Abuse and Neglect (NCCAN). The act authorized the director of NCCAN to compile, analyze, and publish research results regarding child abuse; develop and maintain an information clearinghouse; compile and publish training materials; provide technical assistance (through grants and contracts) to assist public or private nonprofit organizations in the planning, development, and implementation of prevention and treatment programs; and conduct research regarding causes and prevention of child abuse.

To be eligible for CAPTA funding, states had to meet certain criteria, most of which were related to reporting and investigation procedures. In order for states to receive CAPTA funding they had to have a system in place for abuse reporting and investigation, provide criminal and civil immunity for good-faith reporting, ensure that abuse reports and records were kept confidential, and provide guardians *ad litem* for all children. CAPTA also required states to maintain their funding of abuse programming and extend preferential treatment to parental organizations organized to prevent and treat child abuse.

Presumably in response to some of the criticisms presented above, there was discussion of the difficulty in defining such terms as *neglect* and *mental* or *emotional injury* in the House report. However, the bill, as passed, offered the following definition: "This section defines the term 'child abuse and neglect' as the physical or *mental injury,* sexual abuse, *negligent treatment,* or maltreatment of a child under the age of eighteen by a person who is responsible for the child's welfare" (House of Representatives Report No. 685, 1974; emphasis added).

The Child Abuse Prevention and Treatment Act of 1974 has been amended several times so that its scope is now somewhat broader. A number of important amendments were passed in 1984. Public Law 98-457 extended the definition of abuse and neglect to include the sexual exploitation and the withholding of medically indicated treatment (the "Baby Doe" amendment), and expanded CAPTA so that abuse and neglect occurring in residential and out-of-home placements was also covered by the act.

An amendment passed in 1986 (Public Law 99-401) directed the Secretary of Health and Human Services to establish demonstration projects to provide in-home and out-of-home temporary nonmedical child care for handicapped children and children with chronic and terminal illnesses, and to provide crisis nurseries for children at risk for abuse and neglect.

The Children's Justice and Assistance Act (Public Law 99-401) was a 1986 CAPTA amendment which encouraged states to enact reforms designed to improve legal and administrative proceedings in child sexual abuse cases. Such reforms, it was hoped, would protect children from trauma associated with involvement in the abuse investigation and prosecution, and thereby improve the chances of successful prosecutions. The amendment earmarked 24 million dollars for fiscal years 1987 and 1988 (Senate Report No. 123, 1986).

As a funding statute, Public Law 93-247 has had its greatest impact in terms of developing state child abuse reporting and investigation programs. And these reporting requirements appear to have some effect on the identification of abused and neglected children. Studies suggest that mental health professionals have gradually become more knowledgeable of, and increased their compliance with, reporting requirements (cf. Kalichman & Craig, in press; Kalichman, Craig, & Follingstad, 1987; Swoboda, Elwork, Sales, & Levine, 1979). Still, a considerable number of professionals fail to comply with statutory requirements and report suspected abuse or neglect (Maney & Wells, 1988). There has also been a considerable increase in the number of reports made by nonmandated reporters (Melton, 1987b).

OTHER FEDERAL LEGISLATION

In addition to the Child Abuse Prevention and Treatment Act and its amendments, other measures have been enacted by the federal government that are designed to minimize child abuse and neglect, a number of which are reviewed below.

The Parental Kidnapping Prevention Act of 1980 attempts to eliminate some of the legal and practical difficulties occurring in the case of parental kidnapping. The act orders states to honor and enforce any child custody determinations made in the courts of other states and provides assistance to the custodial parent in the case of abduction by the noncustodial parent, including use of state and federal locator services.

The Missing Children Assistance Act of 1984 was enacted as a partial response to the problem of runaway and missing children. The act provided funds for establishment of a toll free hotline to report information about missing children and other projects aimed at locating children or providing services to missing children and their families. The statute also provided funding for research related to missing children.

The Child Sexual Abuse and Pornography Act of 1986 provides for federal prosecution of persons engaged in child pornography, including parents who permit their children to engage in such activities. In addition to fines and imprisonment, the statute also allows for the confiscation of property used in conjunction with the crime. The statute identifies federal district courts as the forums in which civil suits alleging damages to minors engaged in pornography are to be heard, and it sets the minimum award in such cases at $50,000.

As the above review suggests, much of the emphasis at the federal level has remained on reporting, investigation, and prosecution. In contrast to this focus, Children's Trust Funds, which are state mechanisms, place a greater emphasis on prevention and treatment.

CHILDREN'S TRUST FUNDS

Since 1980, advocates for abused and neglected children have established Children's Trust Funds in 44 states (National Committee for the Prevention of Child Abuse [NCPCA], undated). These funds establish a permanent funding mechanism for child abuse and neglect prevention and treatment programs at the community level.

Children's Trust Funds are designed to create continuing funding mechanisms that promote prevention programming for child abuse and neglect at the community level (NCPCA, undated). Revenues are generated from various methods, including: surcharges on marriage licenses and birth certificates, checkoffs on state income tax forms, increases in divorce filing costs, increased fees for death certificates, and heirloom birth certificates. This approach allows for the funding of traditionally neglected prevention programs and insulates them from budget cuts when state monies become scarce.

The governing body of the trust fund creates a public/private partnership. In some states, existing bodies that include representatives from state agencies, the legislature, and the private sector have administered the fund. In other states, public advisory councils consisting of public and private sector representatives have been created.

Trust fund boards oversee program development and implementation, hire program staff, review program proposals, and disburse funds. The major thrust of trust fund programs to date has been in promoting and funding primary and secondary prevention programs at the community level. These include, but are not limited to pre- and postnatal support programs for first-time and recent parents (especially "at risk" families with unhealthy newborns), parent education and training groups, parent self-help and neighborhood support groups, family support services (e.g., crisis babysitters, crisis nurseries, crisis counseling), child care programs, treatment programs for abused and neglected children, and community education on child abuse prevention (NCPCA, undated).

Although the full impact of trust fund programs may not be determined at this point in time, they show promise in that they are nontraditional programs that identify "at risk" populations and attempt to promote cost-effective prevention and treatment programs.

PROCEDURAL AND EVIDENTIARY REFORMS RELATED TO ADJUDICATION

Although nontraditional in approach, the trust funds are consistent with the historic preventive role of the civil child protection system. The initial federal initiatives can be seen in the same light, in that they were intended to uncover maltreatment in order to prevent further harm to children. The most recent wave of legislation in the states (which, as we have already noted, is paralleled in recent federal legislation) appears to be oriented more, though, toward increasing the likelihood of punishment of offenders against children, especially in sexual abuse cases.

Rather than focusing on protection of children from future harm, state legislatures and, indirectly, the Congress (through, for example, the Children's Justice Act) have been active in recent years in establishment of procedural and evidentiary reforms intended to increase the likelihood of successful prosecution of alleged abusers. Most states have enacted new laws providing for special qualification of child victims as witnesses, special hearsay exceptions, exclusion of spectators during testimony by child victims, videotaped depositions, closed circuit television, and special courtrooms (see Bulkley, 1985; Eatman & Bulkley, 1986; Whitcomb, 1985).

The underlying assumption of these reforms is that standard criminal procedure unduly traumatizes the child victim and therefore compromises the ability of the criminal system to identify and sanction those individuals guilty of abuse. All of the proposed reforms are designed to facilitate acceptance of children's statements, often even when not made in court, in order to increase the number of successful child abuse prosecutions.

However noble the intentions of the framers of legislation creating special procedures and hearsay exceptions in abuse cases, such reforms have been controversial and often may have *increased* children's limbo in the criminal justice system by opening the door to appeals. Considerable appellate litigation has resulted from many of the procedural and evidentiary reforms enacted in recent years, because they typically threaten the defendant's sixth-Amendment rights to a public trial and confrontation of witnesses, his fourteenth amendment right to due process, and/or the public's first amendment right to access (through the press) to the trial process (Melton, 1987a).

The Impact of Testifying upon Child Witnesses

Perhaps the most fundamental complaint about the recent wave of legislation is that changes are unneeded and, if needed, may be ineffective or even counterproductive. This point may seem odd to many observers, who conclude intuitively that child victims are further traumatized by their participation in the legal process, particularly testifying at trial. Little is actually known, however, about the impact that testifying has on children (Haugaard & Reppucci, 1988; Melton, 1987a).

In the absence of empirical support, it is premature to conclude that child victims' participation in the criminal process will prove particularly traumatizing. That participation in the criminal process can have positive effects on adult victims' psychological functioning is well-accepted (see, e.g., Kelly, 1987; Kilpatrick & Otto, 1987), and the same may be true for child victims. Staff from two federally funded demonstration projects for the evaluation and treatment of sexual abuse (the Harborview Medical Center, Seattle, and the Children's Hospital National Medical Center, Washington, DC) have published accounts noting the positive impact that participation in the criminal process can have for child victims. Berliner and Barbieri (1984) claim that testifying can be therapeutic for child victims insofar as the experience empowers them and teaches them that their complaints are taken seriously. Rogers (1982) noted that participation in the criminal process provides child victims with a socially sanctioned opportunity for retribution and also may serve as official acknowledgment that the victims were not responsible for their victimization. Preliminary data reported by Runyan and his colleagues (King, Hunter, & Runyan, 1988; Runyan, Everson, Edelsohn, Hunter, & Coulter, 1988) suggest that child victims' adjustment may improve as a function of testifying.

The social psychological literature examining procedural justice and satisfaction lends further credence to these data. Work by Thibaut and Walker (1978) suggests that adults perceive the adversarial method to be the fairest and most satisfactory form of inquiry. At least among older children, then, participation in the adversarial process, even if it is stressful at the time, is likely to heighten their sense of control and perception of justice (Melton, 1983c; Melton & Limber, 1990; Melton & Lind, 1982).

Although it cannot be expected that all child victims will benefit from participation in the criminal process, the theoretical perspectives and data presented above challenge the presumption that participation in criminal proceedings (including testifying) will necessarily traumatize the child victim. Thus, reforms aimed at insulating child victims from the effects of participating in the criminal process may be unnecessary and are likely to be found unconstitutionally overbroad.

CHILDREN'S COMPETENCY TO TESTIFY

At common law, children under the age of 10 were presumed incompetent to testify and the competence of older children was rebuttable (Melton et al., 1987). In evaluating a child's (and adult's) competency to testify, the judge typically examines the person's ability to differentiate the truth from falsehoods, the ability to understand the duty to tell the truth, and the consequences for not doing so. Also evaluated are the witness's ability to avoid suggestion and to have formed a just or valid impression of the facts at the time of the incident in question (Melton, 1987c).

A considerable amount of research examining the competency of child witnesses has been conducted in recent years (see Goodman, 1984; Goodman & Helgeson, 1985; Haugaard & Reppucci, 1988; Melton et al., 1987, for reviews). For the most part, the research literature suggests that the general presumption of children's incompetency is unfounded.

In response to these findings, and in order to facilitate introduction of children's testimony in abuse cases, states have begun to eliminate presumptions of children's incompetency to testify (Melton, 1987b; Whitcomb, 1985). These efforts have been reinforced by the Federal Rules of Evidence (Rule 601) that presume all witnesses to be competent. Although the federal rules only apply to federal proceedings, they serve as model rules which are followed by a large number of states. Thus, whereas the traditional common law system presumed child witnesses to be incompetent to testify, the Federal Rules of Evidence (and the rules in an increasing number of states) presume child witnesses to be competent. In either case the presumption in effect (i.e., competency or incompetency) can be challenged.

Hearsay Exceptions

A number of states have developed special hearsay exceptions for children who are victims/witnesses in sexual abuse cases (Berliner, 1985). These exceptions are designed to allow introduction of out-of-court statements that would otherwise be excluded as hearsay.

Generally, hearsay is not admitted into evidence because it is considered less reliable than court-based testimony subject to cross-examination. Admission of hearsay evidence is considered to violate the defendant's Sixth Amendment right to confront his or her accusers. However, the bar against hearsay testimony in criminal proceedings is not absolute. The Supreme Court has held that hearsay may be admitted against criminal defendants when the prosecuting witness is unavailable and there are "indicia of reliability"—as determined by traditional hearsay exceptions (e.g., complaint of rape exception, statements of medical or physical condition, excited utterances) or other specific "guarantees of trustworthiness" (*Ohio v. Roberts*, 1980).

Under the current system, two tacks may be taken in trying to admit children's out-of-court statements. First, prosecutors may try to fit children's statements regarding abuse into present exceptions such as the excited utterance or medical statement exceptions. Alternatively, some have advocated that another exception be made specifically for child sexual abuse victims. Graham (1985), for example, proposes that the hearsay statements of child victims be allowed (1) if the child also testifies at trial, or (2) if the child is unavailable and the statement is supported by corroborative evidence of some type. Of course, unavailability because of incompetency should serve to bar admission of testimony on the grounds that, on its face, it lacks indicia of reliability. Unavailability resulting from the anticipated trauma associated with testifying may not be assumed (see, e.g., *Connecticut v. Jarzbek*, 1987) and would have to be proven in the particular case.

Among the traditional exceptions, the excited utterance exception allows introduction of out-of-court statements offered immediately following, and in response to the incident in question on the basis that they are highly reliable. Because they frequently are given a considerable amount of time after the alleged act, children's accounts to investigators usually do not appear to meet the general requirement of the excited utterance exception. Some courts have applied this common law exception liberally (Bulkley, 1981), however, and admitted children's hearsay testimony under it (e.g., *Commonwealth v. Adams*, 1987).

The medical statement exception allows introduction of out-of-court statements made to health care professionals during the course of treatment, based upon the assumption that because individuals are unlikely to deceive health care professionals who treat them, their statements are especially trustworthy. Prosecutors may also seek admission of children's allegations gathered by psychologists or physicians but here too, such action does not appear consonant with the intent of the medical exception which requires that the declarant's motive in making the statement to be for the purpose of treatment (*United States v. Iron Shell*, 1980). Again, however, some courts have admitted children's statements made to health care professionals on the basis of the medical exception (e.g., *In re* Freiberger, 1986). The admissibility of 1990 statements made by child victims to health care professionals will be addressed by the Supreme Court in *Idaho v. Wright*, which the court had yet to hear at the time this chapter went to press.

Perhaps the most appropriate hearsay exception through which children's out-of-court statements should be admitted is the general exception noted in Rule 803 of the Federal Rules of Evidence. Section 24 of Rule 803 provides for the introduction of out-of-court statements which do not qualify under any specific exceptions. To be admitted under this exception the statement must have circumstantial guarantees of trustworthiness; be offered as evidence of a material fact; and be more probative than any other evidence which is available to the presenting party. Additionally, it must be determined that the general interest of justice is best served by introduction of the statement.

CLOSED COURTROOMS

In an attempt to minimize potential trauma experienced by the child victim/witness in criminal proceedings, a number of states have passed statutes closing courtrooms to spectators and the press during the child's testimony (Whitcomb, 1985). Such measures are considered by some to violate the defendant's Sixth Amendment right to a public trial and the public's First Amendment right of access to trials through the press. The Supreme Court examined the constitutionality of closed courtrooms in *Globe Newspaper Company v. Superior Court* (1982). In *Globe*, the Court ruled that a Massachusetts statute directing judges to bar the press from *all* trials during the testimony of child sexual assault victims/witnesses was overbroad and in violation of the First Amendment. However, the Court indicated that the courtroom could be closed in some instances. Noting that the state has a compelling interest in protecting child victims from trauma, the Court ruled that, "the trial court can determine on a case-by-case basis whether closure is necessary to protect the welfare of a minor victim" (p. 608).

SPECIAL COURTROOM PROCEDURES

In attempting to increase the likelihood of successful prosecution of child abusers, child advocates also have pressed for reforms in trial and courtroom procedure. In *Kentucky v. Stincer* (1987), the Supreme Court ruled that the state may bar the defendant from children's competency hearings in some sexual abuse cases. In reaching its decision, the Court held that barring the defendant from the hearing did not violate his Sixth or Fourteenth Amendment rights because it did not interfere with his opportunity to cross-examine the witnesses effectively.

The recent Supreme Court decision of *Coy v. Iowa* (1988) suggests, however, that implementation of special procedures designed to protect child witnesses in abuse cases will be examined carefully by the Court. At issue in *Coy* was an Iowa statute permitting use of a screen which could be placed between defendants and child victims/witnesses while they testified. The screen, designed to protect child witnesses from the trauma associated with testifying in front of alleged assailants, blocked the witnesses' view of the defendant, but allowed the defendant to see and hear the witnesses as they testified.

The Court interpreted the meaning of the confrontation clause strictly, holding that it guarantees the defendant a "face-to-face meeting with witnesses appearing before the trier of fact" (p. 2800). Similar to its decision in *Globe*, the Court ruled that the legislatively-imposed presumption of trauma was not sufficient. Such an exception, ruled the Court, is not "firmly rooted" in our system of jurisprudence, and there were no individualized findings that the witnesses in this case were in need of special protection.

Together, the Court's decisions in *Globe Newspapers* and *Coy* suggest that although special procedures may be used in cases where it has been shown that the *specific witness* is at risk for significant trauma without such measures, their mandatory imposition will be barred when a constitutionally protected interest is infringed. How the court may treat similar procedures, such as the presentation of videotaped testimony and the use of closed circuit television, was addressed in the concurring opinion of Justice O'Connor in *Coy* in which she was joined by Justice White. After emphasizing the majority's suggestion that the screen might be justified when the witness was shown to be at special risk, O'Connor went on to discuss the opinion in terms of its applicability to other procedures such as testimony via one- and two-way closed circuit television. Noting that, at the time, 25 states provided for such closed circuit procedures and 33 allowed the presentation of videotaped testimony of child victims, O'Connor wrote that

> nothing in today's decision necessarily dooms such efforts by state legislatures to protect child witnesses. Initially, many such procedures raise no substantial confrontation clause problem since they involve testimony in the presence of the defendant. (p. 2804)

O'Connor's concurrence in *Coy* suggests that the Court may not be as hostile to special procedures in the future. It is possible that O'Connor, White, and Kennedy (who took no part in the decision) will join the *Coy* dissenters (Blackmun and Rehnquist) to form a majority more accepting of special procedures designed to protect witnesses, providing that they are not mandatory and that they allow for "face-to-face" confrontation between the defendant and witness. The Supreme Court will address this issue more specifically in *Craig v. Maryland*, which the court had yet to hear at the time this chapter went to press.

Psychological Testimony about Abuser and Victim Profiles

In the adjudicatory phase of abuse and neglect cases, the state or defense may seek to introduce expert opinion regarding the psychological characteristics of abusers. Through the introduction of this testimony, the state seeks to create the inference that the defendant is like people who abuse children and is, therefore, guilty of the allegations. In a similar vein, the defense might seek to introduce such testimony on the basis that the defendant is not like those individuals who abuse children in order to combat allegations of abuse or neglect. Because such testimony is generally treated as character evidence, it is inadmissible according to Federal Rule of Evidence 404 unless the defendant offers such evidence first.

Mental health professionals may also be asked to testify about the characteristics of abused or neglected children in order to support or diminish the child victim's allegations. The least objectionable testimony of this sort involves the expert explaining to the court aspects of the child's behavior that might be confusing (Haugaard & Reppucci, 1988; Melton & Limber, 1990). Thus, the expert might explain why some child victims fail to report abuse immediately or why they sometimes recant allegations during the investigation. Whether or not such testimony is helpful depends largely upon the knowledge of the lay public (Melton & Limber, 1990).

More problematic is expert testimony regarding "sex abuse syndromes." Testimony about the behavior patterns of abused children is presented in order to create the inference that the child has or has not been abused, depending on whether he or she displays the relevant behaviors. Although such testimony is usually offered by the prosecution in order to buttress allegations of abuse, the defense may sometimes attempt to refute abuse allegations by showing that the child does not fit the abused child profile.

The majority of appellate courts considering this issue have approved of the admission of opinions about the nature of the abuse syndrome, providing that the expert does not offer an opinion about the credibility of the alleged victim. Melton and Limber (1990) argue against admission of such testimony on numerous grounds. First, they note that there is little empirical support for a "sex abuse syndrome," and the purported syndromes are based mainly on clinical intuition. Moreover, many abuse victims display no symptoms at all, and many of the "symptoms" of child abuse are common to other clinical populations (Browne & Finkelhor, 1986; Haugaard & Reppucci, 1988).

Secondly, Melton and Limber (1990) note that introduction of such testimony may mislead the decisionmaker. Even if it could be determined through introduction of expert testimony that the child was abused, it does not prove that the child was abused by the defendant. The decisionmaker may be predisposed, though, to hold the defendant responsible for the abuse.

Finally, Melton and Limber (1990) argue against admission of such testimony on the grounds that it, in some ways, puts the victim "on trial." Such a line of inquiry may result in intrusions into the victim's privacy through extensive evaluations by both the prosecution and defense.

DISCUSSION

The development and implementation of procedural and evidentiary reforms designed to facilitate (and sometimes minimize) children's participation in the criminal process tracks the development of statutory reforms aimed at increasing reports of abuse and neglect. Both sets of reforms were developed with relatively little planning or experimentation and implemented without their efficacy first being demonstrated.

If children are able to testify under standard conditions, it is counterproductive to introduce new procedures that are of questionable utility and constitutional validity (Melton, 1987a). The use of unfounded procedures only provides the defense with firm ground for appeal, the end result being continued involvement by the child witness with no real end or closure in sight. Because of the limitations of evidentiary and procedural reform, the most useful techniques for involving child victims in the criminal process may be a product of the increased resource-fulness of mental health professionals working with children (Melton, 1987b; Melton & Limber, 1990; Whitcomb, 1985).

Mental health professionals skilled in working with children should be able to facilitate communication between the child witness and legal professionals, instruct legal professionals on how to interact with the child, and provide support for children engaged in the criminal process. Because of their expertise in family dynamics and discussing personal matters, child specialists may also be helpful as investigators, especially in the disposition phase, providing the court with information it might not otherwise have (Melton *et al.*, 1987). These and other activities can facilitate the child's participation in the adjudicative process and help ensure that the child is not unduly traumatized.

SUMMARY

The legislature and judiciary have paid increasing attention to the problems of child abuse and neglect over the past 25 years. Numerous reforms have been implemented in an attempt to increase reporting of suspected cases and to facilitate prevention and treatment programs. Additionally, judicial reforms have been instituted in order to facilitate adjudication of sexual abuse and more serious cases of physical abuse.

These efforts have produced mixed results for a variety of reasons. Because no consistent orientation exists among child advocates regarding the nature of child maltreatment, reforms have been based on emotional responses to the problem of abuse as much as empirical analysis or a theoretical basis. Many reforms have been instituted rather hastily, with little foresight and planning. Accordingly, we are left with procedures that are of questionable utility, some of which are also of questionable constitutionality.

The opportunities presented to psychologists are numerous, given the current state of affairs. Most importantly, psychologists must address definitional issues and study the effects of different policies and procedures that are now in use. Additionally, psychologists should apply their expertise and assist child victims and judicial system, while at the same time acknowledging their limitations.

REFERENCES

Alvy, K. T. (1975). Preventing child abuse. *American Psychologist, 30,* 921–928.
Atteberry-Bennett, J. (1987). Child sexual abuse: Definitions and interventions of parents

and professionals. Unpublished doctoral dissertation. University of Virginia, Institute of Clinical Psychology, Charlottesville, Virginia.

Atteberry-Bennett, J., & Reppucci, N. D. (1986, August). *What does child sexual abuse mean?* Paper presented at the meeting of the American Psychological Association, Washington, DC.

Berliner, L. (1985). The child witness: The progress and the emerging limitations. In J. Bulkley (Ed.), *Papers from a national conference on legal reforms in child sexual abuse cases* (pp. 93–108). Washington, DC: American Bar Association.

Berliner, L., & Barbieri, M. K. (1984). The testimony of the child victim of sexual assault. *Journal of Social Issues, 40*(2), 127–137.

Besharov, D. J. (1983). Child abuse: Past progress, present problems, and future directions. *Family Law Quarterly, 17,* 151–172.

Besharov, D. J. (1984). Protecting abused and neglected children: Can law and social work help? In W. Holder & K. Hayes (Eds.), *Malpractice and liability in child protective services* (pp. 29–48). Longmont, CA: Bookmakers Guild.

Bourne, R., & Newberger, E. H. (1977). Family autonomy or coercive intervention? Ambiguity and conflict in the proposed standards for child abuse and neglect. *Boston University Law Review, 57,* 670–706.

Brown, R. H. (1974). Child abuse: Attempts to solve the problem by reporting laws. *Women Lawyers Journal, 60,* 73–78.

Browne, A., & Finkelhor, D. L. (1986). The impact of child sexual abuse: A review of the research. *Psychological Bulletin, 99,* 66–77.

Bulkley, J. (1981). Evidentiary theories for admitting a child's out-of-court statement of sexual abuse at trial. In J. Bulkley (Ed.), *Child sexual abuse and the law* (pp. 153–161). Washington, DC: American Bar Association, National Legal Resource Center for Child Advocacy and Protection.

Bulkley, J. (1985). *State legislative reform efforts and suggested future policy directions to improve legal intervention in child sexual abuse cases.* Washington, DC: American Bar Association, National Legal Resource Center for Child Advocacy and Protection.

Child Abuse Prevention and Treatment Act, 42 U.S.C.S. § 5101–5115 (1979, Cum. Supp. 1988).

Child Sexual Abuse and Pornography Act, 18 U.S.C.S. § 2251–2255 (1979, Cum. Supp. 1988).

Children's Defense Fund. (1987). *A children's defense budget: An analysis of the President's FY 1988 budget and children.* Washington, DC: Author.

Chisolm, B. A. (1978). Questions of social policy—A Canadian perspective. In J. M. Eekelaar & S. N. Katz (Eds.), *Family violence: An international and interdisciplinary study* (pp. 318–328). Toronto: Butterworths.

Clark Foundation. (1985). *Keeping families together: The case for family preservation.* New York: Author.

Cohn, A. H. (1979). Essential elements of successful child abuse and neglect treatment. *Child Abuse and Neglect, 3,* 491–496.

Commonwealth v. Adams, 503 N.E.2d. 1315 (Mass. App. Ct. 1987).

Connecticut v. Jarzbek, 204 Conn. 683, 529 A.2d. 1245 (1987).

Costa, J. J. (1983). *Abuse of women: Legislation, reporting and prevention.* Lexington, MA: Lexington Books.

Costa, J. J., & Nelson, G. K. (1978). *Child abuse and neglect: Legislation, reporting, and prevention.* Lexington, MA: D. C. Heath.

Coy v. Iowa, _____ U.S. _____, 108 S. Ct. 2798 (1988).

Davidson, H. A. (1981). Sexual abuse of children: Effective utilization of the legal systems. Excerpted in H. A. Davidson, R. M. Horowitz, T. B. Marvell, & O. W. Ketcham (Eds.),

Child abuse and neglect litigation: A manual for judges (pp. 145–146). Washington, DC: Department of Health and Human Services.

Davidson, H. A., & Horowitz, R. M. (1984). Protection of children from family maltreatment. In R. M. Horowitz & H. A. Davidson (Eds.), *Legal rights of children* (pp. 262–312). Colorado Springs: Shepard's/McGraw-Hill.

Davidson, H. A., Horowitz, R. M., Marvell, T. B., & Ketcham, O. W. (1981). *Child abuse and neglect litigation: A manual for judges.* Washington, DC: Department of Health and Human Services.

DeConey, J. J. (1975). The legal process: A positive force in the interest of children. In American Humane Association (Ed.), *Fourth national symposium on child abuse* (pp. 62–69). Denver: Author.

Dickens, B. M. (1978). Legal responses to child abuse. In J. M. Eekelaar & S. N. Katz (Eds.), *Family violence: An international and interdisciplinary study* (pp. 338–362). Toronto: Butterworths.

Eatman, R., & Bulkley, J. (1986). *Protecting child victim/witnesses: Sample laws and materials.* Washington, DC: American Bar Association.

Feshbach, N. D., & Feshbach, S. (1976). Punishment: Parent rites versus children's rights. In G. P. Koocher (Ed.), *Children's rights and the mental health professions* (pp. 149–170). New York: Wiley.

Finkelhor, D. (1984). *Child sexual abuse: New theory and research.* New York: Free Press.

Flicker, B. D. (1977). *Standards for juvenile justice: A summary and analysis.* Cambridge, MA: Ballinger.

Fontana, V. J., & Besharov, D. J. (1979). *The maltreated child* (4th ed.). Springfield, IL: Charles C Thomas.

Fraser, B. G. (1979). A glance at the past, a gaze at the present, a glimpse of the future: A critical analysis of the development of child abuse reporting statutes. *Chicago-Kent Law Review, 54,* 641–686.

Garbarino, J. (1977). The price of privacy in the social dynamics of child abuse. *Child Welfare, 56,* 565–575.

Garbarino, J. (1982). *Children and families in the social environment.* New York: Aldine.

Garbarino, J., Gaboury, M. T., Long, F., Grandjean, P., & Asp, E. (1982). Who owns the children? An ecological perspective on public policy affecting children. In G. B. Melton (Ed.), *Legal policies affecting child and youth services* (pp. 43–63). New York: Haworth.

Gelles, R. J. (1982). Problems in defining and labeling child abuse. In R. H. Starr (Ed.), *Child abuse prediction: Policy implications* (pp. 1–30). Cambridge, MA: Ballinger.

Giovannoni, J. M., & Becerra, R. M. (1979). *Defining child abuse.* New York: Free Press.

Globe Newspaper Co. v. Superior Court, 457 U.S. 596 (1982).

Goldstein, J., Freud, A., & Solnit, A. J. (1973). *Beyond the best interests of the child.* New York: Free Press.

Goldstein, J., Freud, A., & Solnit, A. J. (1979). *Before the best interests of the child.* New York: Free Press.

Goodman, G. S. (1984). The child witness: Conclusions and future directions for research and legal practice. *Journal of Social Issues, 40,* 157–175.

Goodman, G. S., & Helgeson, V. S. (1985). Child sexual assault: Children's memory and the law. In J. Bulkley (Ed.), *Papers from a national policy conference in legal reforms in child sexual abuse cases* (pp. 41–60). Washington, DC: American Bar Association, National Legal Resource Center for Child Advocacy and Protection.

Graham, M. H. (1985). Child sex abuse persecutions: Hearsay and confrontation clause issues. In J. Bulkley (Ed.), *Papers from a national policy conference on legal reforms in child sexual abuse cases* (pp. 159–208). Washington, DC: American Bar Association.

Haugaard, J. J., & Reppucci, N. D. (1988). *The sexual abuse of children*. San Francisco: Jossey-Bass.

House of Representatives Report No. 685, 93d Cong., *reprinted in* 1974 U.S. Code Congressional & Administrative News 2663.

Idaho v. Wright, _____ U.S. _____, 110 S. Ct. 883 (1990).

In re Freiberger, 153 Mich. App. 251, 395 N.W.2d 300 (Mich. Ct. App. 1986).

Institute of Judicial Administration/American Bar Association (1981). *Standards relating to abuse and neglect*. Cambridge, MA: Ballinger.

Isaacson, L. B. (1975). Child abuse reporting statutes: The case for holding physicians civilly liable for failure to report. *San Diego Law Review, 12*, 743–777.

Kalichman, S. E., & Craig, M. E. (in press). Victims of incestuous abuse: Mental health professionals' attitudes and tendency to report. *Victimology: An International Journal*.

Kalichman, S. E., Craig, M. E., & Follingstad, D. R. (1987, August). *Factors contributing to mental health professionals' reporting of child abuse*. Paper presented at the meeting of the American Psychological Association, New York.

Kelly, D. P. (1987). Victims. *Wayne Law Review, 37*, 69–86.

Kempe, C. H., Silverman, F. N., Steele, B. F., Droegenmueller, W., & Silver, H. K. (1962). The battered child syndrome. *Journal of the American Medical Association, 181*, 17–24.

Kentucky v. Stincer, 107 S. Ct. 2658 (1987).

Kilpatrick, D. G., & Otto, R. K. (1987). Constitutionally guaranteed participation in criminal proceedings for victims: Potential impact on psychological functioning. *Wayne Law Review, 37*, 7–28.

King, M. P., Hunter, W. M., & Runyan, D. K. (1988). Going to court: The experience of child victims of intrafamilial sexual abuse. *Journal of Health Politics, Policy, and Law, 13*, 705–721.

Lucht, C. L. (1975). Providing a legislative base for reporting child abuse. In American Humane Association (Ed.), *Fourth national symposium on child abuse* (pp. 49–60). Denver: Author.

Maney, A., & Wells, S. (Eds.). (1988). *Professional responsibilities in protecting children: A public health approach to child sexual abuse*. New York: Praeger.

Maryland v. Craig, _____ U.S. _____, 100 S. Ct. 834 (1990).

Melton, G. B. (1982). Children's rights: Where are the children? *American Journal of Orthopsychiatry, 52*, 530–538.

Melton, G. B. (1983a). Toward "personhood" for adolescents: Autonomy and privacy as values in public policy. *American Psychologist, 38*, 99–103.

Melton, G. B. (1983b). Decision making by children: Psychological risks and benefits. In G. B. Melton, G. P. Koocher, & M. J. Saks (Eds.), *Children's competence to consent* (pp. 21–40). New York: Plenum Press.

Melton, G. B. (1987a). Special legal problems in the protection of handicapped children from parental maltreatment. In J. Garbarino, P. E. Brookhouser, & K. J. Authier (Eds.), *Special children-special risks: The maltreatment of children with disabilities* (pp. 179–193). New York: Aldine de Gruyter.

Melton, G. B. (1987b). Children's testimony in cases of alleged sexual abuse. In M. Wolraich & D. K. Routh (Eds.), *Advances in developmental and behavioral pediatrics* (pp. 179–203). Greenwich, CT: JAI Press.

Melton, G. B. (1987c). Law and random events: The state of child mental health policy. *International Journal of Law and Psychiatry, 10*, 81–90.

Melton, G. B., & Corson, J. (1987). Psychological maltreatment and the schools: Problems of law and professional responsibility. *School Psychology Review, 16*, 188–194.

Melton, G. B., & Thompson, R. A. (1987). Legislative approaches to psychological maltreatment: A social policy analysis. In M. R. Brassard, R. Germain, & S. N. Hart (Eds.),

Psychological maltreatment of children and youth (pp. 203–216). New York: Pergamon Press.

Melton, G. B., & Limber, S. (1990). Psychologists' involvement in cases of child maltreatment: Limits of role and expertise. *American Psychologist, 44,* 1225–1233.

Melton, G. B., Petrila, J., Poythress, N. G., & Slobogin, C. (1987). *Psychological evaluations for the courts: A handbook for mental health professionals and lawyers.* New York: Guilford Press.

Midonick, M. L. (1972). *Children, parents and the courts: Juvenile delinquency, ungovernability and neglect.* New York: Practising Law Institute.

Missing Children Assistance Act 42 U.S.C. § 5771–5777 (1982, Supp. 1986).

Mnookin, R. H. (1973). Foster care: In whose best interest? *Harvard Educational Review, 43,* 599–638.

Muehleman, T., & Kimmons, C. (1981). Psychologists' views on child abuse reporting, confidentiality, life, and the law: An exploratory study. *Professional Psychology, 12,* 631–638.

Myers, J. E. B. (1986). A survey of child abuse and neglect reporting statutes. *Journal of Juvenile Law, 10,* 1–72.

National Center for State Courts. (1988). The changing face of child abuse registries. *National Center for State Courts Report, 15*(7), 2.

National Committee for the Prevention of Child Abuse (undated). *Children's trust funds.* Chicago: Author.

Nelson, B. J. (1984). *Making an issue of child abuse: Political agenda setting for social problems.* Chicago: University of Chicago Press.

New York Social Services Law Sec. 413 (McKinney, 1988).

Ohio v. Roberts, 448 U.S. 56 (1980).

Parental Kidnapping Prevention Act 28 U.S.C.S § 1730A (1979, Cum. Supp. 1988).

Paulsen, M. G. (1967). Child abuse reporting laws: The shape of the legislation. *Columbia Law Review, 67,* 1–49.

Pierce v. Society of Sisters, 268 U.S. 510, 45 S.Ct. 571 (1925).

Prince v. Massachusetts, 321 U.S. 158 (1944).

Roe v. Wade, 410 U.S. 113 (1973).

Rogers, C. M. (1982). Child sexual abuse and the court: Preliminary findings. In J. Conte & D. A. Shore (Eds.), *Social work and child sexual abuse* (pp. 145–153). New York: Haworth Press.

Rosenberg, A. H. (1975). The law and child abuse. In N. B. Ebeling & D. A. Hill (Eds.), *Child abuse: Intervention and treatment* (pp. 161–170). Acton, MA: Publishing Sciences Group.

Rosenberg, M. S., & Hunt, R. D. (1984). Child maltreatment: Legal and mental health issues. In N. D. Reppucci, L. A. Weithorn, E. P. Mulvey, & J. Monahan (Eds.), *Children, mental health, and the law* (pp. 79–101). Beverly Hills: Sage.

Runyan, D., Everson, M., Edelsohn, G., Hunter, W., & Coulter, M. L. (1988). Impact of legal intervention on sexually abused children. *Journal of Pediatrics, 113,* 647–653.

Santosky v. Kramer, 455 U.S. 745 (1982).

Senate Report No. 123, 99th Cong. *reprinted in* 1986 U.S. Code Congressional & Administrative News 1967.

Sherman, L. W., & Berk, R. A. (1984). *The Minnesota domestic violence experiment.* Washington, DC: Police Foundation.

Swoboda, J. S., Elwork, A., Sales, B. D., & Levine, D. (1979). Knowledge of and compliance with privileged communication and child-abuse reporting laws. *Professional Psychology, 10,* 448–457.

Thibaut, J., & Walker, L. (1978). A theory of procedure. *California Law Review, 66,* 541–566.

Urzi, T. (1981). *Cooperative approaches to child protection: A community guide.* Excerpted in H. A. Davidson, R. M. Horowitz, T. B. Marvell, & O. W. Ketcham (Eds.), *Child abuse and neglect litigation: A manual for judges.* Washington, DC: Department of Health and Human Services.

United States v. Iron Shell, 633 F.2d. 77 (8th Cir. 1980).

Wald, M. (1975). State interventions on behalf of "neglected" children: A search for realistic standards. *Stanford Law Review, 27,* 985–1040.

Wald, M. S. (1976). State intervention on behalf of "neglected" children: Standards for removal from their homes, monitoring the status of children in foster care, and termination of parental rights. *Stanford Law Review, 28,* 625–706.

Wald, M. S. (1982). State intervention in behalf of neglected children: A proposed legal response. *Child Abuse and Neglect, 6,* 3–45.

Wald, M. S., Carlsmith, J. M., & Leiberman, P. H. (1988). *Protecting abused and neglected children.* Stanford, CA: Stanford University Press.

Whitcomb, D. (1985). Assisting child victims in the courts: The practical side of legislative reform. In J. Bulkley (Ed.), *Papers from a national policy conference on legal reforms in child sexual abuse cases* (pp. 13–29). Washington, DC: American Bar Association, National Legal Resource Center for Child Advocacy and Protection.

Wisconsin v. Yoder, 406 U.S. 205 (1972).

CHAPTER 4

RESEARCH DIRECTIONS RELATED TO CHILD ABUSE AND NEGLECT

Roy C. Herrenkohl

INTRODUCTION

Future directions for research on child abuse and neglect depend on goals for the general area and the role to be played by research in achieving these goals. The goals proposed here are to provide: (1) treatment to abusive families to reduce or remove the likelihood of recurrence, and (2) services to abused children to ameliorate the consequences of abuse and to develop prevention strategies to reduce its incidence. The role of research in meeting these objectives is to obtain information about the incidence and prevalence of abuse, to examine its causes, and to evaluate the effectiveness of treatment and prevention.

Policymakers, the third party to the challenges posed by child abuse, use results from research and the experience of service providers to inform their decisions concerning the provision of resources for treatment, prevention, and research. After two decades of research, the nature and extent of the problem in a descriptive sense is clearer, but

Roy C. Herrenkohl • Center for Social Research, Lehigh University, Bethlehem, Pennsylvania 18015.

key questions for policy (i.e., the causes of abuse and neglect, effective treatment and prevention strategies) remain largely unclear. The inadequacy of relevant findings means that policymakers must develop and implement plans based on informed judgment rather than more objective evidence.

RESEARCH ISSUES

Five research issues concerning child abuse are considered below: incidence/prevalence, causes, consequences, treatment, and prevention. These are interrelated in that what is learned about one often has implications for one or more of the others. There also are important distinctions, depending on which of the four types of abuse (physical, emotional, sexual, or neglect) is involved. These often are mentioned together but are seldom studied or analyzed concurrently. In practice they sometimes occur singly or in combination (E. C. Herrenkohl & R. C. Herrenkohl, 1981). This poses a problem of research strategy. Should research focus on each type of maltreatment separately or on types in combination? The answer may differ depending on the issue under study.

The discussion that follows examines the current state of and possible future directions for research in the aforementioned five areas. Only illustrations from the different types of abuse are offered. For a more comprehensive review of specific projects, the reader is referred to Finkelhor, Hotaling, and Yllo (1988).

INCIDENCE AND PREVALENCE OF ABUSE AND NEGLECT

Information on incidence and prevalence indicates the extent of the problem in society. Accurate data on incidence and prevalence were sought from the early days of research on child abuse. For example, Gil (1970) examined the prevalence of physical abuse (cf. Nagi, 1977), while a comprehensive prevalence study was more recently reported by Straus, Gelles, and Steinmetz (1980). Russell (1983), on the other hand, conducted a prevalence study of sexual abuse. The prevalence of components of neglect have been studied (e.g., poor nutrition: Bassetti, 1974), but a thorough study of the prevalence of neglect has not been conducted, although estimates have been offered (Nagi, 1977; Polansky, Chalmers, Buttenweiser, & Williams, 1981).

The accuracy of incidence/prevalence data for different types of abuse suffers from imprecise conceptualization and inadequate operational definitions (Starr, 1988). For example, definitions of *physical abuse* may specify "intent" to harm, but the occurrence of nonaccidental injury often is taken as sufficient evidence of such intent (Starr, 1988). *Emotional abuse* also has proved very difficult to define. Only the most extreme cases of emotional cruelty are labeled as "abuse" (Hart, Germain, & Brassard, 1987; Garbarino, Guttmann, & Seeley, 1986). Furthermore, strategies for assessing the occurrence of *sexual abuse* are only beginning to be developed (Conerly, 1986). Specific forms of *neglect* have been studied (e.g., malnutrition, medical neglect), but the combination of these conditions has not. The Polansky measure of neglect (Polansky *et al.*, 1981), the Childhood Level of Living Scale (CLL), reflects poverty as well as neglect. For example, a negative response to the CLL Scale item, "mother plans at least one meal consisting of two courses," may indicate neglect or it may indicate poverty. A procedure is needed by which to disentangle neglect from poverty. Such a procedure would distinguish the neglectful quality of the parent's relationship to the child from child care associated with parental level of education and income.

Adequate measures of abuse are the key to obtaining accurate incidence and prevalence data. Such measures can, in turn, serve as the dependent variables for studies of the causes of abuse and as the independent variables in studies of the consequences of abuse. The incidence and prevalence of abuse also are the criteria against which the effectiveness of treatment and prevention strategies are judged.

RESEARCH DIRECTIONS

Generally, a thorough catalogue of manifestations of each type of abuse, including instances that are borderline, is needed. Such a catalogue could provide the basis for developing an index, the reliability and validity of which could then be assessed. Without information on psychometric properties, the accuracy of statistics such as correlations is suspect, and the validity of differentiations between abused and nonabused children is questionable.

Six broad problems confront the development of better measures. First, there is a need for better specification of the differences between: (1) physical abuse and physical discipline, (2) emotional abuse and emotionally oriented discipline, and (3) appropriate touching and sexually abusive touching. In addition, a more comprehensive conception of neglect would bring together the range of features known to comprise neglect.

Second, research to develop more adequate operational measures would follow from clearer definitions. For example, there are operational definitions of physical abuse that emphasize: (1) reported incidents, (2) specific incidents recorded in case records (R. C. Herrenkohl, E. C. Herrenkohl, Egolf, & Seech, 1979), (3) incidents reported as part of discipline (R. C. Herrenkohl & E. C. Herrenkohl, 1988a), and (4) incidents reported as part of family conflict (Straus et al., 1980). Analyses are needed of the psychometric properties of each approach and an assessment of differences and similarities between strategies. The aim would be to develop a more widely agreed on assessment strategy for each type of abuse.

Third, it also is important to consider what represents an incident of maltreatment. For example, Herrenkohl et al. (1979) report that if formal citations for abuse are considered, the rate of recurrence was approximately 25% for a two county area in Pennsylvania. For the same two counties, if incidents recorded in case records are used the rate of recurrence is 55% to 66%. On the other hand, during the same period the official state rate was 8% to 12%. Thus, if abusive incidents reported on a discipline practices measure are used as the criterion, repeated abuse is more frequent and more widespread than child welfare records would indicate (Herrenkohl & Herrenkohl, 1988b).

Fourth, how are valid cases to be identified? Current methods depend on mandated reporters, hot lines, and self-reports, among others. More adequate screening procedures are needed, although their use raises a variety of ethical issues. For example, more accurate information is likely to depend to some degree on self-reports. Adults may be willing to indicate the type of discipline they have used or other reactions they have had to a child's behavior. If such reports are made to persons required by law to make formal notification of abuse, the self-reports can be incriminating (Geffner, Rosenbaum & Hughes, 1988; Finkelhor et al., 1988). Children also can report abusive treatment they have received. Children mature enough to offer such information are old enough to feel responsibility for creating trouble for other family members. Furthermore, a dilemma is raised by identifying more cases while lacking the resources needed to provide treatment. Some states (e.g., Pennsylvania) have narrowed their definition of abuse over the last decade, so as to provide treatment only to more serious cases. Under such circumstances efforts to identify new cases may not be paralleled by increased resources to provide treatment for them.

A fifth issue concerns the prevalence of combinations of maltreatment types. There is little information on how frequently different combinations of abuse occur. Herrenkohl et al. (1981) report that 33% of children experience more than one type of abuse. Moreover, the occurrence of and the relationship between the different types of abuse have not been examined.

Finally, how is the information on incidence and prevalence to be coordinated so that services can be provided to abusive families, policymakers can learn the extent of the problem, and the information can be used in research? This problem points to the need for better coordination and cooperation among service providers, policymakers, and researchers.

CAUSES OF ABUSE AND NEGLECT

Speculation concerning causes of abuse was raised early in the development of research on maltreatment (Steele, 1976). Clearer identification of causes would add to our basic understanding of parenting. It also would give a focus to treatment and prevention because, in order to be effective, treatment and prevention strategies must reduce or remove factors that are assumed to play a causative role in child abuse and neglect.

There have been many causal models of maltreatment (Parke & Collmer, 1975). Some propose that abusive parents have a personality disorder or are mentally ill (McCleer, 1988; Spinetta & Rigler, 1972). Others suggest that abusive parenting styles are learned (Parke & Collmer, 1975; Wolfe, 1987), or that there is an intergenerational transmission of abuse (E. C. Herrenkohl et al., 1983; Egeland, Jacobvitz, & Papatola, 1987). Egeland and Sroufe (1981) examined disruptions in the attachment of parent and child as a possible causative explanation. Others see abusive parents as having inappropriate expectations of their children (Twentyman, Rohrbeck, & Amish, 1984). Still others suggest that abuse is a result of frustration because of stress that leads to excessively aggressive parenting (Elmer, 1979). Some explanations implicate the child in the etiology of abuse; for example, the difficult (handicapped or premature) child has been noted as an elicitor of abuse (de Lissovoy, 1979). Others (Kadushin & Martin, 1981; R. C. Herrenkohl et al., 1983) have suggested that the child's normal behavior can elicit abusive reactions. Societal norms and attitudes that tolerate or condone domestic violence can further influence the occurrence of maltreatment (Straus et al., 1980).

Current explanations for the occurrence of abuse can broadly be characterized as a set of conceptually unrelated propositions or hypotheses; and although most are supported by some empirical data, the consistency and utility of such evidence varies considerably. An early example of such coordination and review was by Spinetta and Rigler (1972) who found many inconsistencies in evidence concerning the hypothesis that personality abnormalities were the cause of physical abuse. A more recent example is the work of Kaufman and Zigler (1987) who examined evidence concerning the intergenerational transmission hypothesis—that abused children will themselves become abusive parents. These authors report that the combined evidence does not lend extensive support to this hypothesis.

Increased efforts are needed to examine etiologic formulations of abuse. These should go beyond simply cataloguing evidence and seek to determine the validity of an hypothesis, taking into consideration variations in the formulation of the hypothesis, methodological strengths and weaknesses of studies which test the hypothesis and variations of the hypothesis that may not have been examined. For example, the proposal that abusive parents have unrealistic expectations for their children's behavior was originally tested by several researchers who questioned parents about developmental norms (e.g., the age at which a child will walk or talk). Differences between abusive and non-abusive parents were not found. There does, however, seem to be validity to the hypothesis, if parental expectations are conceptualized as tolerance for children's misbehavior or what parents consider misbehavior. Work by Kadushin and Martin (1981), Twentyman *et al.* (1984), and R. C. Herrenkohl *et al.* (1983), each from somewhat different perspectives, lend support to the view that abusive parents have inappropriate expectations of their children's behavior as compared to nonabusive parents.

Research is also needed to develop and/or revise current theories or models about the causes of abuse. A valid theory about the occurrence of abuse would involve specification of relevant constructs and their interrelationships. Such a theory also could indicate the constructs or relationships between constructs that must be modified so that recurrence could be avoided or, if modified before the initial occurrence of abuse, so that abuse could be prevented. For example, if simply the overall level of stress on a family were considered the cause of abuse, then casework services to reduce the stress would be the appropriate strategy. If, however, the more specific stresses of child rearing and social isolation were theorized to be responsible for abuse, then services directed at reducing those particular stresses (i.e., the provision of child care services, training in child rearing skills, and participation in a parent support group) would be expected to reduce the stresses and prevent occurrence/recurrence of maltreatment.

The role of social class in general and poverty in particular in the development of abuse has been addressed infrequently (Pelton, 1981). Those who have examined this topic have generally found a relationship between social status and the occurrence of abuse (Elmer, 1981; Straus *et al.*, 1980; Wolfe, 1987). However, the causal implications of this relationship have received little attention.

Many believe that each type of abuse is multidetermined, that is, no single factor will explain its occurrence. Thus, there are several multifactor models. For example, Gelles (1973) described a model in which a network of influences, such as stress, social isolation, parents' child-rearing experience, among other factors was hypothesized to contribute to abuse. On the other hand, Garbarino (1976, 1981) proposed an "ecological model" in which situational factors are given more attention. Belsky (1984) suggested that abusive parenting is considered an extreme on a continuum of general parenting, the quality of which is influenced by a set of factors within the family and community. Wolfe (1987), in contrast, advocated a transitional model in which parent–child interactions change over time into aversive interactions. It should be noted, however, that the complexity of multiconstruct models may require single-construct empirical tests until more is known about each construct.

Existing models are inadequate for several reasons. One is that constructs in the models are not well-defined. Such constructs as "parenting" are not sufficiently explicit to indicate which aspects of inadequate parenting have the more detrimental effect on the child and how different aspects of parenting are interrelated. Because of the inexplicitness of these models, development of operational definitions is difficult. Another difficulty is that there is little differentiation between the causes of one type of abuse and the causes of another and suggested causes of one type of abuse may overlap the proposed causes of a second type.

An additional strategy in constructing more comprehensive models of abuse involves identifying risk factors that are indicators of the potential for abuse. Finkelhor *et al.* (1988) considers this topic one of the better defined research areas. One attraction of this approach is that risk factors, such as being a single-parent family, the child's being handicapped, or having long or multiple separations from parents, are somewhat simpler concepts than stress or social isolation. Consequently, such factors can be identified more readily. Several researchers (Starr, 1982) have examined risk factors (Milner & Wimberlay, 1979; Schneider 1982). Problems beset this approach, however. First, accurate identification of risk factors depends on knowing the "universe" of abusive families. However, the universe of abusive families is unclear. The number of cases continues to increase, and it is likely that even those cases that have been identified are not representative of all cases of abuse. Second, without precise information on the characteristics of all abusive families, identification of risk factors will be based on the characteristics of families known to be abusive. Any biases in those characteristics will be reflected in the identified risk factors. On the one hand, if among identified abusive families there is a disproportionately large number of poverty level families as compared to all abusive families, living in poverty will be identified as a significant risk factor. On the other hand, examination of the characteristics of identified abusive families may fail to pinpoint a characteristic which, in the actual universe, is more salient. A further problem is specifying the level of a factor that constitutes risk. For some possible risk factors, such as prematurity, there are "rules of thumb" about what represents risk. For others, however, such as the level of harsh treatment by a parent of a child, there is no consensus as to what represents risk. The tendency for risk models to predict larger numbers of high risk families than are observed to become abusive is a negative consequence of such sources of bias.

Research Directions

Several steps are needed concerning research on causes. First, problems of conceptualization and measurement of causal constructs are serious. Causal effects cannot be identified unless such constructs are measured reliably and with validity. To develop these measures requires considerable time and skill. Second, there is a need to review and coordinate existing information concerning each causative factor in an effort to narrow the number of possibilities. Those causal explanations that offer the most promise will merit testing in greater depth. Since it is likely that abuse is multidetermined, the smaller the set of likely causal constructs, the more readily they can be tested. Third, given the assumption that variables contributing to abuse are multidetermined, a model or theory is needed that specifies how this multidetermined state operates. This is best developed when more in-depth information on specific causes is available. Care needs to be taken to consider the fact that many abusive families display numerous additional problems, and that a significant number have experienced more than one type of abuse.

CONSEQUENCES OF ABUSE AND NEGLECT

Research on the consequences of abuse can be divided roughly into two parts. One concerns the immediate, often medical, sequelae and the physical trauma of the abuse. The other concerns the longer term, generally psychosocial, consequences of maltreatment.

The medical effects of physical abuse and neglect have been the focus of many studies reported primarily in medical journals. These studies should be catalogued and evaluated for use by those who must determine the etiology of childhood injuries. Such a cataloguing might also provide the basis for indexing injuries with reference to severity which, in turn, could be related to potential for longer term consequences.

Several researchers (e.g., Gray & Kempe, 1976) have described physically abused children's psychological state soon after they were identified as having been abused. Such information can be used to index the degree of psychological trauma manifested by the child at the time the abuse was identified. For example, the short-term consequences of sexual abuse have been described (Wolfe, Wolfe, & Best, 1988) in largely anecdotal terms. Similarly, neglected children's physical and psychological status have been reported by several authors (Polansky et al., 1981; Oates, 1986). Such reports should be coordinated and evaluated. In the case of emotional abuse, however, the short-term consequences have not been differentiated from longer term effects.

The longer term consequences of abuse have been studied by a small group of researchers (e.g., Cicchetti & Rizley, 1981; Egeland & Sroufe, 1981; Elmer, 1977; E. C. Herrenkohl & R. C. Herrenkohl, 1981; Lynch & Roberts, 1982; Martin, 1976; Oates, 1986). To varying degrees, their studies have considered physical abuse, emotional abuse, and neglect. On the other hand, studies of the longer term consequences of sexual abuse have only recently been conducted (Wolfe et al., 1988). Most of this research is longitudinal in nature, although it differs considerably in terms of the time period covered. The reader is referred to more comprehensive reviews of these investigations by Augoustinos (1987) and Toro (1982).

Physical Abuse

Much of the research on consequences of maltreatment has focused on physical abuse. For the roughly 25% (E. C. Herrenkohl & R. C. Herrenkohl, 1981) of abused children who have severe physical injury, the physical damage may result in long-term physical handicaps that, in turn, can lead to problems of social-emotional adjustment (Elmer, 1977; Lynch & Roberts, 1982). For the remaining 75%, the physical injury may be less severe, (i.e., bruises and abrasions), but there still may be longer term developmental difficulties (Martin, 1976). For example, severity of physical abuse can be manifested in the form of injuries that result in lifetime handicaps, injuries that are severe but heal leaving no long-term handicap, and injuries that are not severe. But emotional abuse leaves no observable marks and also can differ in degree. Parents who threaten a young child with abandonment may inflict more serious consequences than parents who tell the same thing to an older child who can judge the likelihood of that happening. Furthermore, less severe but repeated physical or emotional abuse may inflict more physical and/or emotional damage to the child than a single abusive incident.

EMOTIONAL ABUSE

The longer term consequences of emotional abuse are less documented because of difficulties in identifying and measuring emotional abuse. Furthermore, emotional abuse occurs as a separate form of abuse [e.g., threats to abandon or kill a child, or telling a child repeatedly he or she is "stupid" and "worthless" (Navarre, 1987)] or in conjunction with other forms of maltreatment. For example, the effects of emotional abuse are manifested in the helplessness and worthlessness often experienced by physically abused children (Hyman, 1987), the sense of violation and shame found in sexually abused children (Brassard & McNeil, 1987), or the lack of environmental stimulation and support for normal development found by neglected children (Schakel, 1987). The consequences of these different types of emotional abuse, however, have not been empirically examined.

SEXUAL ABUSE

The longer term consequences of sexual abuse are believed to be primarily in the areas of trust and heterosexual relationships (Wolfe *et al.*, 1988). Research on the impact of sexual abuse is currently more in the form of case studies than of empirically controlled studies (Lusk & Waterman, 1986; Tong & Oates, 1987). Consequently, it is difficult to separate the impact of the abuse from the impact of other factors at work in the sexually abusive family context.

CHILD NEGLECT

Research directly on the consequences of child neglect is sparse. Polansky (see Polansky *et al.*, 1981) has studied the neglectful family but has focused more on the characteristics of neglectful parents than on the longer term consequences of neglect in children. Polansky does provide evidence, however, that the cognitive development of neglected children is more retarded than is that of nonneglected children. Oates (1986) examined the longer term consequences of neglect, including an examination of nonorganic failure-to-thrive children. Results from his study found failure-to-thrive children to be significantly lower in social maturity, language development, and verbal ability, and to have more personality abnormalities than a comparison group. Research on areas that comprise child neglect, such as inadequate nutrition (Martin, 1973) and social-emotional understimulation (Schakel, 1987), clearly indicated the negative impact of neglectful parenting on a child's development. These latter studies demonstrate the effects of a particular inadequacy (e.g., malnutrition) on a child, but have not been coordinated in such a manner as to elucidate their combined impact on a neglected child's development.

RESEARCH DIRECTIONS

Several factors render examination of the consequences of abuse a complex and difficult task. First, the reliable and valid measurement of each type of maltreatment is a major problem here as well. Furthermore, improved conceptualization and measurement of consequences are needed. Measures such as that developed by Achenbach (Achenbach & McConaughy, 1987) have proven useful. This instrument assesses cognitive, educational, emotional, social, and physical development, has strong psychometric properties, and has been used with a variety of child and adolescent populations that can provide helpful comparisons.

Second, more adequate formulations of how each type of abuse exerts its effect on the child are needed. This is important for knowing how and when to direct treatment for the consequences of abuse. For example, the act of discipline that injures the child is embedded in an ongoing adult–child relationship. It is possible that the damage to the child's development is determined more by the negative quality of the ongoing interaction than by the abusive act *per se*. Although a number of studies examine the parent–child interaction of abusive and nonabusive families (e.g., Burgess & Conger, 1978; E. C. Herrenkohl, R. C. Herrenkohl, Toedter, & Yanushefski, 1984), none investigate the impact of the combination of discipline and on-going interactions on the child's psychosocial development.

Third, if the various types of abuse have different types of sequelae, it will be necessary to develop hypotheses about consequences for each form of abuse. Further, because some children experience more than one type of abuse, a model or models of how the four types interrelate in various combinations to effect the child are needed.

One strategy to examine how abuse influences psychosocial functioning is to compare abused children who do well developmentally with those who do not. For example, Garmezy (1983) has used this approach to determine why some children who are developmentally at risk do well and others, similarly at risk, do not. It may prove helpful in identifying features in an abusive family or characteristics of an abused child that serve to buffer the child against the impact of abuse (Mrazek & Mrazek, 1987). For example, the abused child who receives nurturance from a parent or parent surrogate or who has sufficient insight to perceive the abusive behavior as due to the perpetrator's problems may not succumb to the most damaging consequences of abuse.

Finally, abuse is related to such factors as poverty, marital discord, and social isolation, and each of these may have an effect on the child's development similar to those stemming from abuse. How to differentiate the contribution of abuse from the effects of other factors with which abuse covaries is an additional research problem that is particularly problematic, because factors, such as poverty, may have a more far-reaching effect than, say, physical abuse, especially, if the physical injuries are endured in the less-severe range.

TREATMENT OF ABUSE AND NEGLECT

The treatment services available for abusive and neglectful families are varied. Reports of treatment approaches generally consider one type of abuse. For example, Starr (1988) summarized treatment forms for physical abuse; Garbarino et al. (1986) considered intervention strategies applicable to emotional abuse; Wolfe et al. (1988) described treatment approaches to sexual abuse; and Polansky et al. (1981) have examined treatment strategies for neglectful families. Sudia (1981) has taken a more comprehensive approach. Noting the multiple problems of many abusive families, she suggests that there is a need to classify families both in terms of the types of problems requiring treatment and in terms of the anticipated duration of interventions before actually providing services.

Another perspective is to consider the recipient of treatment services. The goal of treatment of a perpetrator of abuse or neglect is to prevent recurrence. Frequency of recurrence for perpetrators can range from no recurrence after a first incident to many incidents after a first incident (R. C. Herrenkohl *et al.*, 1979). There is little evidence, however, regarding how effective treatment is when provided to perpetrators. Evidence that does exist suggests that individualized services for cooperative female perpetrators are effective, although there is relatively little evidence pertaining to male perpetrators (Ammerman, 1990). Furthermore, there is little evidence to indicate how frequently and under what circumstances perpetrators cooperate with treatment (Jones, 1987). It is not known how effective different treatment strategies are with perpetrators of different rates of recurrence. It also is unclear whether treatment strategies that are effective with one type of abuse (e.g., physical), also are effective with a second type (e.g., neglect). There are indications that different types of abuse are based on different dynamics (E. C. Herrenkohl *et al.*, 1983), which may mean that different treatment strategies are needed.

Treatment can also be implemented with family members as a group. The family provides a context for the abuse and its members are affected by its occurrence. There is speculation of how a family provides a context for abuse (e.g., Justice & Justice, 1976). However, the way in which the family system contributes to abuse has not been empirically examined.

A third focus of treatment is to reduce or prevent the consequences of abuse for the abused child. Although it is not altogether clear what the consequences are and how they occur, a specific direction for treatment is also unclear. Furthermore, it is unclear whether the child who observes violence, but is not a victim, is as much in need of treatment as the child who is directly maltreated. There is some research on the short-term effects of viewing violence toward a parent (e.g., Hershorn & Rosenbaum, 1985; Hotaling & Sugarman, 1986). Geffner *et al.* (1988), who discuss research needs related to this topic, concluded that "very few conclusions can be drawn regarding child witnesses of parental violence" and that "investigators . . . are probably decades away from being able to specify what type of treatment, under what circumstances, for which types of clients, is most effective" (p. 475–476).

A variety of treatment services are provided to maltreated children and their families (e.g., casework, parent education, individual therapy). Each form of service has an implicit conceptualization of how to prevent recurrence. It assumes a cause or cluster of causes to which the service is addressed, using the assumption that reducing or removing the presumed cause will prevent recurrence. For example, casework to assist families to reduce stresses assumes that stress is a cause of abuse. Family therapy to improve relations between family members assumes that conflicts or distorted relationships between family members contribute to abuse. Counseling to assist an individual in coping more adequately with psychological conflict related to child rearing assumes that such conflict is the cause. A support group to help reduce social isolation or parenting programs to improve parenting skills assumes that these are the causes. The questions that follow from such assumptions are first whether a particular form of treatment can be effective in reducing or removing a presumed cause and, second, whether having removed or reduced the presumed cause recurrence is reduced or stopped.

If the different types of abuse have different etiologies, then treatment strategies that address each of the causes are needed in families involved with more than one type of abuse. The implication of this possibility is that complicated (and costly) treatment strategies may be needed for some families.

When treatment concerns consequences to the child, it is essential that we understand the effects of each type of abuse so that treatment can be directed to the areas of need. For example, the physically abused child, in addition to needing treatment for physical injury, likewise may feel vulnerable and worthless. Group therapy may help such problems, as it may for the emotionally abused or sexually abused child. Treatment for the neglected child may involve medical care, education remediation and other services known to counter the effects of cognitive, social and emotional deprivation. However, assessment of the effectiveness of strategies to reduce the impact of maltreatment of children has not been undertaken.

In some instances, recurrence is prevented because the perpetrator(s) has no access to the child. The perpetrator may voluntarily leave the home, or in those instances of abuse judged to be most severe, children are placed in foster care. This results in the added trauma for the child of separation from family (Goldstein, Freud, & Solnit, 1973). Foster placement introduces the child to a system that has both advantages and disadvantages (Wald, 1976). Although foster placement is widely used, the circumstances under which it is most and least beneficial to the child have not been fully examined (Wald, Carlsmith, Leiderman, French, & Smith, 1985). It also is unclear how foster care may interact with the psychosocial consequences of the abuse, or how circumstances in the foster care system, such as moves from family to family, may influence the child's development.

RESEARCH DIRECTIONS

During the past two decades a number of service/treatment projects have been undertaken to demonstrate the efficacy of the one or a combination of treatment services designed to protect against recurrence. Some of these demonstrations have included evaluations to determine the effectiveness of the service/treatment program (Cohn, 1979a,b; Cohn & Daro, 1987). Some evaluations produced useful results, whereas others did not. Reasons for the lack of useful results were not always evident, although there are some indications. First, the difficulties and complexities of treating abusive individuals and their families have not always been acknowledged. This results in rather unrealistic goals for experimental programs. Second, coordination between service delivery and evaluation staffs in planning and conducting the evaluation was inadequate. There often has been too little joint planning by service providers, researchers, and policymakers with service providers sometimes feeling that they have little to say about the evaluation. As a result, service providers may distrust evaluation specialists and resist the evaluation process, hindering completion of crucial portions of evaluation activities.

Third, clear documentation of the treatment strategy was not developed. This would indicate precisely the treatment components used, how and in what amounts the treatment was provided, and the staff skills needed to carry out the program. Without such information, replication of treatment procedures is not possible.

Fourth, more comprehensive models are needed to indicate how (or why) the phenomenon to be treated (i.e., recurrence, occurrence, or consequences of abuse) developed. An indication is also required as to why occurrence/recurrence can be expected to respond to the treatment program. Such models make it possible to focus treatment in ways that optimize the potential for obtaining the desired results and, where outcomes suggest the need for adjustment, to alter the treatment strategy in a positive way.

Fifth, as noted above, evaluation methods often were not sufficiently rigorous. Time pressures led to inadequate measurement procedures in that reliability and validity characteristics were unknown or determined only after data collection. Research designs often involved serious threats to validity (Cook & Campbell, 1979). Consequently, when results failed to support the effectiveness of a treatment strategy or program, it was unclear whether the reason was the ineffectiveness of the treatment or the inadequacy of the evaluation procedures.

Sixth, cumbersome evaluation procedures were sometimes used placing sizable demands on overworked service delivery staff. As a result, service staff, who were already skeptical of the evaluation undertaking, carried a major portion of the evaluation effort.

Finally, a more comprehensive plan for evaluating treatment effectiveness is needed. In the past, there has been a tendency to depend on one or two large demonstration programs when several smaller projects might have proved more productive. Planning should take into consideration the potential for replicating the treatment procedures and the evaluation since no single evaluation is likely to provide definitive answers.

PREVENTION OF ABUSE AND NEGLECT

Prevention refers to strategies intended to inhibit or deter the occurrence of something undesirable. There have been various suggestions for preventing abuse (Wolfe, 1987). In a formal sense, there are three types of abuse prevention (Goldston, 1977). One type aims at a general population in an effort to reduce or prevent the occurrence of abuse. For example, proposals have been made that the secondary educational system be utilized to teach high school students parenting skills. To implement such a program would require a clear conception of how such a parenting program would work and how it would exert its influence in such a way that would prevent the occurrence of abuse. A second type is prevention aimed at families or children where there is a likelihood of abuse in an effort to prevent its occurrence. An example here is prevention that focuses on identifying children most at risk for abuse and then developing strategies to prevent the risk from actualizing into occurrences of abuse (Wolfe, 1987). A third approach, discussed in the previous section, can be considered prevention in that it aims to prevent recurrence of maltreatment.

RESEARCH DIRECTIONS

The difficulties faced by efforts to prevent abuse derive directly from the problems that have been described. For prevention to have a potential for success, the process by which abuse occurs must be understood well enough to suggest how an effective prevention intervention would be undertaken (Alvy, 1975). This means that from among the wide variety of causes of abuse a smaller number should be apparent as prime candidates for preventive intervention.

The intervention strategy should be spelled out so that its goals are defined and the procedures for achieving those goals are clear. Evaluation then has a dual task. First, to determine if the goal of altering the behavior or circumstances presumed to lead to abuse was actually achieved. For example, did individuals really improve their parenting skills? Second, if there is evidence that the presumed cause was altered, was there evidence that the incidence of abuse was reduced among those who were the target population of the intervention (Rosenberg & Reppucci, 1985)?

Evaluation research has developed rapidly although it has had a relatively small impact on the child abuse/neglect area. The lack of a community of child abuse/neglect evaluators who evaluate child abuse preventive intervention programs and counsel each other on their evaluation activities hinders development of more adequate evaluations of prevention programs. Communities of researchers exist around the other issues considered in this discussion and these groups have played an important role recently. So few evaluations of preventive interventions have been made that each starts largely on its own and tends to operate independently. Campbell (1987), considering evaluations of preventive interventions in the area of mental health, notes that one well-trained scientist or team producing one research report does not result in understanding the effective uses of an intervention. Rather, progress toward such understanding is achieved by a scientific community that stays in close communication on a shared puzzle and that promotes competitive replication and criticism of each other's evaluative activities.

RESEARCH RESULTS AND POLICY CONSIDERATIONS

Thus far, our focus has been on five broad research issues that pertain to child abuse and neglect. Specific questions remain to which answers are needed by policymakers.

INTERGENERATIONAL TRANSMISSION

Is the potential for being abusive passed from generation to generation? Current evidence suggests that some parents who are abused as children become abusive as parents, whereas others do not. What factors enter into an abused child's becoming an abusive parent? Should having been abused as a child be considered, for example, in custody decisions in which judgments about a parent's capacity to care for a child must be made?

ANTISOCIAL BEHAVIOR

Does abuse lead to antisocial or violent behavior? Evidence related to this question is retrospective and suggests that there is a link, but it appears to be conditional (Lane & Davis, 1987). What conditions lead to an abused child's becoming antisocial or violent? Should having been abused as a child be considered as a mitigating circumstance in judgments about penalties for antisocial or violent behavior in juveniles or adults?

Adoption

For some instances of abuse it is necessary to terminate parental rights. What considerations should be taken into account when deciding to terminate parental rights? How much should potential adoptive parents know about the abuse experienced by a child whom they are seeking to adopt? What help is needed by such children, even after adoption, to resolve the consequences of abuse?

Family Dissolution

Particularly with revelations of sexual abuse, a family may be dissolved. What is the effect of such a rupture on the child? Are there considerations that suggest whether a child is better off with the perpetrator leaving the family or remaining in the family and receiving treatment?

Answers to such questions are of interest to society in general. They are of particular concern to policymakers who must set guidelines related to them. Results from research on abuse generally provide equivocal answers and, as a result, lack utility for policymakers. One reason sometimes cited is that research, particularly longitudinal studies, is too time-consuming to obtain results; even though this response begs the question. The results, even after the prescribed wait, may not be sufficiently definitive to be of use. Although the time needed to obtain results is a problem, inadequacies of results are the result of more fundamental issues.

Unrealistic Expectations

There is intense pressure on service providers and policymakers *to do something* about the apparent rise in the incidence of abuse. The pressure on policymakers, as evidenced by the need for short-term results that answer policy questions, has played into some researchers' tendency to oversell potential results in an effort to obtain funding.

Fragmentation of the Research Process

Research on child abuse is conducted in a number of different disciplines and subdisciplines, many of which have distinctive perspectives and research methods. Such diversity is important for progress but also creates a degree of fragmentation that requires concerted effort to transcend. Without continuing coordination in the form of discussion and information exchange between disciplines, service providers, policymakers, and researchers, the context for obtaining the needed information will not exist, nor will the questions to which the research is addressed be those that are relevant to service and policy concerns.

Inadequate Theories

As has been suggested above, our theories and models are inadequate to the demand. The pressure for quick results has tended to steer researchers away from working on conceptual issues and model building that are fundamental to obtaining more definitive results.

Measurement Procedures

A serious need exists for more adequate measurement procedures. For example, conceptualization of the different types of abuse suggests a continuous variable ranging from mild to severe to abusive discipline. Measures most often reflect categorical indicators that are of questionable reliability and validity. In addition, continuous operational definitions are currently being developed.

Adequacy of Designs

Many of the general questions asked regarding research on abuse explicitly or implicitly concern causality. It is generally accepted that unequivocal evidence about causality cannot be obtained (Cook & Campbell, 1979), given the limitations of applied research. The primary aim of research, then, is to come as close as possible to achieve this. In improving research designs the objective is to reduce the number of alternative explanations or, as Cook and Campbell (1979) label them, "plausible rival hypotheses." Much is known about improving quasiexperimental designs that has yet to be applied in this area of research. For example, quasiexperimental designs are subject to selection bias; that is, a nonequivalence of experimental and control or comparison groups on some dimension in addition to the experimental influences under study.

Consequently, an observed effect could be due to the experimental influences or to the additional dimension. In research on abuse, socioeconomic status (SES) can be such a source of selection bias.

Sample Selection

Research to date has tended to use experimental group samples based upon convenience (e.g., hospital patients, clinic patients) and to select control or comparison groups in much the same way. Such samples are important for developing new research areas. As the research becomes more precise, however, issues of generalizability of results increase in importance.

Statistical Procedures

The statistical procedures used in many existing studies are sometimes inadequate to the questions being addressed. Again, this is to be expected in the early stages of developing a research area. However, the models that depict the causes of abuse are likely to be complex, and statistical procedures are currently being tested that are more appropriate to the statistical demands these models create. To date, few studies have used multivariate statistical techniques, even though these are likely to be used with greater frequency in the future. The models proposed to explain the occurrence of abuse or the consequences of abuse are multidetermined and involve a variety of constructs (e.g., Belsky, 1984; Gelles, 1973; Wolfe, 1987). Realistic tests of these models can only be accomplished by using such multivariate procedures as multiple regression, multivariate analysis of variance, factor analysis, or structural equation (LISREL) modeling.

SUMMARY

The preceding discussion has considered current status and future research directions for five issues in the area of child abuse and neglect: incidence/prevalence, causes, consequences, treatment, and prevention. Each issue has a number of problems that require increased attention by the research and clinical community. In particular, major problems to be addressed include the need for more explicit theories and hypotheses, improved measurements and design, and more adequate sampling and statistical procedures. A renewed focus on improved research approaches will significantly enhance our understanding of the development, impact, and treatment of child abuse and neglect.

ACKNOWLEDGMENTS

Preparation of this chapter was supported in part by Grant NO. MH41109 from the National Institute of Mental Health, Program on Anti-Social and Violent Behavior.

REFERENCES

Achenbach, T. M., & McConaughy, S. H. (1987). *Empirically based assessment of child and adolescent psychopathology.* Newbury Park, CA: Sage.

Alvy, K. T. (1975). Preventing child abuse. *American Psychologist, 30,* 921–928.

Ammerman, R. T. (1990). Child abuse and neglect. In M. Hersen (Ed.), *Innovations in child behavior therapy.* New York: Springer.

Augoustinos, M. (1987). Developmental effects of child abuse: Recent findings. *Child Abuse and Neglect, 11,* 15–27.

Bassetti, M. (1974). Nutrition. In K. E. Barnard & H. B. Douglas (Eds.), *Child health assessment* (pp. 59–73). (Part I, USDHEW, Publication No. HRA 75–30). Bethesda, MD: Department of Health, Education, and Welfare.

Belsky, J. (1984). Determinants of parenting: A process model. *Child Development, 55,* 83–96.

Brassard, M. R., & McNeil, L. E. (1987). Child sexual abuse. In H. R. Brassard, R. Germain, & S. N. Hart (Eds.), *Psychological maltreatment of children and youth* (pp. 69–88). New York: Pergamon Press.

Burgess, R. L., & Conger, R. D. (1978). Family interaction in abusive, neglected and normal families. *Child Development, 49,* 1163–1173.

Campbell, D. T. (1987). Guidelines for monitoring the scientific competence of preventive, intervention research centers: An exercise in the sociology of scientific validity. *Knowledge, Creation, Diffusion, Utilization, 8,* 389–430.

Cicchetti, D., & Rizley, R. (1981). Developmental perspectives on the etiology, intergenerational transmission and sequelae of child maltreatment. In R. Rizley & D. Cicchetti (Eds.), *Developmental perspectives on child maltreatment* (pp. 31–55). San Francisco: Jossey-Bass.

Cohn, A. H. (1979a). An evaluation of three demonstration child abuse and neglect treatment programs. *Journal of the American Academy of Child Psychiatry, 18,* 283–291.

Cohn, A. H. (1979b). Essential components of successful child abuse and neglect treatment. *Child Abuse and Neglect, 3,* 491–496.

Cohn, A. H., & Daro, D. (1987). Is treatment too late: What ten years of evaluation research tells us. *Child Abuse and Neglect, 11,* 433–442.

Conerly, S. (1986). Assessment of suspected child sexual abuse. In K. MacFarlane, J. Waterman, S. Conerly, L. Damon, M. Durfee, & S. Long (Eds.), *Sexual abuse of young children* (pp. 30–51). New York: Guilford Press.

Cook, T. D., & Campbell, D. T. (1979). *Quasi-experimentation: Design and analysis issues for field settings.* Boston: Houghton Mifflin.

de Lissovoy, V. (1979). Toward the definition of "abuse provoking child." *Child Abuse and Neglect, 3,* 341–350.

Egeland, B., & Sroufe, A. (1981). Developmental sequelae of maltreatment in infancy. In R. Rizley & D. Cicchetti (Eds.), *Developmental perspectives on child maltreatment* (pp. 77–92). San Francisco: Jossey-Bass.

106   ROY C. HERRENKOHL

Egeland, B., Jacobvitz, D., & Papatola, K. (1987). Intergenerational continuity of abuse. In
    R. J. Gelles & J. B. Lancaster (Eds.), *Child abuse and neglect: Biosocial dimensions* (pp. 255–
    276). New York: Aldine DeGruyter.
Elmer, E. (1977). *Fragile families, troubled children*. Pittsburgh: University of Pittsburgh Press.
Elmer, E. (1979). Child abuse and family stress. *Journal of Social Issues, 35,* 60–71.
Elmer, E. (1981). Traumatized children, chronic illness and poverty. In L. Pelton (Ed.), *The
    social context of child abuse and neglect* (pp. 185–227). New York: Human Sciences Press.
Finkelhor, D., Hotaling, G. T., & Yllo, K. (1988). *Stopping family violence: Research priorities
    for the coming decade*. Newbury Park, CA: Sage.
Garbarino, J. (1976). A preliminary study of some ecological correlates of child abuse: The
    impact of socio-economical stress on mothers. *Child Development, 47,* 178–185.
Garbarino, J. (1981). An ecological approach to child maltreatment. In L. H. Pelton (Ed.),
    The social context of child abuse and neglect (pp. 228–267). New York: Human Sciences
    Press.
Garbarino, J., Guttmann, E., & Seeley, J. W. (1986). *The psychologically battered child*. San
    Francisco: Jossey-Bass.
Garmezy, N. (1983). Stressors of childhood. In N. Garmezy & M. Rutter (Eds.), *Stress,
    coping and development in children* (pp. 43–84). New York: McGraw-Hill.
Geffner, R., Rosenbaum, A., & Hughes, H. (1988). Research issues concerning family
    violence. In V. B. Van Hasselt, R. L. Morrison, A. S. Bellack, & M. Hersen (Eds.),
    Handbook of family violence (pp. 457–481). New York: Plenum Press.
Gelles, R. J. (1973). Child abuse as psychopathology: A sociological critique and reformula-
    tion. *American Journal of Orthopsychiatry, 43,* 611–621.
Gil, D. G. (1970). *Violence against children: Physical abuse in the United States*. Cambridge, MA:
    Harvard University Press.
Goldstein, J., Freud, A., & Solnit, A. (1973). *Beyond the best interests of the child*. New York:
    Free Press.
Goldston, S. E. (1977). Defining primary prevention. In G. W. Albee & J. M. Joffee (Eds.),
    Primary prevention of psychopathology, Vol. I (pp. 18–23). Hanover, NH: University Press
    of New England.
Gray, J., & Kempe, R. (1976). The abused child at time of injury. In H. Martin (Ed.), *The
    abused child* (pp. 57–65). Cambridge, MA: Ballinger.
Hart, S. N., Germain, R. B., & Brassard, M. R. (1987). The challenge: To better understand
    and combat psychological maltreatment of children and youth. In M. R. Brassard, R.
    Germain, & S. N. Hart (Eds.), *Psychological maltreatment of children and youth* (pp. 3–24).
    New York: Pergamon Press.
Herrenkohl, E. C., & Herrenkohl, R. C. (1981). Some antecedents and developmental
    consequences of child maltreatment. In R. Rizley & D. Cicchetti (Eds.), *Developmental
    perspectives on child maltreatment* (pp. 57–76). San Francisco: Jossey-Bass.
Herrenkohl, E. C., Herrenkohl, R. C., & Toedter, L. (1983). Perspectives on the in-
    tergenerational transmission of abuse. In D. Finkelhor, R. J. Gelles, G. T. Hotaling, &
    M. A. Straus (Eds.), *The dark side of families* (pp. 305–316). Beverly Hills, CA: Sage.
Herrenkohl, E. C., Herrenkohl, R. C., Toedter, L., & Yanushefski, A. M. (1984). Parent-
    child interactions in abusive and non-abusive families. *Journal of the American Academy
    of Child Psychiatry, 23,* 641–648.
Herrenkohl, R. C., & Herrenkohl, E. C. (1988a). *Assessing the occurrence of physical and
    emotional maltreatment*. Unpublished manuscript, Lehigh University, Bethlehem, PA.
Herrenkohl, R. C., & Herrenkohl, E. C. (1988b). *Identifying the occurrence of maltreatment in
    comparison groups*. Unpublished manuscript, Lehigh University, Bethlehem, PA.
Herrenkohl, R. C., Herrenkohl, E. C., Egolf, B., & Seech, M. (1979). The repetition of child
    abuse: How frequently does it occur? *Child Abuse and Neglect, 3,* 67–72.

Herrenkohl, R. C., Herrenkohl, E. C., & Egolf, B. (1983). Circumstances surrounding the occurrence of child maltreatment. *Journal of Consulting and Clinical Psychology, 51,* 424–431.

Hershorn, M., & Rosenbaum, A. (1985). Children of marital violence. *American Journal of Orthopsychiatry, 55,* 260–266.

Hotaling, G., & Sugarman, D. (1986). An analysis of risk markers in husband and wife violence: The current state of knowledge. *Violence and Victims, 1,* 101–124.

Hyman, I. A. (1987). Psychological correlates of corporal punishment. In M. R. Brassard, R. Germain, & S. N. Hart (Eds.), *Psychological maltreatment of children and youth* (pp. 59–68). New York: Pergamon Press.

Jones, D. (1987). The untreatable family. *Child Abuse and Neglect, 11,* 409–420.

Justice, B., & Justice, R. (1976). *The abusing family.* New York: Human Sciences Press.

Kadushin, A., & Martin, J. (1981). *Child abuse: An interactional event.* New York: Columbia University Press.

Kaufman, J., & Zigler, E. (1987). Do abused children become abusive parents? *American Journal of Orthopsychiatry, 57,* 186–192.

Lane, T. W., & Davis, G. E. (1987). Child maltreatment and juvenile delinquency: Does a relationship exist: In J. D. Burchard & S. N. Burchard (Eds.), *Prevention of delinquent behavior.* Newbury Park, CA: Sage.

Lusk, R., & Waterman, J. (1986). Effects of sexual abuse on children. In K. MacFarlane, J. Waterman, S. Conerly, L. Damon, M. Durfee, & S. Long (Eds.), *Sexual abuse of young children* (pp. 101–118). New York: Guilford Press.

Lynch, M. A., & Roberts, J. (1982). *The consequences of abuse.* London: Academic Press.

Martin, H. P. (1973). Nutrition: Its relationship to children's physical, mental and emotional development. *American Journal of Clinical Nutrition, 26,* 766–775.

Martin, H. P. (1976). *The abused child.* Cambridge, MA: Ballinger.

McCleer, S. V. (1988). Psychoanalytic perspectives on family violence. In V. B. Van Hassett, R. L. Morrison, A. S. Bellack, & M. Hersen (Eds.), *Handbook of family violence* (pp. 11–30). New York: Plenum Press.

Milner, J. S., & Wimberley, R. C. (1979). An inventory for the identification of child abuse. *Journal of Clinical Psychology, 35,* 95–100.

Mrazek, P., & Mrazek, D. (1987). Resilience in child maltreatment victims: A conceptual exploration. *Child Abuse and Neglect, 11,* 357–366.

Nagi, S. (1977). *Child maltreatment in the United States.* New York: Columbia University Press.

Navarre, E. L. (1987). Psychological maltreatment: The core component of child abuse. In M. R. Brassard, R. Germain, & S. N. Hart (Eds.), *Psychological maltreatment of children and youth* (pp. 45–56). New York: Pergamon Press.

Oates, K. (1986). *Child abuse and neglect, what happens eventually?* New York: Brunner/Mazel.

Parke, R. D., & Collmer, C. (1975). *Child abuse: An interdisciplinary analysis.* Chicago: University of Chicago Press.

Pelton, L. H. (1981). Child abuse and neglect: The myth of classlessness. In L. H. Pelton (Ed.), *The social context of child abuse and neglect* (pp. 23–38). New York: Human Sciences Press.

Polansky, N. A., Chalmers, M. A., Buttenwieser, E., & Williams, D. P. (1981). *Damaged parents: An anatomy of child neglect.* Chicago: University of Chicago Press.

Rosenberg, M. S., & Reppucci, N. D. (1985). Primary prevention of child abuse. *Journal of Consulting and Clinical Psychology, 53,* 576–585.

Russell, D. (1983). The incidence and prevalence of intrafamilial and extrafamilial sexual abuse of female children. *Child Abuse and Neglect, 7,* 133–146.

Schakel, J. A. (1987). Emotional neglect and stimulus deprivation. In M. R. Brassard, R.

Germain, & S. N. Hart (Eds.), *Psychological maltreatment of children and youth* (pp. 100–109). New York: Pergamon Press.

Schneider, C. (1982). The Michigan Screening Profile of Parenting. In R. H. Starr (Ed.), *Child abuse prediction: Policy implications* (pp. 157–174). Cambridge, MA: Ballinger.

Spinetta, J. J., & Rigler, D. (1972). The child abusing parent: A psychological review. *Psychological Bulletin, 77,* 296–304.

Starr, R. H. (1982). *Child abuse prediction: Policy implications.* Cambridge, MA: Ballinger.

Starr, R. H. (1988). Physical abuse of children. In V. B. Van Hasselt, R. L. Morrison, A. S. Bellack, & M. Hersen (Eds.), *Handbook of family violence* (pp. 119–155). New York: Plenum Press.

Steele, B. F. (1976). Violence within the family. In R. E. Helfer & C. H. Kempe (Eds.), *Child abuse and neglect: The family and the community* (pp. 3–23). Cambridge, MA: Ballinger.

Sudia, C. E. (1981). What services do abusive and neglecting families need? In L. H. Pelton (Ed.), *The social context of child abuse and neglect* (pp. 268–290). New York: Human Sciences Press.

Straus, M., Gelles, R., & Steinmetz, S. (1980). *Behind closed doors: Violence in the American family.* Garden City, NY: Anchor Press.

Tong, L., & Oates, K. (1987). Personality development following sexual abuse. *Child Abuse and Neglect, 11,* 371–383.

Toro, P. A. (1982). Developmental effects of child abuse: A review. *Child Abuse and Neglect, 6,* 423–431.

Twentyman, C. T., Rohrbeck, C. A., & Amish, P. L. (1984). A cognitive-behavioral approach to child abuse: Implications for treatment. In S. Saunders, A. M. Anderson, C. A. Hart, & G. M. Rubenstein (Eds.), *Violent individuals and families* (pp. 87–211). Springfield: Charles C Thomas.

Wald, M. S. (1976). State intervention on behalf of "neglected" children: Standards for removal of children from their homes, monitoring the status of children in foster care, and termination of parental rights. *Stanford Law Review, 28,* 623–706.

Wald, M. S., Carlsmith, J. M., Leiderman, P. H., French, R. de S., & Smith, C. (1985). *Protecting abused/neglected children: A comparison of home and foster placement.* Palo Alto, CA: Stanford Center for the Study of Youth Development.

Wolfe, D. A. (1987). *Child abuse: Implications for child development and psychopathology.* Newbury Park, CA: Sage.

Wolfe, D. A., Zak, L., Wilson, S., & Jaffe, P. (1986). Child witnesses to violence between parents: Critical issues in behavioral and social adjustment. *Journal of Abnormal Child Psychology, 14,* 95–104.

Wolfe, D. A., Wolfe, V. V., & Best, C. L. (1988). Child victims of sexual abuse. In V. B. Van Hasselt, R. L. Morrison, A. S. Bellack, & M. Hersen (Eds.), *Handbook of family violence* (pp. 157–185). New York: Plenum Press.

CHAPTER 5

SOCIAL AND EMOTIONAL CONSEQUENCES OF CHILD MALTREATMENT

LISE M. YOUNGBLADE AND JAY BELSKY

INTRODUCTION

More than a quarter of a century ago, Kempe and his colleagues (Kempe, Silverman, Steele, & Droegemueller, 1962) alerted the medical and academic communities to the "battered child syndrome." Ever since, research on, and concern for, child maltreatment has proliferated. Although substantial concern has been directed toward the victims of abuse and neglect, most research has focused upon the perpetrators (see Belsky, 1978, 1980, and Parke & Collmer, 1975, for reviews). There are compelling reasons why etiology rather than consequences of child maltreatment have been the principle focus of empirical inquiry, perhaps the most obvious of which is priorities. The first task of those concerned with child abuse and neglect is to stop it from occurring again or to prevent it from happening in the first place. In order for either remediation or prevention efforts to succeed, understanding of etiology is essential.

LISE M. YOUNGBLADE AND JAY BELSKY • Department of Individual and Family Studies, College of Health and Human Development, Pennsylvania State University, University Park, Pennsylvania 16802.

Despite this humanitarian imperative, there are several important reasons for empirical inquiry into the developmental consequences of child maltreatment to be a central focus of research on this topic. The first, ironically enough, derives directly from concern with etiology. Because both clinical and empirical evidence link a history of maltreatment in one's childhood to its subsequent perpetration as an adult (e.g., Burgess & Youngblade, 1988; Egeland, Jacobvitz, & Papatola, 1987; Kaufman & Zigler, 1987), understanding the effects of child abuse and neglect on the developing child should illuminate processes by which it is intergenerationally transmitted.

A second reason for studying developmental consequences in addition to illuminating etiology is to gain insight into basic processes of human development. As Rutter has stated so cogently:

> Just as knowledge of normal development carries important lessons for those wishing to unravel disease mechanisms, so the investigation of abnormality may shed light on the course of normal development. This is because a focus on the unusual may be crucial for pulling apart elements that ordinarily go together (Rutter, 1982, p. 106; see also Cicchetti, 1984; Cicchetti & Sroufe, 1976).

Our third and final reason for reviewing in this chapter what is known about the developmental effects of being abused or neglected as a child is motivated in part by the results of an investigation reported just a decade ago, indicating that the effects of child maltreatment appear to be indistinguishable from those of economic deprivation more generally. In a study that challenged the field, Elmer (1977) compared three groups of eight-year-olds, two of which has been identified as victims of abuse or of accidents in their first year of life at time of admission to Children's Hospital in Pittsburgh. Broad-based assessments of 17 children from each group, plus an additional 17 control subjects not previously studied, revealed few differences between abused, accident, and control children—a finding that was true whether one looked at physical health, language development, self-concept, intellectual standing, school performance, or self-control. What was most noteworthy was how widespread deficits were in all three samples of children.

The results of the Elmer (1977) study called into question the meaning of virtually all investigations up to that point in time, most of which had been conducted by clinicians not blind to the child's rearing history and without reliance upon appropriate comparison groups (see Aber & Cicchetti, 1984, for review and critique). Thus, Elmer's findings raised the very real possibility that the effects of child abuse might be indistinguishable from that of rearing in an economically deprived family and community setting, contexts which are known to foster maltreatment (Pelton, 1978). In order to determine the extent to which conclusions drawn from Elmer's work have been substantiated in the more rigorous empirical work that has followed publication of her study, it is our plan to review available research on the effects of child maltreatment on socioemotional development. Before doing so, however, several general conceptual, methodological, and theoretical issues must be considered.

ISSUES IN THE STUDY OF CHILD ABUSE AND NEGLECT

What is Child Abuse?

Perhaps the most serious conceptual issue to ponder is what, in fact, is meant by the term *child abuse*. Certainly, this term captures a wide range of behavior, including acts of commission (e.g., physical abuse, sexual abuse, emotional and psychological abuse) and acts of omission (e.g., physical neglect, emotional neglect) (Giovannoni & Becerra, 1979). Moreover, the continuum of child abuse subsumes a wide range of intensity, from repeated slaps or harsh spankings, to one or several blows with an instrument, to vicious verbal attacks, to cigarette burns, and so on. The picture becomes even more clouded when we consider the length of time since the abuse, the duration of abuse, and the developmental period in which the onset of abuse occurred (see Cicchetti & Barnett, in press).

Unfortunately, the majority of studies in the literature fail to operationally define what is meant by child abuse, and do not consider these various qualifiers in their conceptualization and measurement of abuse, relying instead on descriptors such as "officially documented cases of abuse." In all fairness, such an approach reflects the fact that precise documentation of exactly what leads a family to be labeled as abusive or neglectful is not equally clear across cases in the records of child welfare agencies and because, in the ecology of family violence, multiple types of abuse often co-occur (e.g., Cicchetti & Rizley, 1981; Egeland & Sroufe, 1981a). Because the predominant form of abuse perpetrated or the exact mixture of problematical childrearing patterns is not always clearly articulated in case records or research reports, comparison and synthesis across multiple studies can be quite difficult. Grouping together all families that have maltreated their children can lead to confusion and obscure very real differences in etiology, sequelae, cross-generational transmission patterns, and treatment response for different types of maltreatment (Rizley & Cicchetti, 1980; cited in Cicchetti & Rizley, 1981).

Because the lack of conceptual consistency and clarity in the literature, we are forced, for the purposes of this review, to employ a broad definition of the term *child abuse* to refer to acts of commission, regardless of duration, intensity or frequency, and "child neglect" to refer to acts of omission, regardless of duration, frequency or intensity. Where operational definitions are more refined in the research literature, we will draw attention to distinctions made between different types of abuse. However, virtually no study enables us to draw distinctions between groups in terms of duration, frequency, or intensity.

Methodological Issues

In terms of research methodology, there are three issues that must be considered. The first, already alluded to, revolves around the use of comparison/control groups. Although virtually all the research to be cited involves contrast groups of some kind, by no means are all groups (e.g., Gaensbauer, 1982) matched as carefully as were Elmer's (1977). Second, we must consider the developmental sensitivity of the measures used. As we will describe shortly, in infancy the measure used most widely to assess socioemotional "health" involves the assessment of infant–mother attachment security. Even though this assessment has shown adequate reliability and validity properties for use with 12- and 18-month-old infants in "normative" samples (see Waters, 1978), in some of the studies to be reported it has been used to assess maltreated infants ranging from 11 to 24 months, and with minor (Lamb, Gaensbauer, Malkin, & Schulz, 1985) and major (Lewis & Schaeffer, 1981) procedural changes. On the other hand, children of older ages are typically observed in unstructured situations interacting with persons other than their parents—often their peers. And third, although a number of reports emanate from longitudinal research investigations of child abuse in infancy and early childhood—most notably the Minnesota Mother-Child Project (Egeland & Sroufe, 1981a,b) and the Harvard Child Maltreatment Project (e.g., Cicchetti, Carlson, Braunwald, & Aber, 1987; Cicchetti & Braunwald, 1984; Gersten, Coster, Schneider-Rosen, Carlson, & Cicchetti, 1986; Schneider-Rosen, Braunwald, Carlson, & Cicchetti, 1985; Schneider-Rosen & Cicchetti, 1984)—the majority of research, in infancy, preschool, and mid- to late childhood, involves cross-sectional research designs (see Aber & Cicchetti, 1984, for review). All these methodological inconsistencies limit the comparisons that can be made and inferences that can be drawn from this body of research.

Theoretical Issues

A good deal of research on the developmental effects of child maltreatment can be regarded as atheoretical, in that it is guided by little more than the common-sense notion that maltreatment is aversive and thereby bad for children, and thus that children who have been subjected to it should function more poorly than age-mates reared in more considerate ways. Even so, much of the research can be cast in terms of one of two predominant schools of thought—attachment theory (Ainsworth & Wittig, 1969; Bowlby, 1969, 1980; Sroufe, 1977) and social learning theory (Bandura, 1977; Bijou & Baer, 1961; Patterson, 1982). The role that attachment theory plays in guiding empirical inquiry is most evident in the work done on the youngest children who are hypothesized to establish mistrusting or insecure affective bonds with abusive and neglecting parents (e.g., Egeland & Sroufe, 1981a,b). The contribution of social learning theory is most evident in studies of preschoolers and older children, particularly in the study of aggressive behavior (e.g., Reid, Taplin, & Loeber, 1981), because it is hypothesized that children who have been physically abused will be aggressive because they are imitating the behavior they have been subjected to, reinforced for, and/or are reproducing behavior patterns that they have seen rewarded.

Social learning theory and attachment theory are in many ways distinct, in that the former, by tradition, has focused principally upon overt behavior and the role of imitation and rewards and punishment in the generation and maintenance of behavior patterns, whereas the latter has been concerned particularly with affective bonds that influence how individuals view themselves, others, and relationships more generally. With the emergence of a more cognitively oriented social learning approach to behavioral development (Bandura, 1977), it is clear that despite different language systems for explaining human development processes, the two theoretical approaches have much in common (Youngblade, Burgess, & Belsky, 1988). Noteworthy perhaps is the assumption that ways of relating to others result from interpersonal experience and that such experiences not only shape what one does but also what one attends to in the social arena and how social experience is interpreted. Thus, both see the individual as an active agent who, as a result of a social experience, develops expectations that guide interpersonal activity and shape the processing of interpersonal experience. Although it is true that attachment theorists place more emphasis upon how social experience fosters "internal working models" or affective-cognitive processes that affect social functioning than on social skills *per se,* whereas the reverse tends to be true of social learning accounts of social development, it seems to us that differences are more of emphasis and willingness to attribute an inner self to the individual than they are of some fundamental disagreement about behavioral development. Beyond the actual assessment of attachment security *per se,* it is not at all clear what differential predictions the two theoretical approaches would lead to when it comes to considering the behavioral consequences of child abuse and neglect. Indeed, virtually all the differences in the functioning of children who have and have not been subject to maltreatment are consistent with basic tenets of each theoretical orientation.

OVERVIEW

For the remainder of this chapter, we will survey the empirical research that has emerged since the publication of Elmer's (1977) investigation in order to examine the social and emotional consequences of child abuse and neglect. We will review this literature with respect to the developmental period of the dependent variable under investigation. First, we will examine the relationship of child abuse and neglect to children's socioaffective functioning in infancy and toddlerhood, as reflected in the security of infant–mother attachments and toddler–peer interactions. Following, we will consider the relationship of child maltreatment to social interactions in the preschool and elementary school years, both with parents and with peers. We will end with a discussion of consequences for the intergenerational transmission of abusive patterns of parenting in adulthood, before drawing some general conclusions.

SOCIAL AND EMOTIONAL CONSEQUENCES DURING INFANCY AND TODDLERHOOD

Most investigations of the socioemotional consequences of child maltreatment on parent–child relations during the first two years of life rely upon the Strange Situation as a means of assessing the security of infant–parent attachment security. The Strange Situation (Ainsworth, Blehar, Waters, & Wall, 1978; Ainsworth & Wittig, 1969) is an experimental laboratory procedure in which the infant's behavior is studied in response to a series of separations and reunions with a stranger and a parent. Irrespective of whether or not they are overtly distressed by the procedure, infants judged to be secure in their relationship with their

parent (Group "B" infants) greet the parent in an unambiguous manner—by either smiling and vocalizing across a distance or approaching
the parent and establishing physical contact. The attachment bond is
judged to be insecure when the infant's response to the parent is one of
pointed avoidance, either by aborting an approach or averting gaze or
ignoring, or when the infant cannot find comfort in the parent's presence and directs angry resistant behavior at the parent upon reunion
(pushing off, kicking to be put down, refusing a toy). Although develop-
mentalists continue to debate the relative reliability, validity, and utility
of this methodology (Lamb, Thompson, Gardner, Charnov, & Estes,
1984), there is widespread agreement among many that despite its limitations it is one of the most sensitive procedures that is available for
assessing individual differences in infant socioemotional development
(Belsky & Nezworski, 1988; Bretherton & Waters, 1985). Indeed, as shall
become evident, some of the best evidence of the validity of the procedure is to be found in its capacity to distinguish infants and toddlers
who vary in terms of their exposure to abuse and/or neglect.

Beyond the general expectation that maltreated children should be
more at risk for developing insecure attachments, it has been theorized
that because of their exposure to emotionally unavailable parents, and
particularly their experience of physical rejection, children who have
been physically abused should be at particular risk for establishing insecure-avoidant (Group "A" infants) relationships (Ainsworth et al., 1978;
Egeland & Sroufe, 1981b). Infants and toddlers subjected to neglect, on
the other hand, some suggest, should be particularly at risk for developing insecure-resistant attachments (Group "C" infants). The reasoning
here is that the infant's failure to find comfort in the hands of the parent
and the anger that is expressed in the Strange Situation by the insecure-
resistant child is a function of the unresponsive or intermittently/ incon-
sistently responsive care that he or she has received (Egeland & Sroufe,
1981b). Consistent with this line of theorizing is evidence that non-
maltreated infants who are classified as insecure-resistant often have
experienced maternal care that is less contingent upon or responsive to
their own behavior, particularly their distress cries, than is the care
provided by mothers of secure infants (e.g., Belsky, Rovine, & Taylor,
1984; Isabella, Belsky, & Von Eye, 1989). Whereas the insecure-resistant
infant's behavior in the Strange Situation is considered to reflect the
frustration of not having one's needs consistently cared for, that of the
insecure-avoidant infant is presumed to reflect an unwillingness to display and share feelings with the parent and doubt about the parent's
willingness or ability to meet the child's needs for physical contact and
comfort when distressed. Having outlined the general expectations of

attachment theory with regard to child abuse and neglect, we will proceed to summarize the available evidence.

At the most global level, there is general consensus from an empirical standpoint that maltreatment is associated with elevated rates of insecure infant–mother attachments (Cicchetti & Braunwald, 1984; Crittenden, 1985, 1988; Egeland & Sroufe, 1981a,b; Gordon & Jameson, 1979; Lamb et al., 1985; Lyons-Ruth, Connell, Zoll, & Stahl, 1987; Schneider-Rosen, Braunwald, Carlson, & Cicchetti, 1985; Schneider-Rosen & Cicchetti, 1984). The strength of this association is most evident when data obtained from independent samples in separate studies are compiled and subjected to statistical analysis at the aggregate level (see Table 1). Although the data presented in Table 1 derive from investigations that are cross-sectional and longitudinal in design, from studies using standardized or modified Strange Situations, and from research on children of varying ages (see Table 2 for description of study characteristics), it is clear that young children who have been maltreated are far more likely to be classified as insecure in their attachments to their mothers than are agemates from economically similar backgrounds who have not been maltreated. Indeed, this is true even when the data are examined in terms of distinct age groups (12 months, Table 1-2; 18 months, Table 1-3; >18 months, Table 1-4; and mixed ages, Table 1-5).

When it comes to addressing the issue of specificity, that is, whether particular forms of maltreatment are differentially associated with different patterns of attachment, some of the available evidence is consistent with the proposition that infants subject to physical abuse should be more at risk for developing insecure-avoidant attachments, whereas those subject to neglect should be at heightened risk of developing insecure-resistant attachments. Egeland and Sroufe (1981a,b), for example, found that this prediction holds when studying 12-month-olds, and Crittenden (1985, 1988), who studied young children of various ages, reported abuse to be associated with avoidance and neglect with resistance. Inconsistent with the specificity proposition, however, are Egeland's and Sroufe's (1981b) data indicating that by 18 months of age both abused and neglected children are most likely to be classified as insecure-avoidant, a pattern also consistent with the cross-sectional findings of Schneider-Rosen et al. (1985). Exactly why such developmental changes take place in the expression of insecurity in the Strange Situation in the case of maltreated children remains unclear.

As it turns out, there is ever increasing evidence that both abused and neglected children display elevated levels of resistance and of avoidance (Crittenden, 1985, 1988; Lyons-Ruth et al., 1987), a finding which has led to the emergence of a new attachment classification labeled A/C (see also Carlson, Cicchetti, Barnett, & Braunwald, 1989). In fact, Crit-

TABLE 1. The Relation between Maltreatment and Attachment[a,b]

1. All ages; all studies combined[c]

	Maltreatment	Control	Total
Insecure	328 (e = 247)	134 (e = 215)	462
			χ^2 [1] = 112.12, $p < .0000$
Secure	175 (e = 256)	304 (e = 223)	479
	503	438	941

2. At 12 months[d]

	Maltreatment	Control	Total
Insecure	85 (e = 61)	57 (e = 81)	142
			χ^2 [1] = 33.01, $p < .0000$
Secure	37 (e = 61)	106 (e = 82)	143
	122	163	285

3. At 18 months[e]

	Maltreatment	Control	Total
Insecure	60 (e = 41)	40 (e = 59)	100
			χ^2 [1] = 25.49, $p < .0000$
Secure	39 (e = 58)	102 (e = 83)	141
	99	142	241

4. Older than 18 months[f]

	Maltreatment	Control	Total
Insecure	29 (e = 20)	12 (e = 21)	41
			χ^2 [1] = 22.56, $p < .0000$
Secure	14 (e = 23)	32 (e = 23)	46
	43	44	87

(continued)

TABLE 1. (*Continued*)

5. Varying ages in sample[g]			
	Maltreatment	Control	Total
Insecure	154 (*e* = 123)	25 (*e* = 33)	179
Secure	42 (*e* = 73)	64 (*e* = 33)	106
	106	89	285

χ^2 [1] = 67.25, p < .0000

[a]In some cases, the same subjects are reported at more than one time period, because of the fact that they were measured at multiple ages.
[b]Within each cell, data are tabled such that the top value reflects observed/actual frequency and the bottom value (in parentheses) is the expected value.
[c]Egeland & Sroufe (1981a,b); Lyons-Ruth *et al.* (1987); Schneider-Rosen *et al.* (1985); Schneider-Rosen & Cicchetti (1984); Carlson, Braunwald, & Cicchetti (1984); Crittenden (1985, 1988); Lamb *et al.* (1985); Gordon & Jameson (1979).
[d]Egeland & Sroufe (1981a,b); Lyons-Ruth *et al.* (1985); Schneider-Rosen *et al.* (1985).
[e]Egeland & Sroufe (1981a,b); Schneider-Rosen *et al.* (1985).
[f]Schneider-Rosen & Cicchetti (1984)—19 mos.; Schneider-Rosen *et al.* (1985)—24 mos. (*Note*: A separate system to score 24 mos. olds was developed and validated.)
[g]Carlson *et al.* (1984); Crittenden (1985, 1988); Gordon & Jameson (1977); Lamb *et al.* (1985).

tenden (1988) discovered that without the new classification many mal-treated infants were classified, apparently falsely, as secure. Such find-ings raise questions as to whether the data presented in Table 1 might be even more revealing if all studies included this classification category. In fact, the absence of such a category may explain why Lyons-Ruth *et al.* (1987) failed to find an association between attachment classification and maltreatment, even though they discerned elevated levels of resistance and avoidance among infants who were maltreated.

The co-mingling of these two expressions of insecurity in the re-union episodes of the Strange Situation is quite unusual in view of recent findings indicating that avoidance and resistance tend to charac-terize two distinct ends of a behavioral continuum and may even have their origins, to some extent, in temperamental characteristics of the infant (Belsky & Rovine, 1987; Frodi & Thompson, 1985). In view of the possibility that some infants may be inclined to express their insecurity in one form or another (i.e., resistance or avoidance) because of some temperamental or affective proclivity, the behavior of maltreated infants suggests that they may be so distressed and disorganized by their rear-ing experience that they actually run the gamut of affective expression in the search for a pattern of relating that will prove more acceptable to the parent. Although some infants might be predisposed to become avoid-

TABLE 2. Study Characteristics

	Maltreated subjects			Contrast group				
Reseachers	Age (months)	N	Maltreatment	N	Age (months)	Matched on	Attachment assessment	Design
Carlson, Braunwald, & Cicchetti (1984)	13–25	29	Abused/neglected	16	13–25	SES	Standard Strange Situation	Cross-sectional
Crittenden (1985)	2–24; $\bar{x} = 13.7$	17 21 22	Abused Neglected Problematic	13	2–24; $\bar{x} = 13.7$	SES	Standard Strange Situation	Cross-sectional
Crittenden (1985)	2–48; $\bar{x} = 24$	22 31 20 22	Abused Abused/neglected Neglected Marginally maltreated	29	2–48; $\bar{x} = 24$	SES	Standard Strange Situation	Cross-sectional
Egeland & Sroufe (1981a)	12, 18 12, 18 12, 18 12, 18	19 19 24 24	Verbally abused Psychologically abused Neglected Physically abused	85	12, 18	SES	Standard Strange Situation	Longitudinal
Egeland & Sroufe (1981b)	12, 18	33	Abused/neglected	33	12, 18	SES; but received "excellent" care	Standard Strange Situation	Longitudinal
Gaensbauer (1982)	12–19	12	Abused/neglected; low SES	20 20 20	12 15 18	Middle-class sample	Nonclassified	Cross-sectional
Gordon & Jameson (1979)	12–19	12	Nonorganic failure to thrive	12	12–19	SES; hospital experience	Modified Strange Situation	Cross-sectional

(continued)

TABLE 2. (*Continued*)

Reseachers	Maltreated subjects			Contrast group			Attachment assessment	Design
	Age (months)	N	Maltreatment	N	Age (months)	Matched on		
Lamb et al. (1985)	8–32; x̄ = 18.4	32	Abused/neglected	32	8–32; x̄ = 18.7	SES	Modified Strange Situation	Cross-sectional
Lyons-Ruth et al. (1987)	12	10	Abused/neglected	28	12	SES	Standard Strange Situation; and Rating Scales	Cross-sectional
	12	18	Non-maltreated high-risk					
Schneider-Rosen & Cicchetti (1984)	19	18	Abused/neglected	19	19	SES	Standard Strange Situation	Cross-sectional
Schneider-Rosen et al. (1985)	12	17	Abused/neglected	18	12	SES	Standard Strange Situation	Cross-sectional
	18	24	Abused/neglected	24	18	SES		
	24	25	Abused/neglected	25	24	SES		
	Subsample:							
	12, 18	10	Abused/neglected	14	12, 18	SES	Standard Strange Situation	Longitudinal
	12, 18	16	Abused/neglected	16	12, 18	SES		

ant or resistant in their attachment relationship in response to care that is insensitive but not abusive or neglectful, seriously neglected or abused infants may simply be forced to abandon behavioral predispositions in the search for a safer form of expression. Unfortunately, it does not appear that much success is achieved.

The findings reviewed regarding the association between attachment security and child maltreatment clearly indicate that some degree of specificity characterizes the relation between attachment and maltreatment. Consequently, when evidence from all available studies is aggregated to assess the specificity hypothesis, a reasonable degree of empirical support emerges for the propositions that avoidance should be associated with abuse, neglect with resistance, and the combination of avoidance and resistance with maltreatment. As the data displayed in Table 3 indicate, the A/C classification is virtually restricted to children who have been maltreated, particularly abused and abused/neglected children. Infants and toddlers who have been neglected and abused/neglected are over represented among children with insecure-resistant classifications. Finally, although abused and abused/neglected children are over-represented among children classified as insecure-avoidant, so too are neglected children.

In summary, then, a strong association exists between child maltreatment and attachment insecurity. Not only does this theoretically anticipated association emerge across studies and across ages, but to a certain extent specificity of association is also evident in the data. In view of these findings, as well as on the basis of both attachment and social learning theory, there is reason to expect that the young maltreated child's behavior with other social agents should show evidence of disturbance.

Toddler-Peer Relations

Central to attachment theory is the assumption that children's attachment relationships should contribute to their interpersonal relationships outside the family because internal working models, or affective-cognitive processes derived from interactional experience with parent, shape social relations with others. Perhaps the most compelling evidence consistent with this proposition is research showing that toddlers and preschoolers with varying attachment histories (as assessed in the Strange Situation) behave differently toward peers and teachers (Arend, Gove, & Sroufe, 1979; Lieberman, 1977; Sroufe, 1983). Both social learning theory, with its emphasis on social skills and the generalization of behavior patterns, and attachment theory, then, lead to the

TABLE 3. The Relation between Type of Maltreatment
and Quality of Attachment[a,b]

1. All ages; all studies combined[c]

Type of maltreatment

Classification	Abused	Abused/ neglected	Neglected	Marginally maltreated	Control	Total
A	43 ($e = 27$)	62 ($e = 46$)	43 ($e = 32$)	18 ($e = 16$)	74 ($e = 119$)	240
B	22 ($e = 46$)	40 ($e = 76$)	31 ($e = 53$)	24 ($e = 27$)	283 ($e = 198$)	400
C	12 ($e = 15$)	34 ($e = 24$)	30 ($e = 17$)	7 ($e = 9$)	45 ($e = 63$)	128
A/C	18 ($e = 7$)	22 ($e = 12$)	6 ($e = 8$)	7 ($e = 4$)	8 ($e = 30$)	61
Total	95	158	110	56	410	829

$\chi^2 [12] = 176.29, p < .0000$

2. At 12 months[d]

Type of maltreatment

Classification	Abused	Abused/ neglected	Neglected	Marginally maltreated	Control	Total
A	16 ($e = 7$)	17 ($e = 11$)	5 ($e = 9$)	4 ($e = 5$)	32 ($e = 42$)	74
B	8 ($e = 14$)	10 ($e = 22$)	11 ($e = 17$)	8 ($e = 9$)	106 ($e = 82$)	143
C	4 ($e = 5$)	12 ($e = 8$)	17 ($e = 6$)	1 ($e = 3$)	19 ($e = 30$)	53
A/C	0 ($e = 2$)	4 ($e = 2$)	0 ($e = 2$)	5 ($e = 1$)	6 ($e = 9$)	15
Total	28	43	33	18	163	285

$\chi^2 [12] = 88.27, p < .0000$

TABLE 3. (*Continued*)

3. At 18 months[e]

Type of maltreatment

Classification	Abused	Abused/ neglected	Neglected	Control	Total
A	12 (e = 8)	19 (e = 11)	12 (e = 8)	22 (e = 38)	65
B	12 (e = 16)	12 (e = 24)	15 (e = 18)	102 (e = 83)	141
C	4 (e = 4)	10 (e = 6)	3 (e = 4)	18 (e = 21)	35
Total	28	41	30	142	241

χ^2 [6] = 31.76, p < .0000

4. Older than 18 months[f]

Type of maltreatment

Classification	Abused/ neglected	Control	Total
A	18 (e = 11)	5 (e = 12)	23
B	14 (e = 23)	32 (e = 23)	46
C	11 (e = 9)	7 (e = 9)	18
Total	43	44	87

χ^2 [2] = 16.45, p < .0000

5. Varying ages in sample[g]

Type of maltreatment

Classification	Abused	Abused/ neglected	Neglected	Marginally maltreated	Control	Total
A	15 (e = 14)	8 (e = 11)	26 (e = 17)	14 (e = 14)	15 (e = 22)	78

(*continued*)

TABLE 3. (*Continued*)

B	2 (e = 13)	4 (e = 10)	5 (e = 15)	16 (e = 12)	43 (e = 20)	70
C	4 (e = 4)	1 (e = 3)	10 (e = 5)	6 (e = 4)	1 (e = 6)	22
A/C	18 (e = 8)	18 (e = 7)	6 (e = 10)	2 (e = 8)	2 (e = 13)	46
Total	39	31	47	38	61	216

χ^2 [12] = 111.94, p < .0000

[a]In some cases, the same subjects are reported at more than one time period, due to the fact that they were measured at multiple ages.
[b]Within each cell, data are tabled such that the top value reflects observed/actual frequency and the bottom value (in parentheses) is the expected value.
[c]Crittenden (1985, 1988); Egeland & Sroufe (1981a, 1981b); Lamb et al. (1985); Lyons-Ruth et al. (1987); Schneider-Rosen & Cicchetti (1984); Schneider-Rosen et al. (1985).
[d]Egeland & Sroufe (1981b); Lyons-Ruth et al. (1987); Schneider-Rosen et al. (1985).
[e]Egeland & Sroufe (1981b); Schneider-Rosen et al. (1985).
[f]Schneider-Rosen & Cicchetti (1984)—19 mos.; Schneider-Rosen et al. (1985)—24 mos. (*Note:* A separate system was developed and validated to score 24 mos. olds.)
[g]Crittenden (1985; 1988); Lamb et al. (1985).

expectation that children mistreated by their parents should have difficulties in their interactions with their peers. Particularly noteworthy, therefore, is a study by Lewis and Schaefer (1981) that fails to document any differences in the social interactions of abused and non-maltreated children aged 8 to 32 months old in a day-care center.

Indeed, on the basis of their findings, these investigators were led to question the core assumptions of attachment and social learning theory by concluding that parent–child and peer relationship systems are not so much interconnected as they are autonomous. Although there can be little doubt that not all aspects of relations with peers (or with any others, for that matter) are derivative of earlier parent–child relationships, it would seem rather precarious to conclude that no linkage exists. Not only are there serious problems with embracing null findings, but the limits of the Lewis and Schaeffer study, particularly the very short observation periods and the sensitivity of the data obtained, should lead more cautious scientists to question the quality of the data collected and, thus, this particular investigation's capability of assessing the functioning of maltreating toddlers in interaction with age-mates.

Such caution would seem especially appropriate in view of other evidence linking abuse/neglect with problematic behavior with peers. Most noteworthy are three studies of toddlers that show quite clearly, in the aggregate, that maltreated children in interaction with age-mates are more aggressive, less prosocial, and more disturbed in their responses to others' distress, than are children who have not been abused or neglected in the family. Two investigations were based upon detailed narrative observations of 10 abused and 10 control children in four day-care centers, two of which served battered children and two of which served children of families under stress (George & Main, 1979; Main & George, 1985). Conceptualizing child abuse as representing one extreme along a continuum of rejecting maternal behaviors, George and Main (1979) hypothesized that abused children's behavior toward peers and child-care workers would be similar to that displayed in the Strange Situation by children who had been rejected but not abused; thus, abused toddlers were expected to display avoidant, approach-avoidant, and aggressive behavior. A third investigation (Howes & Eldredge, 1985), using a somewhat different observational methodology of 5 physically abused, 4 neglected, and 9 control children, observed during free and structured play, generally replicated the results of the first two studies.

In the George and Main (1979) investigation, abused children were much more likely to avoid other children and caregivers, almost always exhibited approach–avoidance behaviors in response to prosocial initiations, and spontaneously assaulted other children and caregivers significantly more often than the non-maltreated children. In the Howes and Eldredge (1985) study, maltreated children responded to aggression with either aggression or resistance, whereas non-maltreated children generally responded with distress; in response to prosocial behaviors, maltreated children evinced resistance whereas non-maltreated children displayed friendly behavior. Perhaps most interesting, though, was the discovery in both studies that maltreated children responded to distressed peers with aggressive behaviors, whereas control children tended to respond with concern, empathy, and/or sadness. In the Main and George (1985) study, eight of the nine abused toddlers responded with fear, physical attack, nonphysical aggression, or diffuse anger to distress incidents, whereas only one nonabused child reacted in this way.

Because the maltreated and non-maltreated samples of children in the Main and George (1985) study were observed in separate settings, and because it was not possible to control the frequency or intensity of distress which children in either investigation witnessed in their day-care program, some caution is called for in interpreting the findings. Nevertheless, evidence does suggest that exposure to the distress of others, rather than evoking the sympathy or concern that one might expect, may elicit anger and hostility in young children who, presumably, have experienced much distress in their own lives. Perhaps the

negative affect expressed by an age-mate proves contagious to the maltreated child and striking out against its source represents his or her
only way of coping or otherwise achieving some semblance of affective
self-regulation. Conceivably such a response is just what the child has
experienced at the hands of an insensitive parent. In any event, it seems
plausible that the behavior displayed by children in the studies discussed above may be one psychological mechanism through which child
maltreatment is intergenerationally transmitted.

Considered together, these three investigations (George & Main,
1979; Howes & Eldredge, 1985; Main & George, 1985) provide support
for the contention that there is an association between parent–child and
child–peer relations. Not only are maltreated toddlers more likely to be
aggressive—in response to prosocial encounters and to displays of distress—but they are also more likely to avoid interpersonal contacts with
familiar persons who have not mistreated them. There would seem to be
little doubt for concluding, then, at least with respect to the infancy–
toddler years, that child abuse and neglect foster insecure infant–parent
attachments and, perhaps thereby, what can only be regarded as dysfunctional peer relationships.

SOCIAL AND EMOTIONAL CONSEQUENCES DURING CHILDHOOD

In view of the evidence summarized up to this point, indicating that
maltreatment can have profound effects on the infant–parent relationship, as well as upon the toddler's emerging peer relationships,
there is reason to anticipate difficulties, particularly in social relationships, as maltreated children grow older. The general absence of
longitudinal investigations makes it impossible, however, to determine
whether differences between older age children who have and have not
been maltreated are a function of earlier care or their concurrent experience in the family. This reality makes it necessary, before considering the
functioning of preschool and school-aged children who have been maltreated, to examine the ongoing experiences which such children have
in their families. Consideration of parent–child interaction patterns in
particular should alert us to the fact that we should not attribute any
dysfunctional behavior of abused and/or neglected children simply to a
particular episode of parental dysfunction, but rather to ongoing, daily
patterns of interaction in the family. After reviewing what is known
about the daily experiences of maltreated children, attention will be

turned to their own behavioral development and psychological functioning during the preschool and elementary school years.

FAMILY INTERACTION IN MALTREATING HOUSEHOLDS

It is easiest to understand the experiences of abused/neglected children in their families and to gain insight into their development by first
considering Patterson's groundbreaking work on dysfunctional family
interaction processes in households with deviant boys (Patterson, 1976,
1982), as there is all too much consistency between the evidence responsible for his coercion theory of antisocial behavior and the experiences of
abused children. Central to the coercion model of inept family management processes, derived as it is from social learning theory, is the notion
that parents, by being inattentive, erratic, and, thereby, noncontingent
in responding to the child's behavior, essentially—and inadvertently—
teach the child that if he engages in aversive activity or responds in a
sufficiently aversive manner, he will succeed in terminating parental
demands (Patterson & Reid, 1973, 1984). Over time, given a parental
failure to effectively discipline, a setting is generated marked by escalating aversive interchanges, in which the participants, both parents and
children, increase their use of hostile control techniques, including verbal and physical assault (Patterson, 1986).

Consistent with this model is evidence that irritable parent discipline practices and child coercion observed in the home predict more
generalized antisocial behavior, as reported by parents, teachers, peers,
and the child himself (Patterson, 1986; Patterson, Dishion, & Bank, 1984;
Patterson, Reid, & Dishion, in press). Other investigators, too, find that
harsh, erratic, power assertive, and inconsistent parent discipline practices precede aggressive, delinquent, and violent behavior in adolescence (Loeber & Dishion, 1984; Olweus, 1980). Thus, according to this
model, parental failures in family management skills (produce a child
who is antisocial and very likely lacking in social survival skills in such
areas as work, relationships, and academics)(Patterson, 1986).

Upon compositing findings from multiple studies comparing parental attitudes and behavior of abusive and nonabusive parents, it becomes
readily apparent that Patterson's description of relationship dysfunction
is all too evident in maltreating households. For example, maltreating
parents respond to their children in a functionally noncontingent manner
(Dumas & Wahler, 1985; Patterson, 1979; Wahler, Rogers, Collins, &
Dumas, 1984), display substantially more aversive behavior in comparison with not just nonabusive parents, but even in comparison to

parents who experience child-management problems with their children (Reid, 1984; see also Bousha & Twentyman, 1984), and acknowledge using more punitive disciplinary practices and fewer reason-based ones (Trickett & Kuczynski, 1986). They also experience more anger and conflict in the family (Trickett & Sussman, 1988), display less approval (Herrenkohl & Herrenkohl, 1981) and otherwise positive behavior toward their children (Burgess & Conger, 1978; Oldershaw, Waters, & Hall, 1986), and no doubt as a consequence view children and child-related activities less positively than do non-maltreating parents (Disbrow, Doeer, & Caulfield, 1977). Thus, it will come as no surprise to attachment or social-learning theorists that abusive parents are noticeably ineffective when it comes to child management (Reid et al., 1981) and feel more detached in relation to their offspring (E. C. Herrenkohl & R. C. Herrenkohl, 1981).

Behavioral Functioning of Maltreated Children

The family experiences of maltreated children, when considered in light of both attachment and social learning theory, should affect not only the ways in which children behave toward parents and age-mates, but also how they feel about themselves.

Self-Concept

Central to attachment theory is the notion that the child learns more than just social skills or ways of behaving as a function of the way he or she is cared for. In fact, from the standpoint of attachment theory, behavior itself is derivative of the child's internal working model, that is, the child's self-image and views of relationships and the world. From what we have seen, it can be anticipated that maltreated children should feel less positively about themselves than do other children. Evidence from a number of sources provides consistent support for this contention in showing that maltreated children evince deficits in self-esteem (Kaufman & Cicchetti, 1989; Oates, Forrest, & Peacock, 1985), self-adjustment (Perry et al., 1983; Straker & Jacobson, 1981), and emotional development more generally (Kinard, 1980).

In an investigation of 37 6- to 14-year-olds admitted to a hospital with a diagnosis of abuse and 37 matched controls, Oates, Forrest, and Peacock (1985) found that the maltreated children scored significantly lower on a measure of self-concept and, in addition, were less ambitious than nonabused children with respect to occupational goals. Also, they viewed themselves as having fewer friends. Even though Kinard's

(1980) study of 30 legally verified, physically abused children and 30 matched controls failed to discern any significant differences with respect to self-esteem, it did find that abused 5 to 12-year-olds were less trusting of others, just as the findings reviewed earlier pertaining to child maltreatment and attachment security would lead one to anticipate. Despite the fact that it is difficult to reconcile the differences across these two studies on measures of self-esteem, particularly because in the investigation in which an effect of maltreatment on self-concept was discerned (Oates et al., 1985) more time had passed since the abuse report was filed (5.5 years, on average) than in the study in which the differences between abused and control children on self-esteem were not reliable (Kinard, 1980: 1 year), it should be noted that in both investigations maltreated children did score lower than control children. Similarly, in two investigations that relied upon parental as opposed to child report, school-aged children who had been abused were rated by their mothers as having poorer self-concepts (Perry et al., 1983) and lower self-esteem (Kaufman & Cicchetti, 1989) than nonabused children. Noteworthy, too, is the fact that the children in the Perry et al. study were rated by mothers as more poorly adjusted to school, as having more nonnormal behaviors, and as possessing significantly fewer social and communication skills.

Further evidence of emotional and motivational impairment on the part of maltreated children is provided by Aber and Allen (1987; Aber, 1984) in the Harvard Child Maltreatment Project (Cicchetti & Rizley, 1981). Their comparison of 91 maltreated children, 70 children from AFDC families, and 30 children from middle-class households, all between 4 and 8 years of age, revealed that abused children at preschool and schoolage evinced more dependency, less curiosity and, like the aforementioned Perry et al. (1983) investigation, poorer cognitive functioning. Especially important is that these differences remained even after SES background factors were controlled.

The fact, however, that in the Perry et al. (1983) and in the Aber and Allen (1987) investigations, samples that varied as a function of rearing experience on measures related to the self-system differed also in measured intelligence raises the possibility that it is intellectual deficits that are responsible for many of the apparent effects of maltreatment on self-concept and adjustment that have been chronicled (Frodi & Smetana, 1984). Although the results of one investigation is consistent with this reasoning, in showing that group differences in the ability to identify and discriminate other people's emotions disappeared with IQ controlled (Frodi & Smetana, 1984), results of a related inquiry showed that, even with IQ controlled, between-group differences remained significant in labeling feelings and decentering from one's perspective (Baharal, Waterman, & Martin, 1981).

Differences in intelligence, brain damage, and psychosis could not account for perhaps the most disturbing findings in the literature related to self-concept and maltreatment, those pertaining to self-destructive behavior. Upon comparing a clinical sample of 60 school-aged abused children with 30 neglected and 30 control children, Green (1978) found that nearly half of the abused children engaged in acts such as self-mutilation and suicide attempts in response to actual or threatened separation or abandonment from parents or caretakers. Even though such self-destructive behavior should not be regarded as routinely displayed by maltreated children, it does underscore the extent to which abusive care can undermine the integrity and even self-preservative function of the self system.

Relations with Parents and Adults: Aggression/Noncompliance

One of the major difficulties in trying to identify the developmental consequences of child maltreatment involves distinguishing cause from consequence. To what extent might it be the case that the patterns of functioning found to distinguish maltreated from nonmaltreated children actually serve to evoke, or at least maintain their parents' "strategies" of childrearing? The difficulties of interpreting the data are perhaps most apparent when we consider the way maltreated children behave, and are perceived by their parents to function, in the family.

Repeatedly, it has been observed that maltreated children manifest a greater number and frequency of behavior problems of the type that are classified as of the externalizing (as opposed to internalizing) variety, including disobedience, tantrums and aggression directed toward other family members (Aragona & Eyberg, 1981; Kaufman & Cicchetti, in press; E. C. Herrenkohl & R. C. Herrenkohl, 1981; Hoffman-Plotkin & Twentyman, 1984; Oldershaw et al., 1986; Reid et al., 1981; Reidy, 1977; Trickett & Kuczynski, 1986; Wolfe & Mosk, 1983). Four separate investigations of parent–child interaction, using direct behavioral observation data collected in the home (Burgess & Conger, 1978; E. C. Herrenkohl & R. C. Herrenkohl, 1981; Reid et al., 1981) or home simulations (Oldershaw et al., 1986), reveal that children in abusive families exhibit higher rates of aversive behavior to parents and siblings than do nonmaltreated children. Specifically, abused children emit more threatening demands and physically negative behaviors (Reid et al., 1981), are more noncompliant and aggressive (E. C. Herrenkohl & R. C. Herrenkohl, 1981; Oldershaw et al., 1986), and display fewer positive behaviors (Burgess & Conger, 1978; Oldershaw et al., 1986) than do nonabused children. In one study in which behavioral differences did not emerge, questions can be raised about the length of the observation period and the extremely small sample size (Mash, Johnston, & Kovitz, 1983).

It is not just observational studies that highlight externalizing-type behavior on the part of maltreated children. Investigations that rely upon parent reports of behavior problems reveal that the neglected (Aragona & Eyberg, 1981) and the abused children (Mash et al., 1983) are often rated by their mothers as more problematic than other children. Perhaps the most informative parental report study is that designed by Trickett and Kuczynski (1986) in which the abusive and the matched control parents were trained to observe and immediately record naturally occurring incidents of discipline in the home for 5 consecutive days. The evidence so obtained revealed abused children to be more noncompliant and aversive than control children. On the basis of both the observational and parent report data, then, it is difficult to believe that the aggressive, noncompliant and otherwise acting-out/externalizing patterns of behavior discerned, even if initially caused by maltreatment, do not function to maintain such dysfunctional care.

Peer Relations

The research conducted during the preschool and early childhood years, like that already summarized during the toddler years, underscores the apparent effect of maltreatment on relationships with age mates. In one of the earliest relevant studies, Reidy (1977) compared 20 physically abused, 16 neglected, and 22 matched control children in a multimethod assessment of aggressive child characteristics. In play, abused children showed significantly more aggressive behavior than neglected or control children, who rarely exhibited aggressive behavior. Teachers' ratings characterized both abused and neglected children as more aggressive than controls, though not significantly different from each other. And, finally, abused children displayed significantly more fantasy aggression on a projective test than either the neglected or control children. It must be noted that Straker and Jacobson (1981) could not replicate the association between maltreatment and fantasy aggression in their study of 19 abused and 19 control children between 5 and 10 years of age in South Africa.

E. C. Herrenkohl and R. C. Herrenkohl (1981), employing a multi-method approach, also observed that maltreated children (in day-care settings) were more aggressive toward their peers than were children in 3 control groups (all of whom were nonmaltreated, but whose families were receiving either welfare, Head Start services, or day-care programs). A similar day-care-based observational study of physically abused, neglected, and control children, aged 3- to 6-years-old revealed that, overall, neglected children exhibited less prosocial behavior and abused children more aggressive behavior than control children (Hoffman-Plotkin & Twentyman, 1984). Aggressive behaviors were found to occur chiefly in response to difficult tasks or to interfering behavior by peers, suggesting a lower tolerance of frustration.

A follow-up study of the children participating in the Harvard Child Maltreatment Program which assessed 70 maltreated and 67 demographically similar matched comparison school-aged children in a daycamp setting also discerned the now expected relation between maltreatment and aggression, this time using counselor and peer ratings (Kaufman & Cicchetti, 1989). What makes this investigation particularly noteworthy is not only the innovative setting that permitted extensive observations and the large, well-matched sample, but also the attention paid to type of maltreatment. When a variety of subgroups were compared, it was the physically abused children who proved most aggressive.

As it turns out, it is not just acting-out, aggressive, or externalizing behavior that differentiates maltreated and nonmaltreated children in their interactions with their peers. The other standard form in which developmental psychopathology is often manifested, namely internalizing behavior disorders, is hinted at in several investigations. In the aforementioned South African study, Jacobson and Straker (1982) found that their sample of 19 severely physically abused children, aged 5- to 10-years-old engaged in less social interaction and displayed less pleasure, concentration, and imagination in play during 5-min, triadic interactions with 2 matched nonabused children than did these control children. Similarly, observations of maltreated children in the summer camp set up by the Harvard Child Maltreatment Project revealed, according to counselor ratings, that maltreated children were more withdrawn than other children (Kaufman & Cicchetti, 1989). The fact that some of these children also received higher aggression ratings (see above; see also Fagot, Hagan, Youngblade, & Potter, 1989) alerts us to the fact that internalizing and externalizing disorders should not be regarded as mutually exclusive.

The findings summarized earlier pertaining to the way in which toddlers respond to peers who become distressed, along with the results of studies across childhood that now consistently link maltreatment and aggression, lead to the hypothesis that maltreated children do not simply have difficulty with self-control but, perhaps, are limited in a variety of affective and perceptual arenas that are likely to influence their peer interactions. Evidence that this is indeed the case comes from several investigations highlighting deficits in their understanding of the viewpoints of others and in their sensitivity to the affect displayed by others. Consider in this regard Straker and Jacobson's (1981) finding that abused 5- to 10-year-olds were less empathic than matched controls, Frodi and Smetana's (1984) discovery that abused preschoolers were less able to identify and discriminate other people's emotions from picture stories (though group differences disappeared with IQ controlled), and Baharal et al.,'s (1981) report that (even with IQ controlled) abused children were less able than carefully matched controls to label feelings accurately, to cognitively decenter, and to understand complex social roles.

Summary

During the preschool and school-age period there is evidence, just as there was in the case of infants and toddlers, that child abuse in particular is rather consistently, though not universally, associated with problems in parent–child and peer relations as well as in attitudes and feelings about the self. As we have seen, the dysfunctions evident among maltreated children in all too many studies highlight both externalizing and internalizing behavior disorders. And as we have noted, there can be little doubt that although such patterns of behaving are a result of the quality of care the children have received, they also serve to maintain problematic social experiences with parents, teachers/ counselors, and agemates. From the perspective of social-learning theory it would seem that the children have learned maladaptive ways of behaving that function to elicit responses that maintain their problematic behavioral proclivities. From the standpoint of attachment theory, we can speak of behavior patterns that serve to evoke from others responses that confirm internal working models of the self as bad and unworthy of love. To be sure, we need to acknowledge again that these interpretive frames are by no means mutually exclusive and indeed are rather complimentary. Even though one stresses social skills and behavior and the other affective-cognitive processes, both see the maltreated child as a product of his experience who actively contributes and apparently undermines his continuing behavioral and psychological development.

SOCIAL AND EMOTIONAL CONSEQUENCES DURING ADOLESCENCE AND ADULTHOOD

Given the evidence presented thus far regarding the dysfunctional social and emotional consequences of abuse and neglect with respect to child–parent and child–peer relationships during the infancy, preschool and childhood years, we are faced with the obvious question concerning the long-term impact of such experiences beyond these developmental periods. Such impact is hard to document, again given the general lack of prospective, longitudinal research, particularly with respect to discerning whether any long-term consequences are the result of the abuse *per se*, interactive processes characteristic of abusive families, or probabilistic life course trajectories set in motion via the circumstances abused/neglected children find themselves in, both in and outside of the family (Burgess & Youngblade, 1990). In spite of these concerns, there is evidence, nonetheless, to suggest maltreatment can affect adolescent functioning (Garbarino, Sebes, & Schellenbach, 1984) and subsequent parenting, or what is routinely termed "the intergenerational transmission" of child abuse (Egeland *et al.*, 1987; Hunter & Kilstrom, 1979).

Consequences in Adolescence

Several reports indicate that a large portion of parental abuse victims are adolescents. For example, results from the National Study of the Incidence and Severity of Child Abuse and Neglect (Burgdorff, 1982) show that 47% of reported cases of maltreatment involve adolescents between the ages of 12 and 17. Likewise, in a nationwide survey of 2,143 families, Straus, Gelles, and Steinmetz (1980) found that 54% of the 10- to 14-year-olds and 36% of the 15- to 17-year-olds they surveyed had experienced some form of maltreatment. Even so, *very* little research has examined the problem of adolescent maltreatment, particularly in terms of socioemotional consequences. Slightly more attention has been paid to addressing reasons, processes, and conditions leading to the perpetration and continuation of adolescent abuse (see Burgess & Richardson, 1984, and Garbarino & Gilliam, 1980). Nevertheless, one investigation aimed at examining families at risk for destructive parent–child relations in adolescence provides some insight into socioemotional consequences for adolescents.

In this study, Garbarino, Sebes, and Schellenbach (1984) assessed 62 clinically referred families (referred on the basis of adjustment problems of the adolescent), containing at least one child between the ages of 10 and

16, on a battery of questionnaire, interview, and observation instruments. Twenty-seven families were identified, on the basis of a self-report questionnaire tapping attitudes toward and the likelihood of appropriate parental responses to adolescents' actions, as being "high-risk" for having an abusive relationship, whereas 35 families were identified as "low-risk." Using a choice of vignettes to provide an overall conclusion about the family, based on talking with them for several hours, interviewers rated 70% of the high-risk families, and 26% of the low-risk families as abusive (Garbarino, Shellenbach, & Sebes, 1986). The "high-risk" group of families tended to be more chaotic and enmeshed, to include more stepparents (notably, all 8 stepparents in the "high-risk" group were, reportedly, abusive), to be more punishing and less supportive, and to be more stressed by life changes, than the "low-risk" group of families. Adolescents in the "high-risk" families were characterized by significantly more developmental problems (both internalizing and externalizing) and the number of such problems correlated significantly with the risk for destructive parent–child relations.

Admittedly, although this investigation can be faulted for its reliance solely on a clinical sample, without a matched control group, and on grounds of generalizability with respect to documentation and validation of abusive processes or incidences, the results are strikingly consistent with our earlier description of the characteristics of interactions in abusive families and problematic developmental outcomes for maltreated children. Of course, this is an area that merits future investigation.

INTERGENERATIONAL TRANSMISSION

Significantly more attention has been devoted to the most pernicious long-term consequence of a history of maltreatment—the subsequent maltreatment of one's own children. The assertion that abusive parents were maltreated as children not only pervades common knowledge, but is widely reported in child-abuse publications, seemingly without disagreement (Blumberg, 1974; Curtis, 1963; Galdston, 1965; Gibbens & Walker, 1956; Helfer, 1980; Kempe et al., 1962; Silver, Dublin, & Lourie, 1969; Steele & Pollock, 1968). For example, Steele (1983) stated recently that "with few exceptions, parents or other caretakers who maltreat babies were themselves neglected (with or without physical abuse) in their own earliest years" (p. 235). Actually, however, these commonly cited studies are largely clinical and retrospective in design, involve selected case histories, are limited by the use of small, nonrepresentative samples without comparison subjects, routinely lack definitional criteria for "history of abuse" and "current abuse," and rely upon observers who were not blind to the subjects' maltreatment status (Kaufman & Zigler, 1987). Importantly, because these investigations typically do not employ parents who were maltreated but are now providing adequate care to their own children, they tend to overestimate the incidence of intergenerational transmission (Kaufman & Zigler, 1987).

Nevertheless, it is also true that more recent, better-designed, prospective investigations provide support for the link between a history of maltreatment and subsequent maltreatment of one's own children. For example, in an investigation of 282 economically at-risk parents of newborns admitted to an intensive care nursery, 49 parents reported a history of abuse and/or neglect at the initial interview. One year later, 10 of these babies were confirmed as being abused of neglected; nine of the abusing parents had a history of childhood maltreatment (Hunter et al., 1978). In an unrelated study, Egeland et al. (1987) solicited information from nearly 200 impoverished, predominantly single-parent mothers regarding their childhood histories and current disciplinary practices. Using a broad definition of abuse (definite plus borderline or suspected cases), Egeland et al. reported a 70% rate of intergenerational transmission. Using a more conservative estimate (i.e., reported cases only), they found that 34% of the parents who had been abused but only 3% of the parents who had been emotionally supported were mistreating their children. These data are consistent with results from investigations using less extreme samples (see Belsky & Pensky, 1988, for review). For example, in their follow-up of English girls who had been institutionally reared as children, Rutter and his colleagues found that, in comparison to family-reared girls from the same neighborhood, the ex-care girls were much more likely to show insensitivity to their 2- to 4-year-old children, were more prone to exhibit irritability and use frequent spanking and, as a consequence, were far more likely to be categorized as poor parents (Dowdney, Skuse, Rutter, Quinton, & Mrazek, 1985; Quinton & Rutter, 1985; Quinton, Rutter, & Liddle, 1984; Rutter & Quinton, 1984).

On the other hand, in each of the studies just reported, there also is evidence that a significant number of parents, at least during the time of the particular investigation, broke the intergenerational cycle. For example, in the Hunter et al. (1978) investigation, 40 out of 49 parents, at least during infancy, did not mistreat their infants despite their own histories of maltreatment. How might this have happened? Interestingly, these nonabusing parents, as well as the nonrepeaters in the Egeland et al. (1987) sample, reported having more extensive social supports, and were less likely to have been abused by both their parents as children (see also Knutsen, Mehm, & Burger, 1984), were more apt to report a supportive relationship with one parent while growing up, and were more openly angry and better able to give a detailed coherent account of their earlier abuse. Additionally, Egeland *et al.* (1987) found that involvement with a supportive spouse or boyfriend, fewer current stressful life events, and a conscious resolve not to repeat a history of abuse characterized the nonabusing mothers.

Again, these buffering effects are consistent with results from studies using less extreme samples. Rutter and his colleagues, for example, found that ex-care women who spoke warmly of their spouse and/or indicated confiding in him were far more likely to be rated as good parents and far less likely to be rated as poor parents, leading to the conclusion that "the spouse's good qualities exerted a powerful ameliorating effect" on the parental functioning of women known to be at risk as a result of their developmental history (Quinton, Rutter, & Liddle, 1984, p. 115). Similarly, in a study of teenage mothers, Crockenberg (1987) discovered that those who reported a history of parental rejection but experienced good partner support were significantly less likely to be angry and punitive toward their toddlers than those who received comparable care as a child but received limited partner assistance.

In summary, it appears that even though limitations of the data base are widely acknowledged, most reviewers agree that a history of maltreatment in one's own childhood places the person at increased risk of mistreating his or her own offspring (Belsky, 1978; Belsky & Pensky, 1988; Burgess & Youngblade, 1988; Parke & Collmer, 1975). Importantly, however, intergenerational transmission is not inevitable, even if potentially likely. In a recent review, in fact, Kaufman and Zigler (1987) estimated the transmission rate to be around 30%, a figure that underscores the assertion that the focus for researchers and practitioners should not simply be whether transmission across generations occurs but the conditions under which one might expect continuity (Burgess & Youngblade, 1988) or "lawful discontinuity" (Belsky & Pensky, 1988). Although few studies chronicle the factors that enable individuals to escape the intergenerational cycle (but see Egeland, Jacobvitz, & Sroufe, 1988; Hunter & Kilstrom, 1979), it is generally acknowledged that it is principally in interaction with other etiological factors (e.g., child temperament, marital quality, social support) that the risk associated with child-rearing history is or is not "realized" (Belsky & Pensky, 1988; Cicchetti & Rizley, 1981). Thus, we might conceptualize the risk of perpetuating the abused-abusing cycle as being akin to the latent vulnerability of a brittle bone. In and of itself, the property of being brittle will not cause the bone to break, but to the extent pressure is put on the bone, the prospect of breakage increases. Likewise, to the extent "pressure" (e.g., no social or spousal support, low income) is put on the parent who experienced abuse as a child, might the parent succumb to maltreating his or her own child.

SUMMARY

We began this chapter by considering Elmer's (1977) findings indicating that the developmental functioning of impoverished children who were maltreated was indistinguishable from that of non-maltreated children from equally impoverished households. Such results clearly brought into question the assumed negative impact of child abuse and neglect on child development. Our review of the evidence that has become available since the publication of the Elmer study, framed as it was in terms of attachment and social-learning theory, leads us to conclude that there are indeed serious socioemotional consequences of being maltreated in childhood above and beyond those that emanate from growing up in an economically disadvantaged household. Although clearly not inevitable, we consistently found a history of abuse and/or neglect to be linked to negative consequences.

More specifically, three relatively coherent and interconnected patterns of socioemotional effects emerged. First, from infancy through adolescence, we found maltreatment to be accompanied by dysfunctional parent–child relations, marked by the increased likelihood of forming an insecure attachment in infancy, coercive interpersonal exchanges in the childhood years, and chaotic, punishing and enmeshed family life during adolescence. Second, the effects of child maltreatment were not limited to familial relations, as there was repeated indication that maltreatment is associated with dysfunctional peer relations. Several studies reveal maltreated children to be more aggressive, less prosocial, and more disturbed in interaction with age mates than are comparison children. Particularly noteworthy was the discovery that in response to displays of distress—as well as prosocial overtures—maltreated toddlers were more likely to be aggressive. Moreover, they were more likely to avoid interpersonal contacts with familiar persons who have not mistreated them (e.g., preschool teachers). Third, data from multiple investigations also indicated that abused and neglected children tend to have lower self-esteem and to display significantly more internalizing and externalizing behavior problems than non-maltreated children. Most importantly, although such patterns of behaving are almost certainly a result of the quality of care the children have received, they also serve to maintain problematic social experiences with parents, teachers, counselors, and agemates (see also Johnson & Morse, 1968).

Not only does the experience of maltreatment have potentially profound effects on the individual, but as we have seen, the effects of such a history can manifest themselves in the next generation, insofar as that individual is at risk of mistreating his or her offspring. Such intergenerational transmission is certainly congruent with the argument that cognitive-affective information about self, others, and relationships, as well as behavioral skills relevant to those domains, derived from experience in the family, is "not only internalized but carried forward to new relationships" (Sroufe & Fleeson, 1986, p. 61). It is by no means the case, however, that all maltreated children grow up to mistreat their own children. When discontinuity characterizes the developmental process, it appears that some compensatory relationship experiences have taken place with spouses, schoolmates, or some nonparental adult, which presumably enhanced the individual's feelings of worthiness while, at the same time, providing behavioral models of consideration and caring (Belsky & Pensky, 1988; Burgess & Youngblade, 1988).

This last set of findings should not be taken to mean that one should not be concerned about the long-term developmental consequences of child abuse and neglect. Even if, as Kaufman and Zigler (1987) estimate, only 30% of maltreated individuals grow up and abuse and/or neglect their own offspring, one should wonder whether parental behavior is influenced in less extreme, yet still adverse ways by a history of maltreatment in one's own childhood. What the findings on intergenerational discontinuity do indicate, however, is that even an experience as disconcerting as child maltreatment need not inevitably doom a child to a life of psychological and behavioral dysfunction. If therapeutic experiences can be provided which instill a sense of trust, of self-worth, while providing behavioral skills to deal with others, particularly in affectively charged situations, then there is every reason to expect that the effects of child maltreatment can be ameliorated. For a fortunate few, and for reasons that remain unclear, such experiences are provided in the course of growing up and mating. For others it is likely that concerted efforts by a caring community will need to be made to structure such growth-promoting opportunities into their lives. In light of the widespread psychological and behavioral deficits that maltreated children are at heightened risk for displaying, there is every reason for such intervention efforts to be instituted at the earliest possible time.

ACKNOWLEDGMENTS

Work on this chapter was supported by a grant from the National Institute of Child Health and Human Development (R01HD15496) and by an NIMH Research Scientist Development Award (K02MH00486) to the second author. Authors' address: College of Health and Human Development, The Pennsylvania State University, University Park, PA 16802.

REFERENCES

Aber, J. L. (1984, August). *Environmental influences on the social emotional and cognitive development of maltreated children*. Paper presented at the 92nd Annual Meeting of the American Psychological Association, Toronto.

Aber, J. L., & Allen, J. P. (1987). Effects of maltreatment on young children's socioemotional development: An attachment theory perspective. *Developmental Psychology, 23,* 406–414.

Aber, J. L., & Cicchetti, D. (1984). The socio-emotional development of maltreated children: An empirical and theoretical analysis. In H. Fitzgerald, B. Lester, & M. Yogman (Eds.), *Theory and research in behavioral pediatrics* (Vol. 2, pp. 147–205). New York: Plenum Press.

Ainsworth, M. D. S., Blehar, M. C., Waters, E., & Wall, S. (1978). *Patterns of attachment*. Hillsdale, NJ: Lawrence Erlbaum.

Ainsworth, M. D. S., & Wittig, B. A. (1969). Attachment and exploratory behavior of one-year-olds in a strange situation. In B. M. Foss (Ed.), *Determinants of infant behavior* (Vol. 4, pp. 113–136). London: Methuen.

Aragona, J. A., & Eyberg, S. M. (1981). Neglected children: Mother's report of child behavior problems and observed verbal behavior. *Child Development, 52,* 596–602.

Arend, R., Gove, F., & Sroufe, L. A. (1979). Continuity of individual adaption from infancy to kindergarten: A predictive study of ego resiliency and curiosity in preschoolers. *Child Development, 50,* 950–959.

Beharal, R., Waterman, J., & Martin, H. (1981). The social-cognitive development of abused children. *Journal of Consulting and Clinical Psychology, 49,* 508–516.

Bandura, A. (1977). *Social learning theory.* Englewood Cliffs, NJ: Prentice Hall.

Belsky, J. (1978). Three theoretical models of child abuse: A critical review. *Child Abuse and Neglect, 2,* 27–49.

Belsky, J. (1980). Child maltreatment: An ecological integration. *American Psychologist, 35,* 320–335.

Belsky, J., & Nezworski, T. (Eds.). (1988). *Clinical implications of attachment.* Hillsdale, NJ: Lawrence Erlbaum.

Belsky, J., & Pensky, E. (1988). Developmental history, personality and family relationships: Toward an emergent family system. In R. Hinde & J. Stevenson-Hinde (Eds.), *The interrelation of family relationships* (pp. 193–217). London: Cambridge University Press.

Belsky, J., & Rovine, M. (1987). Temperament and attachment security in the Strange Situation: An empirical rapproachment. *Child Development, 58,* 787–795.

Belsky, J., Rovine, M., & Taylor, D. (1984). The Pennsylvania infant and family development project III: The origins of individual differences in infant-mother attachment: Maternal and infant contributions. *Child Development, 55,* 718–728.

Bijou, S. W., & Baer, D. M. (1961). *Child development, Vol. 1: A systematic and empirical theory.* New York: Appleton-Century-Crofts.

Blumberg, M. L. (1974). Psychopathology of the abusive parent. *American Journal of Psychopathology, 28*, 21–29.

Bowlby, J. B. (1969). *Attachment and loss, Vol. 1: Attachment.* New York: Basic Books.

Bowlby, J. (1980). *Attachment and loss, Vol. 3: Loss, sadness and depression.* New York: Basic Books.

Bousha, D. M., & Twentyman, C. I. (1984). Mother-child interactional style in abuse, neglect, and control groups: Naturalistic observations in the home. *Journal of Abnormal Psychology, 93*, 106–114.

Bretherton, I., & Waters, E. (Eds.). (1985). *Growing points in attachment theory and research. Monographs of the Society for Research in Child Development 49* (6, Serial No. 209).

Burgdorff, K. (1982, December). *Recognition and reporting of child maltreatment: Findings from the national study of the incidence and severity of child abuse and neglect.* Prepared for the National Center on Child Abuse and Neglect, Washington, D.C.

Burgess, R. L., & Conger, R. (1978). Family interaction in abusive, neglectful, and normal families. *Child Development, 49*, 1163–1173.

Burgess, R. L., & Richardson, R. A. (1984). Child abuse during adolescence. In R. M. Lerner & N. L. Galambos (Eds.), *Experiencing adolescents: A sourcebook for parents, teachers, and teens* (pp. 119–151). New York: Garland Publishing.

Burgess, R. L., & Youngblade, L. M. (1989). Social incompetence and the intergenerational transmission of abusive parental-behavior. In R. J. Gelles, G. Hotaling, D. Finkelhor, & M. Strauss (Eds.), *New directions in family violence research* (pp. 38–60). Beverly Hills: Sage.

Carlson, V., Braunwald, K. G., & Cicchetti, D. (1984, August). *Maternal history, family environment and history of child maltreatment: Their effects on security of attachment.* Paper presented at the 92nd Annual Meeting of the American Psychological Association, Toronto, Ontario, Canada.

Carlson, V., Cicchetti, D., Barnett, D., & Braunwald, K. (1989). Finding order in disorganization: Lessons from research on maltreated infants' attachments to their caregivers. In D. Cicchetti & V. Carlson (Eds.), *Child maltreatment: Theory and research on the causes and consequences of child maltreatment.* New York: Cambridge University Press.

Cicchetti, D. (1984). The emergence of developmental psychopathology. *Child Development, 55*, 1–7.

Cicchetti, D., & Barnett, D. (in press). Toward the development of a scientific nosology of child maltreatment. In D. Cicchetti & W. Grove (Eds.), *Thinking clearly about psychology.* New York: Cambridge University Press.

Cicchetti, D., & Braunwald, K. (1984). An organizational approach to the study of emotional development in maltreated infants. *Infant Mental Health Journal, 5*, 172–183.

Cicchetti, D., Carlson, V., Braunwald, K. G., & Aber, J. L. (1987). The sequelae of child maltreatment. In R. Gelles & J. Lancaster (Eds.), *Child abuse and neglect: Biosocial dimensions.* New York: Aldine Gruyter.

Cicchetti, D., & Rizley, R. (1981). Developmental perspectives on the etiology, intergenerational transmission and sequelae of child maltreatment. *New Directions for Child Development, 11*, 31–55.

Cicchetti, D., & Sroufe, L. A. (1976). The relationship between affective and cognitive development in Down's Syndrome infants. *Child Development, 47*, 920–929.

Crittenden, P. M. (1985). Maltreated infants: Vulnerability and resilience. *Journal of Child Psychology and Psychiatry, 26*, 85–96.

Crittenden, P. M. (1988). Relationships at risk. In J. Belsky & T. Nezworski (Eds.), *Clinical implications of attachment* (pp. 136–174). Hillsdale, NJ: Lawrence Erlbaum.

Crockenberg, S. (1987). Predictors and correlates of anger toward and punitive control of toddlers by adolescent mothers. *Child Development, 58,* 964–975.

Curtis, G. (1963). Violence breeds violence—perhaps. *American Journal of Psychiatry, 120,* 386–387.

Disbrow, M. A., & Doeer, H., & Caulfield, C. (1977). Measuring the components of parents' potential for child abuse and neglect. *Child Abuse and Neglect, 1,* 279–296.

Dowdney, L., Skuse, D., Rutter, M., Quinton, D., & Mrazek, D. (1985). The nature and qualities of parenting provided by women raised in institutions. *Journal of Child Psychology and Psychiatry, 26,* 599–625.

Dumas, J. E., & Wahler, R. G. (1985). Indiscriminate mothering as a contextual factor in aggressive-oppositional child behavior. *Journal of Abnormal Child Psychology, 13,* 1–18.

Egeland, B., Jacobvitz, D., & Papatola, K. (1987). Intergenerational continuity of abuse. In R. Gelles & J. Lancaster (Eds.), *Child abuse and neglect: Biosocial dimensions* (pp. 255–276). New York: Aldine Gruyter.

Egeland, B., Jacobvitz, D., & Sroufe, L. A. (1988). Breaking the cycle of abuse. *Child Develoment, 59,* 1080–1088.

Egeland, B., & Sroufe, L. A. (1981a). Developmental sequelae of maltreatment in infancy. *New Directions for Child Development, 11,* 77–92.

Egeland, B., & Sroufe, L. A. (1981b). Attachment and early maltreatment. *Child Development, 52,* 44–52.

Elmer, E. (1977). A follow-up study of traumatized children. *Pediatrics, 59,* 273–279.

Fagot, B. I., Hagan, R., Youngblade, L. M., & Potter, L. (1989). A comparison of the play behaviors of sexually abused, physically abused, and normal preschool children. *Topics in Early Childhood Special Education, 9*(2), 88–100.

Frodi, A., & Smetana, J. (1984). Abused, neglected, and nonmaltreated preschoolers' ability to discriminate emotions in others: The effects of IQ. *Child Abuse and Neglect, 8,* 459–465.

Frodi, A., & Thompson, R. (1985). Infants' affective responses in the Strange Situation: Effects of prematurity and of quality of attachment. *Child Development, 56,* 1280–1291.

Gaensbauer, T. J. (1982). Regulation of emotional expression in infants from two contrasting caretaking environments. *Journal of the American Academy of Child Psychiatry, 21,* 163–171.

Galdston, R. (1965). Observations on children who have been physically abused and their parents. *American Journal of Psychiatry, 122,* 440–443.

Garbarino, J., & Gilliam, G. (1980). *Understanding abusive families.* Lexington, MA: Heath Publishing.

Garbarino, J., Sebes, J., & Schellenbach, C. (1984). Families at risk for destructive parent-child relations in adolescence. *Child Development, 55,* 174–183.

Garbarino, J., Schellenbach, C., & Sebes, J. (1986). *Troubled youth, troubled families.* New York: Aldine.

George, C., & Main, M. (1979). Social interactions of young abused children: Approach, avoidance, and aggression. *Child Development, 50,* 306–318.

Gersten, M., Coster, W., Schneider-Rosen, K., Carlson, V., & Cicchetti, D. (1986). A socioemotional basis of communicative functioning: Quality of attachment, language development, and early maltreatment. In M. E. Lamb, A. L. Brown, & B. Rogoff (Eds.), *Advances in developmental psychology* (Vol. 4, pp. 105–151). Hillsdale, NJ: Lawrence Erlbaum.

Gibbens, T. E. N., & Walker, A. (1956). Violent cruelty to children. *British Journal of Delinquency, 6,* 260–277.

Giovannoni, J., & Becerra, R. (1979). *Defining child abuse.* New York: Free Press.

Gordon, A. H., & Jameson, J. C. (1979). Infant-mother attachment in patients with non-organic failure to thrive syndrome. *Journal of the American Academy of Child Psychiatry, 18*, 251–259.

Green, A. H. (1978). Psychopathology of abused children. *Journal of the American Academy of Child Psychiatry, 17*, 92–103.

Helfer, R. E. (1980). Developmental deficits which limit interpersonal skills. In C. H. Kempe & R. E. Helfer (Eds.), *The battered child* (3rd ed., pp. 36–48). Chicago: University of Chicago Press.

Herrenkohl, E. C., & Herrenkohl, R. C. (1981). Some antecedents and developmental consequences of child maltreatment. *New Directions for Child Development, 11*, 57–76.

Hoffman-Plotkin, D., & Twentyman, C. T. (1984). A multi-modal assessment of behavioral and cognitive deficits in abused and neglected preschoolers. *Child Development, 55*, 794–802.

Howes, C., & Eldredge, R. (1985). Responses of abused, neglected and non-maltreated children to the behaviors of their peers. *Journal of Applied Developmental Psychology, 6*, 261–270.

Hunter, R., & Kilstrom, N. (1979). Breaking the cycle in abusive families. *American Journal of Psychiatry, 136*, 1320–1322.

Isabella, R., Belsky, J., & Von Eye, A. (1989). Origin of infant-mother attachment: Examination of interaction synchrony during the infant's first year. *Developmental Psychology, 25(1)*, 12–21.

Jacobson, R. S., & Straker, G. (1982). Peer group interaction of physically abused children. *Child Abuse and Neglect, 6*, 261–270.

Johnson, B., & Morse, H. A. (1968). Injured children and their parents. *Children, 15*, 147–152.

Kaufman, J., & Cicchetti, D. (1989). The effects of maltreatment on school-aged children's socioemotional development: Assessments in a day-camp setting. *Developmental Psychology, 25(4)*, 516–524.

Kaufman, J., & Zigler, E. (1987). Do abused children become abusive parents? *American Journal of Orthopsychiatry, 57*, 186–197.

Kempe, C., Silverman, F., Steele, B., & Droegemueller, W. (1962). The battered child syndrome. *Journal of the American Medical Association, 181*, 17–24.

Kinard, E. M. (1980). Emotional development in physically abused children. *American Journal of Orthopsychiatry, 50*, 686–696.

Knutsen, J. F., Mehm, J. G., & Burger, A. M. (1984). *Is violence in the family passed from generation to generation?* Unpublished manuscript, University of Iowa, Iowa City.

Lamb, M. E., Gaensbauer, T. J., Malkin, C. M., & Schulz, L. (1985). The effects of child abuse and neglect on security of infant-adult attachment. *Infant Behavior and Development, 8*, 35–45.

Lamb, M. E., Thompson, R. A., Gardner, W. P., Charnov, E. L., & Estes, D. (1984). Security of infantile attachment as assessed in the Strange Situation: Its study and biological interpretation. *The Behavioral and Brain Sciences, 7*, 127–171.

Lewis, M., & Schaeffer, S. (1981). Peer behavior and mother-infant interaction in maltreated children. In M. Lewis & L. A. Rosenblum (Eds.), *The uncommon child.* (pp. 193–223). New York: Plenum Press.

Lieberman, A. (1977). Preschoolers' competence with a peer: Relationships with attachment and peer experience. *Child Development, 48*, 1277–1287.

Loeber, R., & Dishion, T. J. (1984). Boys who fight at home and school: Family conditions influencing cross-setting consistency. *Journal of Consulting and Clinical Psychology, 52*, 759–768.

Lyons-Ruth, K., Connell, D. B., Zoll, D., & Stahl, J. (1987). Infants at social risk: Relations among infant maltreatment, maternal behavior, and infant attachment behavior. *Developmental Psychology, 23,* 223–232.

Main, M., & George, C. (1985). Responses of abused and disadvantaged toddlers to distress in age-mates: A study in the day-care setting. *Developmental Psychology, 21,* 407–412.

Mash, E. J., Johnston, C., & Kovitz, K. (1983). A comparison of the mother-child interactions of physically abused and non-abused children during play and task situations. *Journal of Clinical Child Psychology, 12,* 337–341.

Oates, R. K., Forrest, D., & Peacock, A. (1985). Self-esteem of abused children. *Child Abuse and Neglect, 9,* 159–163.

Oldershaw, L., Waters, G., & Hall, D. K. (1986). Control strategies and noncompliance in abusive mother-child dyads: An observational study. *Child Development, 57,* 722–732.

Olweus, D. (1980). Familial and temperamental determinants of aggressive behavior in adolescent boys: A causal analysis. *Developmental Psychology, 16,* 644–660.

Parke, R., & Collmer, C. (1975). Child abuse: An interdisciplinary review. In E. M. Hetherington (Ed.), *Review of child development research* (Vol. 5, pp. 509–590). Chicago: University of Chicago Press.

Patterson, G. R. (1976). The aggressive child: Victim and architect of a coercive system. In E. Mash, L. Hamerlynck, & L. Handy (Eds.), *Behavior modification and families* (pp. 267–316). New York: Brunner/Mazel.

Patterson, G. R. (1979). A performance theory for coercive family interaction. In R. B. Cairns (Ed.), *The analysis of social interactions: Methods, issues, and illustrations* (pp. 117–162). Hillsdale, NJ: Lawrence Erlbaum.

Patterson, G. R. (1982). *Coercive family process.* Eugene, OR: Castalia.

Patterson, G. R. (1986). The contribution of siblings to training for fighting: A microsocial analysis. In D. Olweus, J. Block, & M. Radke-Yarrow (Eds.), *Development of antisocial and prosocial behavior: Research, theories, and issues* (pp. 235–261). Orlando, FL: Academic Press.

Patterson, G. R., Dishion, T. J., & Bank, L. (1984). Family interaction: A process model of deviancy training. *Aggressive Behavior, 10,* 253–267.

Patterson, G. R., & Reid, J. B. (1973). Intervention for families of aggressive boys: A replication study. *Behaviour Research and Therapy, 11,* 383–394.

Patterson, G. R., & Reid, J. B. (1984). Social interactional processes within the family: The study of moment-by-moment family transaction in which human social development is embedded. *Journal of Applied Developmental Psychology, 5,* 237–262.

Patterson, G. R., Reid, J. B., & Dishion, T. J. (in press). *Antisocial boys.* Eugene, OR: Castalia.

Pelton, L. (1978). Child abuse and neglect: The myth of classlessness. *American Journal of Orthopsychiatry, 48,* 608–617.

Perry, M. A., Doran, L. D., & Wells, E. A. (1983). Developmental and behavioral characteristics of the physically abused child. *Journal of Clinical and Child Psychology, 12,* 320–324.

Quinton, D., & Rutter, M. (1985). Parenting behaviors of mothers raised "in care." In A. Nichol (Ed.), *Longitudinal studies in child psychology and psychiatry* (pp. 157–210). London: Wiley.

Quinton, D., Rutter, M., & Liddle, C. (1984). Institutional rearing, parenting difficulties, and marital support. *Psychological Medicine, 14,* 107–124.

Reid, J. B. (1984). Socio-interactional patterns in families of abused and nonabused children. In C. Zahn-Waxler, M. Cummings, & M. Radke-Yarrow (Eds.), *Social and biological origins of altruism and aggression*. Cambridge: Cambridge University Press.

Reid, J. B., Taplin, P. S., & Loeber, R. (1981). A social-interactional approach to the treatment of abusive families. In R. Stuart (Ed.), *Violent behavior: Social learning approaches to prediction, management and treatment* (pp. 83–100). New York: Brunner/Mazel.

Reidy, T. J. (1977). The aggressive characteristics of abused and neglected children. *Journal of Clinical Psychology, 33,* 1140–1145.

Rizley, R., & Cicchetti, D. (1980). *Heterogeneity in the etiology, type, sequelae, and treatment of child maltreatment*. Unpublished manuscript, Harvard University, Cambridge.

Rutter, M. (1982). Epidemiological-longitudinal approaches to the study of development. In W. Collins (Ed.), *Minnesota symposium of child development: Vol. 15. The concept of development* (pp. 105–144). Hillsdale, NJ: Lawrence Erlbaum.

Rutter, M., & Quinton, D. (1984). Long-term follow-up of women institutionalized in childhood: Factors promoting good functioning in adult life. *British Journal of Development and Psychology, 2,* 191–204.

Schneider-Rosen, K., Braunwald, K. G., Carlson, V., & Cicchetti, D. (1985). Current perspectives in attachment theory: Illustration from the study of maltreated infants. In I. Bretherton & E. Waters (Eds.), *Growing points in attachment theory and research: Monographs of the Society for Research in Child Development* (pp. 194–210). Chicago: University of Chicago Press.

Schneider-Rosen, K., & Cicchetti, D. (1984). The relationship between affect and cognition in maltreated infants: Quality of attachment and the development of visual self-recognition. *Child Development, 55,* 648–658.

Silver, L. B., Dublin, C. C., & Lourie, R. S. (1969). Does violence breed violence? Contributions from a study of the child abuse syndrome. *American Journal of Psychiatry, 126,* 404–407.

Sroufe, L. A. (1977). Wariness of strangers and the study of infant development. *Child Development, 48,* 731–746.

Sroufe, L. A. (1983). Infant-caregiver attachment and patterns of adaptation in preschool: The roots of maladaptation and competence. In M. Perlmutter (Ed.), *Minnesota symposium in child psychology* (Vol. 16, pp. 41–83). Hillsdale, NJ: Lawrence Erlbaum.

Sroufe, L. A., & Fleeson, J. (1986). Attachment and the construction of relationships. In W. Hartup & Z. Rubin (Eds.), *Relationships and development*. Hillsdale, NJ: Lawrence Erlbaum.

Steele, B. F. (1983). Child abuse and neglect. In J. D. Call, E. Galenson, & R. L. Tyson (Eds.), *Frontiers of infant psychiatry.* New York: Basic Books.

Steele, B. F., & Pollock, C. (1968). A psychiatric study of parents who abuse infants and small children. In R. Helfer & C. Kempe (Eds.), *The battered child syndrome* (pp. 89–131). Chicago: University of Chicago Press.

Straker, G., & Jacobson, R. S. (1981). Aggression, emotional maladjustment and empathy in the abused child.*Developmental Psychology, 17,* 762–765.

Straus, M. A., Gelles, R. J., & Steinmetz, S. K. (1980). *Behind closed doors: Violence in the American family.* Garden City, NY: Anchor Press.

Trickett, P. K., & Kuczynski, L. (1986). Children's misbehaviors and parental discipline strategies in abusive and nonabusive families. *Developmental Psychology, 22,* 115–123.

Trickett, P. K., & Sussman, E. J. (1988). Parental perceptions of child-rearing practices in physically abusive and nonabusive families. *Developmental Psychology, 24,* 270–276.

Wahler, R. G., Rogers, D., Collins, B., & Dumas, J. E. (1984, November). *Maintenance factors in abusive mother-child interactions: The compliance and uncertainty hypotheses*. Paper presented at the 18th Annual Convention of the Association for Advancement of Behavior Therapy, Philadelphia.

Waters, E. (1978). The stability of individual differences in infant-mother attachment. *Child Development, 49*, 483–494.

Wolfe, D. A., & Mosk, M. D. (1983). Behavioral comparisons of children from abusive and distressed families. *Journal of Consulting and Clinical Psychology, 51*, 702–708.

Youngblade, L. M., Burgess, R. L., & Belsky, J. (1988, May). *Are social skills enough? A multilevel view of the ecology of peer rejection*. Paper presented at the 5th Biennial Waterloo Conference on Child Development, Waterloo, Ontario.

Part III

RISK FACTORS ASSOCIATED WITH CHILD ABUSE AND NEGLECT

CHAPTER 6

SOCIOLOGICAL AND ECOLOGICAL FACTORS

JOAN I. VONDRA

INTRODUCTION

Understanding how child maltreatment evolves—whether it is characterized by violent confrontations between parent and child, inattention to a child's needs for adequate nutrition or supervision, chronic emotional belittlement and/or withdrawal of affection, or some combination of these—is inherently a task of integration. Knowledge from developmental psychology about what children need for healthy psychological development, knowledge from clinical psychology about the origins and manifestations of child and/or adult psychopathology, knowledge from family disciplines about the dynamics that underlie day-to-day family functioning and crisis situations, and knowledge from sociology about social and economic forces that foster or undermine the well-being of the family, each make a vital contribution to our understanding of both normal and dysfunctional parenting. Thus, the study of parental care and its effects on child development is, or should be, by its very nature

JOAN I. VONDRA • Department of Psychology in Education, University of Pittsburgh, Pittsburgh, Pennsylvania 15260.

interdisciplinary in its perspective. Without integrating these complementary sources of information, we are left with an incomplete portrait of parenting—its origins, its expression, and its impact on subsequent generations of children and parents. Indeed, nowhere is this more apparent than in the case of child maltreatment.

Emerging understanding of both the necessary and sufficient causes of maltreatment points to broad and interacting sets of factors that contribute to individual instances of abusive behavior or, more commonly, a pattern of chronic emotional maltreatment and neglect of the physical and/or psychological needs of the developing infant, child, or adolescent. These factors arise from within and outside the family and, more often than not, converge to create a family situation characterized by both extreme need and an inability to develop or maintain the external supports that could help bolster this very fragile system. Indeed, if research has accomplished little else, it has demonstrated again and again that recurrent maltreatment is *not* the outcome of any single factor—whether parental psychopathology or the experience of maltreatment in childhood, child temperamental or behavioral deviance, marital conflict or violence, economic hardship and job stress, inadequate and ineffective social supports, or sociocultural mores that encourage punitive, authoritarian parenting.

Nevertheless, by examining each factor in turn, it becomes clearer how these multiple factors interact and coalesce to produce circumstances that are ripe for abusive and/or neglectful parenting. In this sense, we are discussing an "ecology" of child maltreatment—an integrative approach to the etiology of maltreatment that focuses on the interaction of both individual and environmental characteristics.

Given this perspective, it stands to reason that any compelling intervention model must incorporate this multifactor model in its selection and organization of services for families. Interventions that fail to address the *multiple* problems confronting these families are unlikely to provide for the full range of services necessary to help these families to get back on their feet and in control of their lives. It will become increasingly apparent throughout this chapter that there are as many combinations of inadequate resources and dysfunctioning individuals as there are families, but that the patterns of need, distress, and disturbance repeat themselves over and over, and offer a consistent message about the nature and scope of the interventions we are challenged to provide. By examining these problems with care, we are better equipped to suggest strategies for effective, long-term change.

THE MULTIPLE DETERMINANTS OF PARENTING

A Model of Influences

In the decade since Bronfenbrenner (1977) proposed his integrative "ecological" model of influences on development, much progress has been made linking work from different fields and broadening theoretical perspectives in order to formulate comprehensive models of the determinants of parenting. Models describing normative samples (Belsky, 1984; Elder, Caspi, & Downey, 1986; Elder, Liker, & Cross, 1984; Sameroff, 1975; Sameroff & Chandler, 1975) and maltreating samples (Belsky & Vondra, 1989; Cicchetti & Rizley, 1981; Engfer & Schneewind, 1982) challenge simplistic notions of main effects and unidirectional influence. Not only do multiple factors operate cumulatively and interactively, but many may have multiple paths of influence and may serve to modify or ameliorate the impact of other contributing factors.

Although it is always possible to focus on a single source of influence and to measure its relation to parenting variables, the truth is that every factor is embedded in an entire network of influences, and each factor's relation to parenting is, in part, a consequence of its relations with many other relevant influences. Ignoring these relations descriptively, or failing to examine or control for them methodologically, leads to misleading overemphasis of the importance of individual factors. Certain conditions or circumstances may play a central role in influencing other resources or risk conditions. Nevertheless, it is the cumulative balance of stress and supports (Belsky, 1984) or "protective" and "vulnerability" factors (Cicchetti & Rizley, 1981) that determines individual differences in parental care.

FACTORS WITHIN THE FAMILY

Childrearing History

Parents bring with them a long history of experiences within their family of origin and in interaction with peers, teachers, and other adults and children loosely comprising their social network. Attachment theory (Ainsworth, Blehar, Waters, & Wall, 1978; Bretherton, 1985; Sroufe & Fleeson, 1986) provides persuasive argument for the enduring influence of the quality of relationship established and maintained with one's primary attachment figure(s). According to attachment theory, infants construct an "internal working model" of relationships based on the quality of their primary attachment relationship. When this model is derived from and *maintained over time* in the context of a troubled attachment relationship, the working model a child—and later adult—applies to subsequent relationships is unlikely to foster secure, mutually satisfying, enduring interpersonal relations (see Belsky & Nezworski, 1988).

The validity of this argument is evident in research on college students and adults (Hazan & Shaver, 1987; Kobak & Sceery, 1988) that links self-described attachment status or retrospective reports of attachment history with current psychological adjustment, social functioning, and attitudes about relationships. Individuals evidencing insecure attachment relationships from childhood are described by peers as less flexible and resourceful, more anxious, and more hostile. They express less positive expectations of love relationships and maintain their "most important love relationship" over a shorter period of time. They also describe themselves as more lonely, having more distress symptoms, and having less supportive peer and family relationships. In other words, cumulative attachment experiences begun early in life would appear to exercise considerable influence over the quality and perception of close interpersonal relationships established over the course of later childhood and adulthood.

Other data in support of the existence and impact of attachment "working models" are emerging from recent intergenerational attachment studies (see Ricks, 1985). There is growing evidence that mothers who experience unresolved anger and distress over troubled childhood relations with their own parents tend to have "insecure" relationships with their infants and young children. Fraiberg (1980; Fraiberg, Adelson, & Shapiro, 1975) provided clinical case studies illustrating this same pattern among maltreating mothers. In her casework, Fraiberg found that abusive and neglectful mothers could not mobilize resources in support of their infants' development until their own history of attachment disturbances was acknowledged and addressed. The same observation has been reported by Greenspan and his colleagues (Greenspan, Wieder, Nover, Lieberman, Lourie, & Robinson, 1987) in their intervention work with maltreating mothers.

Within the maltreating family, interpersonal difficulties and/or disturbances characterize multiple family members as well as multiple family relationships. A pattern of troubled relationships, without necessarily involving overt physical abuse or neglect, has often been established long before maltreatment evolves in the family system. Kaufman and Zigler (1990) reported an incidence rate for physical maltreatment of 33% among parents *similarly* maltreated in childhood. At the same time, there is ample evidence that a high proportion of parents who maltreat and/or who have a child removed from their care have experienced disturbances and disruptions in relations with their own parents, without necessarily having suffered the identical form of maltreatment they themselves perpetrate (Altemeier, O'Connor, Vietze, Sandler, & Sherrod, 1982; Engfer & Schneewind, 1982; Kotelchuck, 1982; Newberger, Reed, Daniels, Hyde, & Kotelchuck, 1977; Rutter, Quinton, & Liddle, 1983).

When considering the broad spectrum of troubled parent–child relations, maltreating adults appear to share a common history characterized by insecure, unstable, and/or pathological relations with their parents. Given what we know from attachment research, it is significant that these impoverished relations are typically reflected in their other intimate relationships as well. For example, recent data indicate that the vast majority of maltreated infants exhibit insecure attachment relations with their caregivers (Cicchetti & Olsen, 1990; Crittenden & Ainsworth, 1989). Studies described later in the chapter will highlight deficiencies in relations of maltreating parents with partners and peers as well. Taken together, these findings strongly suggest that attachment issues form the crux of the maltreating family's interpersonal problems. Attachment issues can apparently predispose vulnerable parents to maltreat their own children, who then carry forward the socioemotional legacies of another generation of disturbed attachment relationships.

This is not to say that every child who experiences even severe attachment disruptions or disturbances will maltreat or even have troubled relations with his or her own children. Retrospective prediction to maltreatment is invariably more accurate than is prospective prediction. A childhood history of pathogenic attachment relations can, for example, serve as the basis for *rejecting* harsh parental attitudes and practices. Indeed, data suggest that open acknowledgment and criticism of painful attachment experiences may be the "decoupling" mechanism that halts the progression of disturbed parent–child relations (including official "maltreatment") across the generations (Main & Goldwyn, 1984). Considered from another standpoint, however, defensively positive or idealistic descriptions of childhood attachment experiences on the part of parents maltreated in childhood may preclude discerning real group differences between maltreating and comparison parents. Methodologically, this implies careful attention to the measures used to assess retrospectively the quality of childhood experiences (see Main & Goldwyn, 1985).

Despite variations in its expression from one generation to the next, then, the disturbed attachment relations and emotional suffering that underlie all maltreatment are, in all probability, passed down from parents to children. The mechanism of transmission may be dysfunctional working models of relationships, reactive personality characteristics (e.g., low self-esteem, frustration tolerance, and/or impulse control), modeling and internalization of parenting roles and behaviors, or a combination of all three. In any event, the underlying emotional messages of rejection and worthlessness based in disturbed parent–child relationships seem to be the common factor in child maltreatment across families and generations. It has already been pointed out that the legacy of emotional maltreatment may be especially difficult to overcome (Garbarino & Vondra, 1987; Hart & Brassard, 1987). Attachment theory provides the theoretical underpinning for this observation. Physical maltreatment may not be passed down in the majority of families, but attachment disturbances and emotional maltreatment may very well be.

ADULT PSYCHOLOGICAL RESOURCES

With this psychological background, it is understandable why the maltreating parent has typically been characterized in terms of psychological disorders and deficits (Altemeier, Vietze, Sherrod, Sandler, Falsey, & O'Connor, 1979; Brunnquell, Crichton, & Egeland, 1981; Estroff, Herrera, Gaines, Shaffer, Gould, & Green, 1984; Spinetta, 1978). Gilbreath and Cicchetti (1990; see also Kaplan, Pelcovitz, Salzinger, & Ganeles, 1983), for example, report a rate of clinically defined depression among maltreating mothers (47%) that is twice that of low-income comparison mothers (22%). The deficits exhibited by depressed mothers in the care of their infants and children have been well documented (Billings & Moos, 1983; Coletta, 1983; Field, 1984; Hops, Sherman, & Biglan, in press; Tronick & Field, 1986).

In fact, qualitative differences in parenting have been linked to a wide variety of individual and personality characteristics, including age, emotional maturity, ego-strength, and mental health (see Belsky, 1984; Belsky & Vondra, 1989). In each case, studies can be cited reporting poorer status or functioning of maltreating families in these domains (e.g., Brunnquell et al., 1981; Melnick & Hurley, 1969). On the average, maltreating parents tend to be younger when they have their children, more simplistic and egocentric in their thinking about themselves and their children, less mature in their emotional expression and regulation, and more likely to exhibit symptoms of mental distress or illness.

Depression, negative affectivity (Watson & Clark, 1984), poor ego-control and ego-resiliency (Block & Block, 1980), low self-esteem, and a host of other impairments in ego functioning may well have their roots in the early family environment. With or without the contribution of genetic endowment, the kind of troubled parent–child relations described earlier among maltreating families no doubt increases greatly the degree of subsequent adult psychopathology. Data are already accumulating that demonstrate relations among both high-risk (Erickson, Sroufe, & Egeland, 1985) and nonclinical populations (Lewis, Feiring, McGuffog, & Jaskir, 1984; Sroufe, 1983) between insecurity of early attachment and both psychological deficits and behavior problems in childhood. Thus, childrearing history—through the channel of attachment security—has indirect implications for child maltreatment via adult psychological resources and functioning.

Dubow, Huesmann, and Eron (1987) provide an important direct link in this regard by relating childhood experiences of rejection and authoritarian punishment to subsequent ego development in adulthood. Their data, like those of Rohner and Rohner (1980) in their cross-cultural study of parental rejection and those of Elder *et al.* (1986) in their intergenerational study of families during the Depression, help support a model of effects whereby childhood experiences shape adult psychological resources which, in turn, influence differences in parental care. To the extent, then, that childhood experiences undermine subsequent adult psychological well-being, they play an additional, albeit indirect, role in shaping parental behavior.

Here, then, is an example of one source of influence—childrearing history—that affects parenting outcomes via multiple pathways. On the one hand, childhood experiences of parental care are hypothesized to have a direct impact on the quality of relations established with one's own children. On the other hand, experiences of early care influence parenting outcomes indirectly by promoting or undermining parental psychological resources. To ignore either factor—childrearing history *or* parental personality—is to leave the picture incomplete and the intervention model potentially weakened.

THE MARITAL RELATIONSHIP

Another critical pathway by which childrearing history and parental personality—and factors outside the family as well—have an impact on parenting is through the presence/absence and quality of relationships established with friends, neighbors, and, of particular relevance to this section, spouse or partner. Both psychological background and current functioning are strongly implicated in determining the quality of and satisfaction with social network support, including that provided by the spouse(s) or partner(s) one selects.

As the evidence reviewed here and reported in diverse fields of study indicates, childhood experiences translate into differences in social skills and relationship "working models" that, no doubt, contribute to the quality of intimate relationships established in adulthood. By the age of two to four years, for example, it is already possible to distinguish maltreated children by abnormalities and deficits in their social interactions with both peers and adults (George & Main, 1979, 1980; Gaensbauer & Sands, 1979; Hoffman-Plotkin & Twentyman, 1984). Social deficits are cited in studies of older maltreated children as well (Howes & Espinosa, 1985; Kaufman & Cicchetti, 1990).

These deficits, established in childhood, help account for consistent findings demonstrating a poverty of both intimate and extrafamilial supportive social relationships among maltreating parents (Crittenden, 1985). Social isolation is perhaps the single most common finding of studies comparing maltreating families with low-income comparisons (Egeland & Brunnquell, 1979; Kotelchuck, 1982; Rosario, Salzinger, Feldman, & Hammer, 1987; Starr, 1982; see also Garbarino & Gilliam, 1980). Crittenden's (1985) work suggests, however, that social *isolation* may be more characteristic of neglectful parents, whereas social *conflict*—arising from enmeshed, asymmetric relationships—may be more characteristic of abusive parents. In any case, maltreating mothers are more likely than their low-income comparisons to be unmarried at the time of study (Egeland & Brunnquell, 1979; Kotelchuck, 1982; Rosario *et al.*, 1987), suggesting that stable, long-term support from an intimate partnership may be lacking.

Further inferences about the quality of relationships established by maltreating parents may be drawn from the observed association between interspousal violence and child maltreatment (Rosenbaum & O'Leary, 1981; Straus, Gelles, & Steinmetz, 1980). Violence between partners and violence between parent and child are likely to co-occur. From the standpoint of indirect child-rearing effects, it is interesting to note the correlation Gwartney-Gibbs, Stockard, and Bohmer (1987) found among undergraduates between self-reports of witnessing parents in violent confrontations and reports of aggressing against and sustaining violence from dating partners. Whether or not these young adults also *sustained* violence from their parents, there is evidence linking violence in the family of origin to violence in early dating relationships (see also Kalmuss, 1984).

Cummings, Zahn-Waxler, and Radke-Yarrow (1981) have begun elucidating one probable pathway of effects in their work on young children's responses to the expression of anger by family members and strangers. Observing physical aggression in the context of anger episodes and/or frequent interparental fighting seems especially to elicit emotional arousal and affective responses among young children and to sensitize these children to conflict. In the researchers' view, such experiences act as "socioenvironmental stressors" that could, when they involve individuals of importance to the child, threaten his or her sense of social security. These results and interpretation offer potential explanatory power about the link between violence in childhood and in later adulthood that is distinct from the conceptual positions of both attachment and observational learning theory.

In conjunction with data presented earlier on the effects of early maltreatment, it is probable that troubled, emotionally abusive relationships in childhood (perhaps observed as well as experienced) jeopardize the quality of later adult relationships, particularly the critical marital relationship. Correlational data reported by Crockenberg (1987) are consistent with this hypothesis. Mothers in her low-SES sample who perceived their own mothers to be less accepting reported receiving less *current* social support both from them and from their own partners. These mothers were especially likely to appear angry and punitive toward their 2-year olds. Similarly, in their study of middle-class mothers in Germany, Engfer and Gavranidou (1985, 1988) found that maternal developmental history predicted marital satisfaction, which itself was associated with both maternal sensitivity to their infants and later use of extreme physical punishment.

The central importance of conjugal relationships as a source of social support for parents is by now well-established. Intimate support of this kind is associated with less maternal depression (Bromet & Cornely, 1984; Colletta, 1983), greater psychological well-being (Levitt, Weber, & Clark, 1986), more positive parenting attitudes and more developmentally supportive parenting (Cotterell, 1986; Crnic, Greenberg, Ragozin, Robinson, & Basham, 1983; Crnic, Greenberg, Robinson, & Ragozin, 1984; Engfer & Gavranidou, 1985; Goldberg & Easterbrooks, 1984; Weinraub & Wolf, 1983).

Pianta, Egeland, and Hyatt (1986), in particular, noted that when disadvantaged mothers engaged in unstable, intimate relationships during their children's first four years, initially maternal sensitivity and, ultimately child functioning, was jeopardized. The same was not true of low-income mothers who were able to maintain stable relationships with their partner. Evidence, then, that maltreating parents are especially likely to be deficient in social skills and supportive social relationships is very much in keeping with the hypothesized role of intimate social support in the parenting model. Whatever strengths these adults may possess as parents—likely to be meager from the outset—their inability to garner the support of a stable, intimate partner will undermine their functioning as caregivers.

CHILD CHARACTERISTICS

The role that the child plays in eliciting patterns of parental care is accorded special attention in the case of child maltreatment. Nevertheless, a growing body of research exists that demonstrates relations between child factors and parental care within the general population as well. Factors during infancy, such as gender, prematurity, congenital handicaps, and temperament, have all been cited as correlates of the quality of care received. With age, differences in care are increasingly related to the cognitive status and to observable behaviors of the child. However, the bidirectional nature of these relations is apparent even at birth. Parents shape their children's behavior and development which, in turn, influences subsequent caregiving, and so on.

One finding within the child maltreatment literature is that maltreated infants tend to be ill more often (Sherrod, O'Connor, Vietze, & Altemeier, 1984) and that their mothers experience somewhat more pregnancy and birth complications (Egeland & Brunnquell, 1979). This is tempered by the fact, however, that abusive mothers have been found to express more negative feelings about their pregnancy, to be delivering more unplanned and unwanted infants, and to have made fewer preparations for the infant in terms of prenatal and infant care than low-income comparison mothers (Altemeier et al., 1982, 1984; Egeland & Brunnquell, 1979). The extent to which these latter findings also reflect unstable and/or conflicted relations with the father of the child has not been examined.

Similarly, although neglected infants have been observed to withdraw socially and affectively in response to their social environment (Fraiberg, 1980; Gaensbauer & Sands, 1979; Provence & Lipton, 1962), maltreating mothers have been found to respond adversely to videotapes of smiling or crying infants, and to exhibit greater hostility and intrusiveness, and less responsivity, in their interactions with their infants during the first year of life (Crittenden, 1981; Dietrich, Starr, & Kaplan, 1980; Frodi & Lamb, 1980; Lyons-Ruth, Connell, Zoll, & Stahl, 1987). Using prospective observational data from six infants later identified as victims of extreme physical punishment, Engfer and Gavranidou

(1988) were able to document that, as newborns, these infants did not differ in irritability or social responsiveness from demographically matched controls. As early as 8 months, however, they found these youngsters to be significantly unhappier and more negative in mood and, by 33 months, less cooperative and compliant than comparison children. Importantly, the mothers of these children appeared less sensitive in their interactions even on the maternity ward, and later appeared more negative, angry, and coercive with their children. Furthermore, they described their youngsters as more difficult at every age of assessment, ratings found to correlate more with characteristics of the mothers themselves than with observed infant behavior. There is certainly reason to suspect that the majority of behavioral differences observed in maltreated children have their foundation in the poor care and/or disturbed relationships the children share with their caregivers.

The same may be noted for older children. Maltreating parents report that their school-aged children exhibit a clinical rate of behavior problems, and investigators observe that maltreated preschoolers engage in less "positive self-directed activity" in the home, exhibit low self-esteem, ego-control, persistence, and compliance in the laboratory, more behavior problems, dependency, and psychopathology in preschool, and perform more poorly on intelligence tests than low-income comparisons (Aragona & Eyberg, 1981; Barahal, Waterman, & Martin, 1981; DiLalla & Crittenden, 1987; Egeland, Sroufe, & Erickson, 1983; Estroff et al., 1984; Green, 1978; Sandgrund, Gaines, & Green, 1974). This is countered by findings that abusive parents are less positive and more negative and hostile, and that neglecting parents are less positive, more critical, and more controlling in social interactions with their children (Aragona & Eyberg, 1981; Burgess, Anderson, Schellenbach, & Conger, 1981; DiLalla & Crittenden, 1987; Mash, Johnston, & Kovitz, 1983). In addition, maltreating parents provide, in general, a poorer quality home environment as a context for development than do low-income controls (Rosario et al., 1987; Trickett & Susman, 1988).

Obviously, there is a problem with untangling cause and effect in these observations. Starr, Deitrich, Fischhoff, Ceresnie, and Zweier (1984) discuss this same issue in reference to the finding that maltreated children are more likely to be physically or mentally handicapped. Characteristics that make maltreated infants and children less appealing and more difficult to care for very likely evolve, at least in part, from the quality of care received . . . even in the prenatal period. By the time they reach preschool and school age, maltreated youngsters are actively contributing to a destructive cycle of aversive interactions (Burgess & Conger, 1978; Trickett & Kuczynski, 1986). Trying to assign responsibility either to parents *or* children for the problematic relationship at this point becomes a meaningless endeavor.

FACTORS OUTSIDE THE FAMILY

Social Network Support

The significance and probable etiology of maltreating parents' social isolation and/or interpersonal difficulties have already been pointed out. Dissatisfaction with social network support, less contact with friends and more exclusive contact with relatives who are likely to be needy themselves, and greater reliance on institutional support agencies are common patterns in at-risk and/or actively maltreating families (Colletta, 1983; Crittenden, 1985; Rosario *et al.*, 1987; Starr, 1982). Egeland and his colleagues (Egeland, Breitenbucher, & Rosenberg, 1980) put it this way:

> These [mothers who provide inadequate care] were reported to be easily frustrated and annoyed and quick to respond to their frustration in a hostile and aggressive fashion. They tended to annoy and alienate their families and friends rather than using these relationships to help in dealing with problems and crises. (p. 203)

The impact on children of parental social network deficits is at least twofold. On the one hand, inadequate social support undermines the functioning of parents, both as individuals and as caregivers. Parents need the emotional support and instrumental assistance furnished by social networks for their own day-to-day functioning and feelings of well-being (Colletta, 1983; Levitt *et al.*, 1986; Whittaker & Garbarino, 1983). These needs are compounded when childcare demands add to the burden of meeting personal and familial needs. Parents who report dissatisfaction with the support provided by friends, neighbors, and relatives tend to be dissatisfied with their caregiving role, to engage in less optimal parent–child interaction, and to provide a poorer quality home environment for child development (Cotterell, 1986; Crnic *et al.*, 1983, 1984; Stevens, 1988; Weinraub & Wolf, 1983).

At the same time, relations that are conflicted, enmeshed, or otherwise self-limiting, affect children directly via the observations and experiences they furnish (Cochran & Brassard, 1979). Garbarino (Garbarino & Gilliam, 1980; Garbarino & Sherman, 1980) further pointed out that the social networks maltreating families establish typically fail to provide the social control functions what would normally set limits on extremes of parental behavior. Thus, these impoverished social relations offer neither positive standards or role models nor any lifeline or safety net to these families in need. Combined with the fact that maltreating families are especially likely to be stressed by extreme poverty, unstable job and marital arrangements, family addictions and psychopathology, and traumatic life events (Egeland *et al.*, 1980; Greenspan *et al.*, 1987; Kotelchuck, 1982), these social support deficits take on added significance.

SOCIOECONOMIC CONSIDERATIONS

That the majority of chronically maltreating families fall within the lowest social echelons is no coincidence. Economic, sociocultural, and interpersonal factors act jointly in these families to create a situation of severe economic stress, hardship, and dependency that has been cited as the single greatest threat to adequate family functioning (Gil, 1970; Siegal, 1982; see also Garbarino & Gilliam, 1980).

Decades of research support the link between low socioeconomic status and styles of child-rearing that emphasize authoritarian control, encouragement of conformity, and punitive disciplinary techniques, all of which increase the probability of child maltreatment. Engfer and Gavranidou (1988) note three general clusters of attitudes toward child-rearing that are common among maltreating families: (1) a quest for emotional gratification from one's own children, (2) impatience and helplessness in the face of negative child behaviors, and (3) rigid authoritarianism. The first is typical of a history of attachment disturbances, the second of an insecure parent–child relationship, and the third of lower-class families in general.

Lower-class mothers of below-average education are consistently found to provide home environments and to employ child-rearing strategies that are associated with poorer developmental functioning and lower educational achievement among children (e.g., Bradley & Caldwell, 1984; Bronfenbrenner, 1958; Gecas, 1979; Gottfried & Gottfried, 1984; Kohn, 1975; 1977). Children from such backgrounds are at increased risk for poor school performance and low educational attainment (Garbarino & Asp, 1981), critical links to subsequent occupational status and economic resources.

Parental job characteristics and work conditions have also been related to styles of parenting that are, themselves, likely to contribute to the perpetuation of low-status employment across generations (Mortimer, 1974, 1976; Mortimer & Kumka, 1982; Piotrkowski & Katz, 1982; see also Bronfenbrenner & Crouter, 1982). In particular, when parents hold jobs that emphasize subordination to authority and offer little self-direction, they tend to emphasize authoritarian values of compliance, conformity, and physical punishment with their children at home.

For parents who experienced troubled relationships during childhood, the problems attendant with low SES may be exacerbated by personal and interpersonal deficits that make it difficult to maintain good job relations and consistent work performance. Job loss and economic instability, circumstances likely to befall maltreating families (Siegal, 1982; Steinberg, Catalano, & Dooley, 1981), may be especially detrimental to family functioning (Elder et al., 1984; Elder, Nguyen, & Caspi, 1985; Moen, Kain, & Elder, 1981). Increased irritability, arbitrary discipline, conflict, and physical punishment are common parental responses to these economic stressors.

When economic difficulties are combined with impoverished social relations, and both evolve in the context of a parent vulnerable to depression or chemical dependency (from a history of troubled relations with parents), and without positive parental role models, the prognosis for parenting is poor. Thus, we may view sociological risk conditions as both a cause and outcome of child maltreatment. Socioeconomic status influences childrearing practices that help shape adult psychological and sociological circumstances which, in turn, contribute to the quality of parental care in the next generation. As Siegal (1982) noted, "Perhaps there is no better single example of the importance of studying the socioeconomic conditions underlying parent-child relations than child abuse" (p. 16). Child maltreatment and family social and economic impoverishment go hand in hand (Garbarino & Sherman, 1980; Straus et al., 1980; Vondra, 1986).

THE SOCIOCULTURAL MILIEU

Many have argued persuasively that maltreatment of children at the rates observed in this country must, furthermore, be predicated on sociocultural mores that condone the use of physical force and the view of children as private property (Garbarino, Stocking, & Associates, 1980; Gil, 1970; Talbot, 1976; Zigler, 1981). The notion that parents have the right to rear children as they see fit, in the privacy of their home, is a deeply rooted tradition in American history. Public scrutiny and, worse, public intervention into private lives are almost universally frowned upon. However, the combination of this zealous defense of family privacy with the belief that children are the property of their parents, opens the way for child-rearing practices that victimize children (Garbarino, 1977b). In the context of lower-class attitudes about the nature of children and child-rearing, the probability that childcare will drift into child maltreatment increases proportionately. With social isolation, economic hardship, parental psychological deficits, spousal conflict, and child behavior problems factored into the equation, whatever social forces exist in support of children are unlikely to provide them with adequate protection, in light of "private property" and "physical force" principles of childrearing. Ignoring "macrosystem" forces such as these, which are filtered down to families from larger social and cultural institutions, denies a significant and pervasive ecological contribution to the quality of parenting and of family life (Bronfenbrenner, 1977; Garbarino, 1977a).

SUMMARY

Given the multiple and interacting factors that contribute to inadequate and abusive parental practices, it is apparent that any one parenting outcome may be the result of very different patterns of resources and stressors. A single, adolescent, black mother raising two children in her mother's small, inner-city apartment—already shared by married and unmarried siblings—may display some of the same forms of maltreatment as the wife of an abusive husband, enlisted in the military, who moves his wife and four children from base to base in rapid succession. In each case, different ecological factors are likely to be contributing to family dynamics. In both cases, however, the balance of supportive resources to undermining stressors is insufficient to sustain adequate parental care.

Crockenberg (1987) found that it was only when low-SES mothers felt rejected by their own mothers in childhood *and* reported a lack of support from their partners that they acted in an angry, punitive way toward their toddlers. Carroll (1977) reported that it was the *combination* of low family warmth and high parental punishment during childhood that predicted family violence in adult clinic patients. Egeland, Breitenbucher, and Rosenberg (1980) noted that high life event stress predicted child maltreatment *only* when it was experienced by mothers who exhibited a cluster of personality deficits indicating poor coping skills. And Sameroff and Chandler (1975) have demonstrated that prematurity only predicts developmental delay and/or disability when child-rearing occurs in the context of family social and economic impoverishment.

Belsky (1984; Belsky & Vondra, 1989) conceptualized this balance in terms of "stresses and supports," describing parenting as a "buffered" system. Cicchetti and Rizley (1981) referred to "potentiating and compensatory factors" of short- and long-term duration that jointly contribute to parenting outcomes. Both argue that maltreatment is not the outcome of any single condition or circumstance. Rather, it evolves when the factors working to ameliorate the impact of risk conditions are insufficient to overcome the cumulative effects of those stressors. In fact, Belsky assembles data in support of his argument that the quality of parental care is directly proportional to the relative balance of stresses to supports. As stresses increase, parenting quality is increasingly jeopardized, to the point where inadequate care becomes active maltreatment.

The ecology of child maltreatment, in other words, may be different only quantitatively—not qualitatively—from the ecology of adequate and superior childcare. In theory, then, prevention, intervention, and enhancement services for parents should be sensitive to many of the same ecological issues, because they operate for all parents—as risk conditions for some, and as supportive resources for others. In any case, these services should all be implemented in recognition of the full spectrum of stresses and supports that will be operating in each individual case.

Providing quality parental care is a great enough challenge in and of itself. Providing such care without having experienced it oneself, without the self-confidence, self-esteem, and adaptability such a role demands, without a loving spouse to share the burden, without the knowledge and skills to overcome difficult child characteristics, without supportive family and friends to help out when the path grows bumpy, without the educational and economic resources to ensure financial stability, and in the context of a society that sanctions violent solutions to conflict, "ownership" of children, and privacy before safety, requires more than can be expected of any individual. Child maltreatment, in this sense, is an *over*determined outcome. So many factors conspire against adequate parenting at this point that the only question left unanswered is how the system failed to intervene earlier. This is the question that risk research is now seeking to answer.

REFERENCES

Ainsworth, M. D. S., Blehar, M. C., Waters, E., & Wall, S. (1978). *Patterns of attachment.* Hillsdale, NJ: Lawrence Erlbaum.

Altemeier, W. A., Vietze, P. M., Sherrod, K. A., Sandler, H. M., Falsey, S., & O'Connor, S. M. (1979). Prediction of child maltreatment during pregnancy. *Journal of the American Academy of Child Psychiatry, 18,* 205–218.

Altemeier, W. A., O'Connor, S., Vietze, P. M., Sandler, H. M., & Sherrod, K. B. (1982). Antecedents of child abuse. *Journal of Pediatrics, 100,* 823–829.

Aragona, J. A., & Eyberg, S. M. (1981). Neglected children: Mothers' report of child behavior problems and observed verbal behavior. *Child Development, 52,* 596–602.

Barahal, R. M., Waterman, J., & Martin, H. P. (1981). The social cognitive development of abused children. *Journal of Consulting and Clinical Psychology, 49,* 508–516.

Belsky, J. (1984). The determinants of parenting: A process model. *Child Development, 55,* 83–96.

Belsky, J., & Nezworski, T. (Eds.). (1988). *Clinical implications of attachment.* Hillsdale, NJ: Lawrence Erlbaum.

Belsky, J., & Vondra, J. (1989). Lessons from child abuse: The determinants of parenting. In D. Cicchetti & V. Carlson (Eds.), *Child maltreatment: Research and theory on the consequences of abuse and neglect* (pp. 153–202). New York: Cambridge University Press.

Billings, A. G., & Moos, R. H. (1983). Comparison of children of depressed and nondepressed parents: A social-environmental perspective. *Journal of Abnormal Child Psychology, 11,* 463–486.

Block, J. H., & Block, J. (1980). The role of ego-control and ego-resiliency in the organization of behavior. In W. A. Collins (Ed.), *Minnesota Symposia on Child Psychology* (Vol. 13). Hillsdale, NJ: Lawrence Erlbaum.

Bradley, R. H., & Caldwell, B. M. (1984). 174 children: A study of the relationship between home environment and cognitive development during the first five years. In A. W. Gottfried (Ed.), *Home environment and early cognitive development.* New York: Academic Press.

Bretherton, I. (1985). Attachment theory: Retrospect and prospect. *Monographs of the Society for Research in Child Development, 50* (1–2, Serial No. 209).

Bromet, E. J., & Cornely, P. J. (1984). Correlates of depression in mothers of young children. *Journal of the American Academy of Child Psychiatry, 23,* 335–342.

Bronfenbrenner, U. (1958). Socialization and social class through time and space. In E. E. Maccoby, T. M. Newcomb, & E. L. Hartley (Eds.), *Readings in social psychology.* New York: Henry Holt.

Bronfenbrenner, U. (1977). Toward an experimental ecology of human development. *American Psychologist, 32,* 513–530.

Bronfenbrenner, U., & Crouter, A. C. (1982). Work and family through time and space. In S. B. Kammerman & C. D. Hayes (Eds.), *Families that work: Children in a changing world.* Washington, DC: National Academy Press, 1982.

Brunnquell, D., Crichton, L., & Egeland, B. (1981). Maternal personality and attitude in disturbances of child rearing. *American Journal of Orthopsychiatry, 51,* 680–691.

Burgess, R. L., & Conger, R. D. (1978). Family interaction in abusive, neglectful, and normal families. *Child Development, 49,* 1163–1173.

Burgess, R. L., Anderson, E. S., Schellenbach, C. J., & Conger, R. D. (1981). A social interactional approach to the study of abusive families. In J. P. Vincent (Ed.), *Advances in family intervention, assessment, and theory: An annual compilation of research* (Vol. 2). Greenwich, CT: JAI Press.

Carroll, J. C. (1977). The intergenerational transmission of family violence: The long-term effects of aggressive behavior. In *Aggressive Behavior* (Vol. 3, pp. 289–299). Alan R. Liss, Inc.

Cicchetti, D., & Olsen, K. (1990). The developmental psychopathology of child maltreatment. In M. Lewis & S. Miller (Eds.), *Handbook of developmental psychopathology.* New York: Plenum Press.

Cicchetti, D., & Rizley, R. (1981). Developmental perspectives on the etiology, intergenerational transmission, and sequelae of child maltreatment. In R. Rizley & D. Cicchetti (Eds.), *Developmental perspectives on child maltreatment.* San Francisco: Jossey-Bass.

Cochran, M., & Brassard, J. (1979). Child development and personal social networks. *Child Development, 50,* 601–616.

Colletta, N. D. (1983). At risk for depression: A study of young mothers. *Journal of Genetic Psychology, 142,* 301–310.

Cotterell, J. L. (1986). Work and community influences on the quality of childrearing. *Child Development, 57,* 362–374.

Crittenden, P. M. (1981). Abusing, neglecting, problematic, and adequate dyads: Differentiating by patterns of interaction. *Merrill-Palmer Quarterly, 27,* 201–218.

Crittenden, P. M. (1985). Social networks, quality of childrearing, and child development. *Child Development, 56,* 1299–1313.

Crittenden, P. M., & Ainsworth, M. D. S. (1989). Attachment and child abuse. In D. Cicchetti & V. Carlson (Eds.), *Child maltreatment: Research and theory on the consequences of abuse and neglect* (pp. 432–463). New York: Cambridge University Press.

Crnic, K. A., Greenberg, M. T., Ragozin, A. S., Robinson, N. M., & Basham, R. B. (1983). Effects of stress and social support on mothers and premature and full-term infants. *Child Development, 54,* 209–217.

Crnic, K. A., Greenberg, M. T., Robinson, N. M., & Ragozin, A. S. (1984). Maternal stress and social support: Effects on the mother-infant relationship from birth to eighteen months. *American Journal of Orthopsychiatry, 54,* 224–234.

Crockenberg, S. (1987). Predictors and correlates of anger toward and punitive control of toddlers by adolescent mothers. *Child Development, 58,* 964–975.

Cummings, E. M., Zahn-Waxler, C., & Radke-Yarrow, M. (1981). Young children's responses to expressions of anger and affection by others in the family. *Child Development, 52,* 1274–1282.

Dietrich, K. N., Starr, R. H., & Kaplan, M. G. (1980). Maternal stimulation and care of abused infants. In T. M. Field, S. Goldberg, D. Stern, & A. M. Sostek (Eds.), *High-risk infants and children: Adult and peer interactions.* New York: Academic Press.

DiLalla, D. L., & Crittenden, P. M. (1987). *A factor analytic study of maltreated children's home behavior.* Research presented at the Biennial Meeting of the Society for Research in Child Development, Baltimore, April.

Dubow, E. F., Huesmann, L. R., & Eron, L. D. (1987). Childhood correlates of adult ego development. *Child Development, 58,* 859–869.

Egeland, B., & Brunnquell, D. (1979). An at-risk approach to the study of child abuse: Some preliminary findings. *Journal of the American Academy of Child Psychiatry, 18,* 219–235.

Egeland, B., Breitenbucher, M., & Rosenberg, D. (1980). Prospective study of the significance of life stress in the etiology of child abuse. *Journal of Consulting and Clinical Psychology, 48,* 195–205.

Egeland, B., Sroufe, L. A., & Erickson, M. (1983). The developmental consequence of different patterns of maltreatment. *Child Abuse and Neglect, 7,* 459–469.

Elder, G. H., Jr., Liker, J. K., & Cross, C. E. (1984). Parent-child behavior in hard times and the life course: A multi-generational perspective. In P. Baltes & B. Brim (Eds.), *Lifespan development and behavior* (Vol. 6). New York: Academic Press.

Elder, G. H., Jr., Nguyen, T. V., & Caspi, A. (1985). Linking family hardship to children's lives. *Child Development, 56,* 361–375.

Elder, G. H., Jr., Caspi, A., & Downey, G. (1986). Problem behavior and family relationships: A multigenerational analysis. In A. Sorensen, F. Weinert, & L. Sherrod (Eds.), *Human development and the life course.* Hillsdale, NJ: Lawrence Erlbaum.

Engfer, A., & Gavranidou, M. (1985, January). *Antecedents and consequences of observed maternal sensitivity: A longitudinal study.* Paper presented at the International Symposium on Psychobiology and Early Development, Free University, Berlin, West Germany.

Engfer, A., & Gavranidou, M. (1988, June). *Prospective identification of violent mother-child relationships*. Paper presented at the Third European Conference on Developmental Research, Budapest.

Engfer, A., & Schneewind, K. A. (1982). Causes and consequences of harsh parental punishment. *Child Abuse and Neglect, 6,* 129–139.

Erickson, M. F., Sroufe, L. A., & Egeland, B. (1985). The relationship between quality of attachment and behavior problems in preschool in a high-risk sample. *Monographs of the Society for Research in Child Development, 50* (Serial No. 209).

Estroff, T. W., Herrera, C., Gaines, R., Shaffer, D., Gould, M., & Green, A. H. (1984). Maternal psychopathology and perception of child behavior in psychiatrically referred and child maltreatment families. *Journal of the American Academy of Child Psychiatry, 23,* 649–652.

Field, T. M. (1984). Follow-up developmental status of infants hospitalized for nonorganic failure to thrive. *Journal of Pediatric Psychology, 9,* 241–256.

Fraiberg, S. (1980). *Clinical studies in infant mental health: The first year.* New York: Basic Books.

Fraiberg, S., Adelson, E., & Shapiro, V. (1975). Ghosts in the nursery: A psychoanalytic approach to the problems of impaired infant-mother relationships. *Journal of the American Academy of Child Psychiatry, 14,* 387–421.

Frodi, A. M., & Lamb, M. E. (1980). Child abusers' responses to infant smiles and cries. *Child Development, 51,* 238–241.

Gaensbauer, T. J., & Sands, S. K. (1979). Distorted affective communications in abused/neglected infants and their potential impact on caretakers. *Journal of the American Academy of Child Psychiatry, 18,* 236–250.

Garbarino, J. (1977a). The human ecology of child maltreatment: A conceptual model for research. *Journal of Marriage and the Family, 39,* 721–727.

Garbarino, J. (1977b). The price of privacy in the social dynamics of child abuse. *Child Welfare, 56,* 565–575.

Garbarino, J., & Asp, E. (1981). *Successful schools and competent students.* Lexington, MA: Lexington Books.

Garbarino, J., & Gilliam, G. (1980). *Understanding abusive families.* Lexington, MA: D.C. Heath.

Garbarino, J., & Sherman, D. (1980). High-risk neighborhoods and high-risk families: The human ecology of child maltreatment. *Child Development, 51,* 188–198.

Garbarino, J., Stocking, S. H., & Associates (1980). *Protecting children from abuse and neglect: Developing and maintaining effective support systems for families.* San Francisco, CA: Jossey-Bass.

Garbarino, J., & Vondra, J. (1987). Psychological maltreatment of children and youth. In M. A. Brassard, R. Germain, & S. N. Hart (Eds.), *The psychological maltreatment of children and youth* (pp. 25–44). New York: Pergamon Press.

Gecas, V. (1979). The influence of social class on socialization. In W. R. Burr, R. Hill, F. I. Nye, & I. L. Reiss (Eds.), *Contemporary theories about the family* (Vol. 1). New York: Free Press.

George, C., & Main, M. (1979). Social interactions of young abused children: Approach, avoidance, and aggression. *Child Development, 50,* 306–318.

George, C., & Main, M. (1980). Abused children: Their rejection of peers and caregivers. In T. M. Field (Ed.), *High-risk infants and children: Adult and peer interactions.* New York: Academic Press.

Gil, D. (1970). *Violence against children: Physical child abuse in the United States.* Cambridge, MA: Harvard University Press.

168   JOAN I. VONDRA

Gilbreath, B., & Cicchetti, D. (1990). *Psychopathology in maltreating mothers.* Manuscript submitted for publication.
Goldberg, W. A., & Easterbrooks, M. A. (1984). Role of marital quality in toddler development. *Developmental Psychology, 20,* 504–514.
Gottfried, A. W., & Gottfried, A. E. (1984). Home environment and mental development in young children. In A. W. Gottfried (Ed.), *Home environment and early mental development: Longitudinal research.* New York: Academic Press.
Green, A. (1978). Psychopathology of abused children. *Journal of the American Academy of Child Psychiatry, 17,* 92–103.
Greenspan, S. I., Wieder, S., Nover, R., Lieberman, A., Lourie, R., & Robinson, M. G. (Eds.) (1987). *Infants in multirisk families.* Madison, WI: International Universities Press.
Gwartney-Gibbs, P. A., Stockard, J., & Bohmer, S. (1987). Learning courtship aggression: The influence of parents, peers, and personal experiences. *Family Relations, 36,* 276–282.
Hart, S. N., & Brassard, M. R. (1987). A major threat to children's mental health: Psychological maltreatment. *American Psychologist, 42,* 160–165.
Hazan, C., & Shaver, P. (1987). Romantic love conceptualized as an attachment process. *Journal of Personality and Social Psychology, 52,* 511–524.
Hoffman-Plotkin, D., & Twentyman, C. T. (1984). A multimodal assessment of behavioral and cognitive deficits in abused and neglected preschoolers. *Child Development, 55,* 794–802.
Hops, H., Sherman, L., & Biglan, A. (1990). Maternal depression, marital discord, and children's behavior: A developmental perspective. In G. R. Patterson (Ed.), *Depression and aggression: Two facets of family interactions.* Hillsdale, NJ: Lawrence Erlbaum.
Howes, C., & Espinosa, M. P. (1985). The consequences of child abuse for the formation of relationships with peers. *Child Abuse and Neglect, 9,* 397–404.
Kalmuss, D. (1984). The intergenerational transmission of marital aggression. *Journal of Marriage and the Family, 46,* 11–19.
Kaplan, S. J., Pelcovitz, D., Salzinger, S., & Ganeles, D. (1983). Psychopathology of parents of abused and neglected children and adolescents. *Journal of the American Academy of Child Psychiatry, 22,* 238–244.
Kaufman, J., & Cicchetti, D. (1989). The effects of maltreatment on school-aged children's socioemotional development: Assessments in a day camp setting. *Developmental Psychology, 25,* 516–524.
Kaufman, J., & Zigler, E. (1990). The intergenerational transmission of child abuse and the prospect of predicting future abusers. In D. Cicchetti & V. Carlson (Eds.), *Child maltreatment: Research and theory on the consequences of child abuse and neglect* (pp. 129–150). Cambridge, MA: Harvard University Press.
Kobak, R. R., & Sceery, A. (1988). Attachment in late adolescence: Working models, affect regulation, and representations of self and others. *Child Development, 59,* 135–146.
Kohn, M. L. (1975). Social class and parent-child relationships: An interpretation. In U. Bronfenbrenner & M. Mahoney (Eds.), *Influences on human development.* Hinsdale, IL: Dryden Press.
Kohn, M. L. (1977). *Class and conformity: A study in values.* Chicago, IL: University of Chicago Press.
Kotelchuck, M. (1982). Child abuse and neglect: Prediction and misclassification. In R. H. Starr, Jr. (Ed.), *Child abuse prediction.* Cambridge, MA: Ballinger.
Levitt, M. J., Weber, R. A., & Clark, M. C. (1986). Social network relationships as sources of maternal support and well-being. *Developmental Psychology, 22,* 310–316.

Lewis, M., Feiring, C., McGuffog, C., & Jaskir, J. (1984). Predicting psychopathology in six-year-olds from early social relations. *Child Development, 55*, 123–136.

Lyons-Ruth, KI., Connell, D. B., Zoll, D., & Stahl, J. (1987). Infants at social risk: Relations among infant maltreatment, maternal behavior, and infant attachment behavior. *Developmental Psychology, 23*, 223–232.

Main, M., & Goldwyn, R. (1984). Predicting rejection of her infant from mother's representation of her own experience: Implications for the abused-abusing intergenerational cycle. *Child Abuse and Neglect, 8*, 203–217.

Main, M., & Goldwyn, R. (1985). *Adult attachment classification system*. Unpublished manuscript, University of California, Berkeley.

Mash, E. J., Johnston, C., & Kovitz, K. (1983). A comparison of the mother-child interactions of physically abused and non-abused children during play and task situations. *Journal of Clinical Child Psychology, 12*, 337–346.

Melnick, B., & Hurley, J. (1969). Distinctive personality attributes of child-abusing mothers. *Journal of Consulting and Clinical Psychology, 33*, 746–749.

Moen, P., Kain, E. L., & Elder, G. H., Jr. (1981). *Economic conditions and family life: Contemporary and historical perspectives*. Paper presented for the National Academy of Sciences Assembly of Behavioral and Social Sciences, Committee on Child Development Research and Public Policy, December.

Mortimer, J. T. (1974). Patterns of intergenerational occupational movements: A smallest space analysis. *American Journal of Sociology, 79*, 1278–1299.

Mortimer, J. T. (1976). Social class, work, and the family: Some implications of the father's career for familial relationships and sons' career decisions. *Journal of Marriage and the Family, 38*, 241–256.

Mortimer, J. T., & Kumka, D. (1982). A further examination of the "occupational linkage hypothesis." *The Sociological Quarterly, 23*, 3–16.

Newberger, E. H., Reed, R. B., Daniels, J. H., Hyde, J. N., & Kotelchuck, M. (1977). Pediatric social illness: Toward an etiological classification. *Pediatrics, 60*, 175–185.

Pianta, R. C., Egeland, B., & Hyatt, A. (1986). Maternal relationship history as an indicator of developmental risk. *American Journal of Orthopsychiatry, 56*, 385–398.

Piotrkowski, C. S., & Katz, M. H. (1982). Indirect socialization of children: The effects of mothers' jobs on academic behaviors. *Child Development, 53*, 1520–1529.

Provence, S., & Lipton, R. (1962). *Infants in institutions*. New York: International Universities Press.

Ricks, M. H. (1985). The social transmission of parental behavior: Attachment across generations. *Monographs of the Society for Research in Child Development, 50* (1–2, Serial No. 209).

Rohner, R. P., & Rohner, E. C. (1980). Antecedents and consequences of parental rejection: A theory of emotional abuse. *Child Abuse and Neglect, 4*, 189–198.

Rosario, M., Salzinger, S., Feldman, R., & Hammer, M. (1987, April). *Home environments of physically abused and control school-age children*. Research presented at the Biennial Meeting of the Society for Research in Child Development, Baltimore.

Rosenbaum, A., & O'Leary, D. (1981). Marital violence: Characteristics of abusive couples. *Journal of Consulting and Clinical Psychology, 49*, 63–71.

Rutter, M., Quinton, D., & Liddle, C. (1983). Parenting in two generations: Looking backwards and looking forwards. In N. Madge (Ed.), *Families at risk* (pp. 60–98). London: Heinemann.

Sameroff, A. J. (1975). Early influences on development: Fact or fancy? *Merrill-Palmer Quarterly, 21*, 267–294.

Sameroff, A. J. & Chandler, M. (1975). Reproductive risk and the continuum of caretaking casualty. In F. Horowitz, E. Hetherington, & G. Siegel (Eds.), *Review of child develop-ment research* (Vol. 4). Chicago, IL: University of Chicago Press.

Sandgrund, A., Gaines, R. W., & Green, A. H. (1974). Child abuse and mental retardation: A problem of cause and effect. *American Journal of Mental Deficiency, 79,* 327–330.

Sherrod, K. B., O'Connor, S., Vietze, P. M., & Altemeier, W. A. (1984). Child health and maltreatment. *Child Development, 55,* 1174–1183.

Siegal, M. (1982). Economic deprivation and the quality of parent-child relations. In *Fairness in children.* New York: Academic Press.

Spinetta, J. J. (1978). Parental personality factors in child abuse. *Journal of Consulting and Clinical Psychology, 46,* 1409–1414.

Sroufe, L. A. (1983). Infant-caregiver attachment and patterns of adaptation in preschool: The roots of maladaptation and competence. In M. Perlmutter (Ed.), *Minnesota Symposia in Child Psychology* (Vol. 16). Hillsdale, NJ: Lawrence Erlbaum.

Sroufe, L. A., & Fleeson, J. (in press). Attachment and the construction of relationships. In W. Hartup & K. Rubin (Eds.), *The nature and development of relationships.* Hillsdale, NJ: Lawrence Erlbaum.

Starr, R. H., Jr. (1982). A research-based approach to the prediction of child abuse. In R. H. Starr, Jr. (Ed.), *Child abuse prediction.* Cambridge, MA: Ballinger.

Starr, R. H., Jr., Dietrich, K. N., Fischhoff, J., Ceresnie, S., & Zweier, D. (1984). The contribution of handicapping conditions to child abuse. *Topics in Early Childhood Special Education, 4,* 55–69.

Steinberg, L., Catalano, R., & Dooley, D. (1981). Economic antecedents of child abuse and neglect. *Child Development, 52,* 975–985.

Stevens, J. H. (1988). Social support, locus of control, and parenting in three low-income groups of mothers: Black teenagers, black adults, and white adults. *Child Development, 59,* 635–642.

Straus, M. A., Gelles, R. J., & Steinmetz, S. K. (1980). *Behind closed doors: Violence in the American family.* New York: Anchor Press.

Talbot, N. E. (Ed.). (1976). *Raising children in modern America: What parents and society should be doing for their children.* Boston: Little, Brown.

Trickett, P. K., & Kuczynski, L. (1986). Children's misbehaviors and parental discipline strategies in abusive and nonabusive families. *Developmental Psychology, 22,* 115–123.

Trickett, P. K., & Susman, E. J. (1988). Parental perceptions of childrearing practices in physically abusive and nonabusive families. *Developmental Psychology, 24,* 270–276.

Tronick, E. Z., & Field, T. M. (Eds.) (1986). *Maternal depression and infant disturbance.* San Francisco: Jossey-Bass.

Vondra, J. I. (1986). Socioeconomic considerations: The family economy. In J. Garbarino & Associates, *Troubled youth, troubled families.* New York: Aldine.

Watson, D., & Clark, L. A. (1984). Negative affectivity: The disposition to experience aversive emotional states. *Psychological Bulletin, 96,* 465–490.

Weinraub, M., & Wolf, B. M. (1983). Effects of stress and social supports on mother-child interaction in single- and two-parent families. *Child Development, 54,* 1297–1311.

Whittaker, J. K. & Garbarino, J. (1983). *Social support networks: Informal helping in the human services.* New York: Aldine.

Zigler, E. (1981). Controlling child abuse: Do we have the knowledge or the will? In G. Gerbner, K. Ross, & E. Zigler (Eds.), *Child abuse: An agenda for action.* New York: Oxford University Press.

CHAPTER 7

PARENTAL PSYCHOPATHOLOGY AND HIGH-RISK CHILDREN

DAVID C. FACTOR AND DAVID A. WOLFE

INTRODUCTION

Interest in the relationship between parental behavior and children's developmental outcome has long been a fundamental concern of social scientists. This is a fact regardless of the direction of a person's basic developmental orientation—genetic or environmental—because the two orientations place significant weight on parental characteristics and influence. Furthermore, it is now widely recognized that parents and children influence each other in a reciprocal fashion (e.g., Bell & Harper, 1977), rather than in a unidirectional, parent-to-child fashion as was originally assumed by many investigators. Understanding of the manner in which parental psychological characteristics can affect the developing child's emotional and behavioral adjustment has grown immensely over the past decade, and these recent findings form the foundation for the discussion in this chapter.

Numerous explanations have been given as to why children of psychologically disturbed parents may be affected by their parents' psychopathology. These arguments range from the heritability of specific disor-

DAVID C. FACTOR • TRE-ADD Program, Thistledown Regional Center for Children and Adolescents, Rexdale, Ontario, Canada M9V 4L8.   DAVID A. WOLFE • Department of Psychology, University of Western Ontario, London, Ontario, Canada N6A 5B8.

ders and genetic predispositions to the environmental contingencies and learning opportunities made available throughout the child's development. Because of the significance to children's mental and early intervention programming, our attention is primarily on the recent findings from the study of subsamples of parents who have been diagnosed with a specific psychiatric disturbance (e.g., affective disorder) or an identifiable adjustment problem (e.g., child abuse). We assume that children may be affected by their parent's psychopathology on the basis of factors that may directly and indirectly impair or limit the course of a child's normal development. These factors include, for example, the well-documented effects of parental modeling of inappropriate behavior, the effects of the individual's pathology on the marital relationship and family functioning, and the direct and indirect effects resulting from inconsistent or inappropriate child-rearing methods and unpredictability in mood or behavior.

Our assumption is that children of parents who are suffering from psychological disturbances or who exhibit extreme behavior in the presence of the child are vulnerable and at-risk of developing mental health problems. Such problems are caused, at least in part, to the important influences of modeling, marital conflict, family dysfunction, and inappropriate child-rearing methods. Accordingly, various forms of parental pathology can be viewed as significant "risk factors" that contribute to a higher probability for the development of a disorder (Masten & Garmezy, 1985). In fact, longitudinal research has shown that mental illness and substance abuse in parents increase the risk of impairment in their offspring, and children who accumulate four or more risk factors frequently exhibit learning and behavioral problems, delinquency, and/or psychiatric disturbance (Rutter, 1979; Werner, 1989).

CHILD-REARING PATTERNS AND THEIR SUSPECTED INFLUENCE ON CHILD DEVELOPMENT

Social learning theory provides a sound and widely supported theoretical basis for explaining the preponderance of correlational data linking disorders in parents to increased developmental risk in their offspring. This theory, which accomodates behavioral, emotional, cognitive, and physiological mechanisms of behavior acquisition and maintenance, places a heavy emphasis on children's abilities to learn a contingency, or relationship, between their actions and consequences. Once children learn the association between their behavior and the consequences for that behavior, they form a cognitive understanding of the probability, or expectation, of such consequences in choosing to engage in the behavior in the future.

Therefore, according to social learning theory, children of disturbed parents may be at-risk of developmental deviation or delay, at least in part, because of their exposure to inappropriate learning opportunities (e.g., witnessing seemingly positive consequences for parental violence or criminal behavior), the lack of consistent, appropriate consequences for normal variations in child behavior (e.g., harsh parental punishment for minor transgressions, curiosity, and distorted expectations of themselves and others. Because a parent or caregiver exerts the major influence on the developing child's sense of self and of others, awareness of moral values, and the learning of basic social and self-control skills (to name but a few), deviant socialization practices can find a number of possible routes by which to disrupt the child's ongoing development.

One of the more prominent routes or mechanisms by which parental behavior is believed to influence child development directly is through variations in family socialization practices, or "parenting styles." Variations in socialization practices occur normally in relation to child, family, and situational events. Yet, the erroneous assumption is often made that there are two "types" of parents: those who naturally possess the motivation to raise their children in a positive, supportive fashion, and those who presumably do not possess this desire or ability (a conclusion often based on a small, but significant, aspect of their child-rearing, such as abuse, neglect, or rejection). Parents who fall into this latter group are labeled "abnormal" or "disturbed," and a false dichotomy is easily formed between "good" and "bad" parenting. Alternatively, parenting practices can be viewed along a continuum, whereby one extreme represents practices that are severe and potentially harmful to the child, and at the other extreme are methods that promote many aspects of the child's development. Viewing parental behavior toward the child along a continuum, rather than a dichotomy, helps to draw attention to the fact that even "disturbed" or "abusive" parents may highly resemble "typical" child-rearing practices except in terms of their degree or frequency of engaging in some of the more extreme methods (Wolfe, 1987).

The mechanisms by which parenting style may influence child development are represented by the intersection of two fundamental dimensions of parenting: *demandingness* and *responsiveness.* Demandingness is described as the amount or degree of control the parent attempts to exert over the child, whereas responsiveness is defined as the frequency of interactions with the child (both positive and negative) that are child-centered versus parent-centered (Maccoby & Martin,

1983). Throughout the discussion of parental disorders that follows, regardless of the specific topology of the disorder (i.e., depression, criminal behavior, immaturity), a common element that emerges is the extent to which each disorder is associated with an impairment of the parent's age-appropriate demands on the child (i.e., demands for mature behavior, independence, and clear communication) and the parent's sensitivity or responsiveness to the child's capabilities.

As a point of reference, the most healthy, appropriate parenting style is one in which parents are both demanding and child-centered in their responsiveness, a style that is referred to as *authoritative*. This style is considered to be most effective in terms of desirable developmental outcome and in reducing parent–child conflict, because authoritative parents place age-appropriate demands on their children, are more consistent in their discipline, and rely on a wide choice of techniques to teach their children (Baumrind, 1971). In contrast to this healthy parenting style, three other styles can be identified on the basis of the degree of demandingness versus responsiveness that the parent displays toward the child, each of which has been associated with less desirable developmental outcomes for the child (Maccoby & Martin, 1983). For example, parents who are demanding of their child but who are rejecting or unresponsive to their child's needs have been labeled "authoritarian"; those who demand little of their children yet are extremely child-centered are referred to as "indulgent"; and those who are both undemanding as well as unresponsive to their children are described as "neglecting." Thus, the mechanisms whereby parental disorders influence child development can be understood in terms of the extent to which a given disorder affects parents' *demandingness* and *responsiveness* towards their child. The resultant disruption in the balance of these two important dimensions is subsequently reflected in parents' socialization practices, often with negative consequences to their child's development. In the following discussion of parental disorders and their relationship to negative developmental changes, we highlight the advances that have been made in recent years in our understanding of these processes.

PARENTAL DISORDERS AND CHILD ADJUSTMENT: AN OVERVIEW OF THE LITERATURE

Based on the above argument linking children's developmental risk status to parental and family functioning, some discussion is warranted of several of the more well-known situational conditions that have been associated with children's adjustment. In reviewing these relationships, it should be kept in mind that none of these identified conditions or situations has been found to be fully or even largely responsible for a given child's developmental outcome; rather each serves as a "marker" variable that may indicate a significant factor that has been shown to influence the course of development. Because of the immense literature in this area, only psychological phenomena affecting developmental progress will be treated (interested readers may wish to pursue other studies dealing with biological, genetic, and sociological factors related to parental adjustment and child development). Accordingly, after an overview of the more significant psychological factors, a more in-depth look at children of depressed parents will illustrate the major implications that are currently emerging from this field.

PARENTAL IMMATURITY

Although not a specific psychiatric disorder *per se*, parental immaturity (i.e., a young adult's development of independent living skills, cognitive problem-solving, or emotional development) has long been suspected to play a role in the developmental status of the offspring. Specifically, children of adolescent parents have been described as being more at-risk for developmental and behavioral disorders than children of adult parents, because of the inability of the adolescent parent to meet the demanding needs, consistently or effectively, of a young infant or a child. Investigations of this relationship between adolescent parents and developmental risk status in their offspring have confirmed that these children display more cognitive, emotional, and physical problems than do children of more mature parents (Phipps-Yonas, 1980). In particular, infants of adolescent parents have more physical health problems and higher mortality rates when mothers were younger than 15 years of age. Moreover, there is a high (negative) correlation between the rate of child abuse and the age of the mother when she gave birth to her first child (Wolfe, 1987). Important situational factors, such as income and housing stability, education, social and economic resources, conjugal violence, and many others, play a role in impairing the child-rearing effectiveness of the adolescent parent, which together lead to a significant increase in the developmental risk to the infant (Schwartz, 1979).

Although maturity of the adolescent *mother* has been the primary focus of attention to date, more effort must be directed as well toward an improved understanding of the role of the father/partner in contributing to developmental risk. Male immaturity in relation to child-rearing responsibility is commonly expressed as a pattern of poor job history, violence (toward partner as well as in the community), substance abuse, financial irresponsibility, and minimal contact or involvement with the infant or toddler (Scott, Field, & Robertson, 1981). Although it is difficult to establish an underlying causal mechanism for such patterns among very young male and female parents, the notion of developmental immaturity (perhaps associated with previous lack of proper childcare and family life in their own families of origin) seems to describe adequately the existing relationship between adolescent parents and developmental risk.

PARENTAL CRIMINALITY

Criminal involvement on the part of one or both parents has also been identified as a significant developmental risk factor, although the mechanisms by which such patterns are transmitted are poorly understood. A recent study provides a clear example of data that support this relationship between increased risk of antisocial acts in children and the criminal history of the father, in particular. Kandel *et al.* (1988) examined the sons of fathers who had engaged in criminal behavior that was deemed to be "severely sanctioned" or the sons who were free from any "registration from criminal behavior." These authors developed four groups of offspring based on their classification of the fathers: (1) high-risk, severely sanctioned; (2) high-risk, no registration; (3) low-risk, severely sanctioned; and (4) low-risk, no registration. By matching these samples on socioeconomic status, several hypotheses were confirmed. Most significantly, sons with severely sanctioned fathers had an elevated risk of criminal involvement that was 5.6 times greater than it was for the low-risk sons. Interestingly, serious criminal offenders in the youth sample evidenced lower IQ scores than did subjects who did not engage in criminal behavior, although this finding was true only for high-risk subjects. In fact, boys in the high-risk group who did not engage in any criminal activity had relatively higher intelligence test scores.

CHRONIC PARENTAL ILLNESS AND FAMILY FUNCTIONING

Chronic illness on the part of one or both parents has also been associated with greater risk of developmental impairment. Blackford (1988) argued that such children have a greater incidence of depression and psychosomatic disorders, and that antisocial behavior and poor school performance are common associated features. Interestingly, females of chronically ill parents appear to be less noticeably affected by this situation than are males, a finding that Blackford (1988) and Rutter (1971) explained in terms of the development of increased sensitivity to others and the greater resistance to stress among girls than among boys. Although it is accepted that chronic parental illness is linked with undesirable developmental outcomes in the children, several authors do differentiate between loss of a parent through natural events (i.e., death, divorce) and the diminution of child-rearing responsibilities, as evidenced by chronic illness and other impairments affecting family functioning; that is, a loss of the parent does not necessarily lead to impairments in the child's development, but that developmental outcome can be predicted more or less on the basis of the presence of other compensatory factors in the child's family, such as the support of family members, availability of the other parent, and the absence of conflict and discord in the child's presence (Emery, 1982; Hetherington & Martin, 1986).

Along these same lines, several researchers have looked more generally at family functioning and its relationship to children's development. Drawing from Olson, Sprenkle, and Russell's (1979) work with family cohesion and adaptability, Smets and Hartup (1988) explored the family systems in which child behavior problems seem to emerge. "Cohesion" is defined as the "connectedness of relationships within the family or the extent to which family members are 'bonded' to one another," whereas adaptability refers to "the capacity of the family system to change its power structure, role relations, and rules in response to situational and developmental stress" (p. 239). According to family systems theory, a "balanced" family system is described as one in which members are both moderately cohesive and adaptable, rather than falling at an extreme of one or both dimensions. In their review of previous studies, Smets and Hartup (1988) highlighted the finding that families of juvenile offenders often score more frequently in the extreme regions of family functioning (i.e., showing either too high or too low cohesion and/or adaptability). Similar results are found among families who have referred their children to clinics because of problematic child behavior. These researchers concluded, on the basis of previous work as well as on the basis of their own study involving 120 clinic families, that extreme forms of family functioning tend to be associated with abnormal child behavior. These findings concur, as well, with the studies by Minuchin (1974; Minuchin, Rossman, & Baker, 1978) involving psychosomatic families.

CHILDREN OF PARENTS WITH PSYCHIATRIC ILLNESSES

In further exploring the relationships between parental disorders and developmental deviations among their offspring, there is a vast literature that focuses on specific psychiatric diagnoses. Although admittedly incomplete, Goldstein (1988) summarized the views of much of the field when he stated that "the best risk marker for most mental disorders is still the rather crude index of being an offspring of a parent with that disorder" (p. 285). This familial link was explored in one of the earliest studies conducted by Rutter (1966). Following the rationale that children are affected by their parents' psychopathology on the basis of the disturbance such disorders may create in family functioning as well as in child behavior, Rutter's study demonstrated that children with psychiatrically disturbed parents were more likely (than control children) to suffer from a diagnosable disorder. Similar findings were reported by Cooper, Leach, Storer, and Tonge (1977), in which the rate of psychiatric disorders among children of adult patients was 45%, compared to 26% in the control group of children from organically ill parents.

Additional support for the additive influence of generic parental psychopathology follows from a study by Cantwell and Baker (1984), in which they compared subsamples of children with two healthy parents, one psychiatrically ill parent, and two parents with psychiatric illness. Their results indicated that when children had two disturbed parents, there was a significantly greater probability that they would suffer developmental problems, in comparison to both of the other groups. Interestingly, no significant differences emerged between the two subsamples in which one or both parents were healthy; however, children with one or two ill parents experienced more psychosocial stress (e.g., changes in schools, residence, income) than did the children of healthy parents, which may partially account for the mechanisms whereby parental behavior disrupts child development. Furthermore, more behavior problems were found among those children having two psychiatrically disturbed parents if one of the parents was diagnosed as having an antisocial disorder (compared to any other diagnosis). Similar to the findings presented above on children of criminal parents, Cantwell and Baker (1984) stressed the significance of the relationship between developmental deviation and the presence of antisocial behavior in one or both parents.

The sex of the parent may also play a role in the expression of developmental problems in the offspring. Schore (1988) reported that in families in which only one parent was psychiatrically disturbed, 47% of the children had received psychiatric diagnoses when that parent was the father, compared to 66% when the diagnosed parent was the mother. Thus, with the exception of the diagnosis of antisocial behavior, the mother's psychopathology was suspected to be even more influential than that of the father.

Although few studies have been conducted to date, the emerging literature on children of anxiety-disordered parents merits some discussion. Generally, these studies have focused on parents who exhibited signs of panic disorder, generalized anxiety disorder, obsessive-compulsive disorder, agoraphobia, or some specific phobic pattern. In an exemplary study of this issue, Turner, Beidel, and Costello (1987) investigated 59 children between the ages of 7 and 12 years. Sixteen of these children had a parent with a known anxiety disorder (agoraphobic or obsessive-compulsive), 14 had a parent with a dysthymic or depressive disorder, and 13 came from families with nonpsychiatrically ill parents. The remaining 16 children were from families with no known psychiatric illness. Based on the Child Assessment Schedule, children who had parents with anxiety disorders were significantly different from the normal control group on 9 of the 12 comparison areas: they had more difficulties at school and in making friends, more specific fears and worries, and experienced more symptoms of depression, anxiety, and somatic complaints. However, only two differences emerged between the children of anxiety-disordered parents and children of depressed parents, with the former stating more problems at school and spending more time in solitary activities than the children of depressed parents.

In addition, the above-named study found that 44% (7 out of 16) of the children of anxiety-disordered parents met the criteria for a psychiatric diagnosis on the basis of test results, compared to 22% of the children of depressed parents, 8% of the first control group, and none of the normal control group. Hence, children of anxiety-disordered parents were found to be more than two times as likely to have a DSM-III disorder as the children of dysthymic parents, and were twice as likely to show signs of an anxiety disorder. Similar findings, using other measures and samples, have confirmed a link between the presence of anxiety disorders in the parents and psychiatric disturbance (and symptoms of anxiety) in the offspring (Silverman, Cerny, Nelles, & Burke, 1988; Sylvester, Hyde, & Reichler, 1987).

In commenting on these findings relating various psychiatric problems in the parents to developmental abnormalities in the offspring, we should note that the data are not conclusive or explanatory. More particularly, the data do not support the notion of specific, diagnostically relevant problems being replicated in the offspring. The findings certainly support the belief that having two psychiatrically ill parents means a greater likelihood that the child will receive a psychiatric diagnosis, and a somewhat diminished (but still clinically significant) likelihood of receiving a diagnosis if only one parent suffers from a disturbance. Yet, there is little evidence to demonstrate that having a parent with a particular diagnosis implies that the child will have a similar or predictable diagnostic pattern. Most of the literature to date exploring specific psychiatric diagnostic categories has focused on children of either thought-disordered parents (i.e., schizophrenic adults) or children of parents with major affective disorders (i.e., uni- or bipolar depression). To illustrate the psychological processes involved, as well as the developmental implications for the child, we now turn to the expansive literature on children of depressed parents.

PARENTAL DEPRESSION AND ITS INFLUENCE ON CHILD DEVELOPMENT

Adult depression is the most common psychiatric disorder, affecting approximately 10% of the population. According to Anderson (1987), 20% of women and 11% of men will experience a serious depressive episode at some time in their lives. Because a depressive disorder usually affects self-esteem and behavior as well as mood, its impact on family functioning in general, and childrearing in particular, has long been suspected to be pervasive and severe (see Barnett & Gotlib, 1988, for further discussion of adult depression).

Reviews of the literature examining the suspected link between adult depression and childhood disorders began to emerge in the 1970s, and have generally confirmed the existence of a correlational relationship. However, several additional findings have simultaneously emerged from these studies, which have helped to clarify the nature and extent of this relationship.

One of the first reviews of this literature was reported by Orvaschel, Weissman, and Kidd (1980). Reviewing the major studies conducted at the time, these investigators noted that the majority of children of depressed parents evinced developmental abnormalities, such as depression, interpersonal problems, acting out behavior, and school and attentional difficulties. Although the authors felt assured that having a depressed parent led to greater risk of developmental deviation, they also recognized that adequate control groups had rarely been used in these early studies and that methods of assessment were quite varied and inexact.

Shortly after this review was published, Sameroff, Seifer, and Zax (1982) reported several significant findings from their longitudinal work with children at-risk for schizophrenia and major psychiatric disorders. Comparing infants and toddlers of a "neurotic depression" group with normal controls, these researchers noted that at all ages studied (pre-

natal through 30 months) the depressed mothers appeared more anxious and lower in social competence, and their newborns had the lowest
obstetric status. At 4 months of age, depressed mothers were showing
less involvement with their newborns, although these differences were
less pronounced by 1 year. By the time the children were 30 months old,
they were found to have acquired fewer adaptive behaviors in the home,
and their mothers reported them to be "less cooperative with family
members, less cooperative with others, more bizarre, more depressed,
and more often engaged in imaginary play" (p. 43).

Orvaschel (1983) concluded that, in the aggregate, these early studies strongly suggest a causal relationship between parents with depression and problems exhibited by their children, citing problematic communication, less affection, and maladaptive coping techniques learned
from their parents. Another review to emerge at the same time examined 24 studies of children who were considered to be at-risk because of
the presence of an affective disorder in one or both parents (Beardslee,
Bemporad, Keller, & Klerman, 1983). Similar to the findings of Orvaschel (1983), these researchers pointed out that children with depressed parents did not necessarily exhibit symptoms of childhood depression, but rather showed a wide array of difficulties, such as neurotic
or behavioral disturbances, attentional problems, drug abuse, and conflict with the law.

Thus, researchers in this area noted early on that depression in the
offspring of depressed parents is not necessarily a common or even
probable observed diagnosis, but that such children appear to display a
variety of symptoms indicative of developmental deviation or delay.
Unfortunately, the prognosis of such impairments is not known, because this area is too new to have produced information on long-term
effects among targeted samples.

Commenting on these preliminary conclusions, Coyne, Kahn, and
Gotlib (1987) suggested that the expression of developmental deviation
in the offspring may be accounted for to a large extent on the basis of
disturbance in childrearing methods associated with depression. Rather
than a unilateral, causal relationship between parental depression and
childhood disturbance, however, these researchers pointed to the major
role depression plays in the marital relationship and in similar aspects of
family functioning. Furthermore, they noted that most of the data to
emerge from studies in this area are generalizable to mothers only, since
the influence of depressed males in the family has not been as thor-
oughly investigated. Finally, Coyne et al. (1987) pointed out that few
observations of the daily interactions between depressed parents and
their children have been conducted, which might help to explain the

mechanisms whereby parental depression and its associated behavioral manifestation may influence ongoing child development.

In the review of recent studies in this area that follows, the literature is divided into three subsections reflecting the major directions taken in the field to understand the relationship between parental depression and development. The first subsection explores in greater detail the behavioral problems reported among this child population. These studies are followed by a close look at the cognitive and affective disturbances exhibited among children of depressed parents. The final subsection presents findings regarding the observed parent–child interactions in such families, in an attempt to outline the major processes that may explain the negative developmental sequelae that have been observed to date.

Behavioral Problems among Children of Depressed Parents

To aid in clarification and specificity, two distinctions are typically made in the literature on adult depression: (1) the presence of a unipolar versus bipolar (i.e., manic/depressive episodes) form of mood disorder, and (2) whether or not the adult is receiving inpatient versus outpatient treatment for the disorder, because the presence of one or the other form or severity of depressive symptomatology is predictive of the course and prognosis of the disorder. Accordingly, Kashani, Burk, Horowitz, and Reid (1985) were interested in comparing 41 children (from 19 different families) who had parents with unipolar disorder with 9 children (from 5 families), whose parents suffered from bipolar depression. All parents were inpatients at the time the study was conducted, with a ratio of 3 mothers to every one father in the study. Among these two small samples of children (who ranged in age from 7 to 17 years, with a mean age of 12.4), the researchers found that children in the unipolar sample reported significantly more symptoms of somatization and separation anxiety than did children in the bipolar group. In contrast, children in the bipolar sample reported significantly more symptoms of alcohol use/abuse than the comparison sample. Despite these important differences, however, it should be noted that the researchers failed to find very many significant differences between the two at-risk groups overall on formal measures of child adjustment (e.g., diagnostic interviews and parent-report questionnaires), a finding that was repeated in a similar study reported by Hammen, Adrian, Gordon, Burge, Jaenicke, and Hiroto (1987).

Zahn-Waxler *et al.* (1988) reported on a unique investigation in which they were able to follow the development of seven 5- and 6-year-old male children who each had a depressed parent (4 mothers and 3 fathers suffered from bipolar depression, and 5 of their spouses were diagnosed as having a unipolar depression disorder). The researchers noted that from a very early age, these children were likely to display insecure attachment with their caregivers and to have problems in regulation of affect. In addition, as infants and small children, these subjects had difficulties in the appropriate expression of prosocial behavior and the control of aggression. When compared to 12 male controls of the same age, the children of depressed parents displayed a higher frequency and severity of problematic behaviors, a finding that was sustained at least over the preschool period in which these children were followed.

Using an older sample, Lee and Gotlib (1989) compared 7- to 13-year-old children of unipolar depressed mothers ($N = 20$), children of nondepressed, psychiatric patients ($N = 13$), children of nondepressed medical patients ($N = 8$), and children of nondepressed, nonpatient mothers in the community ($N = 30$). Based on the Child Behavior Checklist, the researchers reported that the highest proportion of scores in the clinically disturbed range (both internalizing and externalizing problems) were found among children of depressed mothers (i.e., two-thirds of these children had elevated scores falling in the clinical range on this instrument). Based on clinician ratings, children of both psychiatric patient subgroups exhibited more symptomatology and poorer adjustment overall when compared to the other two groups of children. Interestingly, the authors noted that both groups of children of psychiatric patients were behaving at a level comparable to children who have been referred to outpatient clinics for behavior problems.

These recent findings on the adjustment problems among children of depressed parents illustrate some of the general disturbances in behavior that have been observed, and generally support the view that parental depression is associated with greater adjustment problems among their offspring. However, mention should be made that a particular pattern or diagnostic cluster of symptoms has not been identified which corresponds wholly or in major part to the parental diagnosis of depression. Similar to other situational and familial factors (such as child maltreatment) associated with developmental risk (e.g., Wolfe, 1987), the presence of parental depression appears to disrupt the child's normal, ongoing development in a pervasive manner that cannot be predicted or described in a unidimensional fashion. Rather, parental depression, and perhaps other forms of psychiatric disturbance as well, interferes with the child's normal development of behavioral, cognitive, and affective abilities, and such interference carries with it an unpredict-able developmental course. Further support for such interference and negative influence is found in the following studies on children's cog-nitive delays or impairments associated with major depression in the caregiver.

COGNITIVE AND AFFECTIVE DISTURBANCES AMONG CHILDREN OF DEPRESSED PARENTS

In addition to the increased risk of behavior problems, investigators have been concerned with other developmental impairments that might result from parental psychopathology, but that might be less detectable or disruptive to the untrained observer. Worland, Weeks, Janes, and Strock (1984) were among the first to note the preponderance of cog-nitive and affective symptomatology among children of disturbed par-ents. These researchers studied 158 6- to 12-year-old children who had parents who were diagnosed as either schizophrenic, manic-depressive, or suffering from chronic physical illness, along with a nondiagnosed control group. Using path analysis to determine the best fit to their data, they looked at such variables as children's intelligence, classroom behav-ior, achievement in school, and emotional functioning. The effect of parental depression seemed to be most pronounced in terms of its influ-ence on cognitive development, followed by impairments in emotional-behavioral adjustment; that is, children's classroom behavior was medi-ated by intelligence and by academic achievement—cognitive variables that are believed to be most vulnerable among children of depressed parents.

The greater preponderance of developmental psychopathology among children of depressed parents is further confirmed in studies looking at the frequency of various psychiatric diagnoses among this population. Weissman et al. (1984), in an investigation of school-aged children (ages 6–18), found that the rate of psychiatric diagnosis among the children of depressed parents was three times greater than that of the normal sample. Major depression accounted for approximately 13% of the diagnoses, and was the most frequently occurring single diag-nosis among the sample of 44 children of parents with major depression and 89 children of parents with mild depression. Attention deficit disor-der and separation anxiety each accounted for 10% of the diagnoses, and multiple diagnoses in these children often appeared. Orvaschel, Walsh-Allis, and Ye (1988) found further support for the relationship between parental depression and cognitive/affective disturbance among a sample of 61 children of depressed parents and 40 children of nondepressed parents. Their data revealed that 41% of the children of depressed parents met the criteria for at least one psychiatric disorder during the course of their childhood, in comparison to 15% of the normative sample. In addition, the high-risk target group received more outpatient treatment services, and were described as receiving significantly more diagnoses for affective disorders and attention deficit disorder than the comparison group. Not only did they find higher rates of these disorders among the proband's children, the results indicated that these problems were more severe and long-term.

A growing consensus among researchers does support a small but significant continuity between parents and their children in terms of symptoms of affective disturbance. As noted previously, research has not supported the simple notion that children of depressed parents become depressed themselves, yet this is one of the more prominent developmental outcomes that is gaining recognition in recent studies. For example, Hammen et al. (1987a) and Hammen, Gordon, Burge, Adrian, Jaenicke, & Hiroto (1987b) looked at frequency of diagnoses among school-aged children of depressed mothers (including both unipolar and bipolar subsamples) in addition to medical and normal comparison groups. They discovered that rates of affective disturbances among the children of depressed parents differed only from the normal, and not the medical, controls. However, it is revealing to note that slightly less than one half of the children in the unipolar group (9 out of 19) had high rates of depression, whereas only one quarter (3 out of 12) of the bipolar group exhibited such problems. The researchers concluded that although a complicated risk path is involved, children with parents who suffer from affective disturbances are at a significantly higher risk of receiving a psychiatric diagnosis and impairment in social and cognitive functioning. Similar results and conclusions are reported by Klein, Clark, Dansky, and Margolis (1988), with the added finding of a higher rate of dysthymia in the female offspring of patients with unipolar depression than in the offspring of parents with medical problems or those who did not evidence any history of psychiatric or medical disorders.

One major study did not find support for this relationship between maternal depression and affective disorders among child/adolescent offspring, although the findings raise important questions for future research in this area. Forehand et al. (1988) studied young adolescents (mean age = 13.5 years) who were assessed along with their parents on two measures of depression involving self-report and behavioral ratings. Over time, they found that maternal depression self-ratings were highly correlated, yet this was not found for the adolescents on either measure. However, they discovered that maternal depression increased in association with an increase in marital conflict, a finding that mirrors the literature on wife battering and maternal effectiveness (e.g., Wolfe, Jaffe, Wilson, & Zak, 1985). That is, marital conflict and violence are suspected to influence negatively maternal effectiveness and depressive symptomatology directly, and these impairments in turn have an indirect impact on parenting abilities. Thus, the study by Forehand *et al.* (1988) has several implications for the type of measures used to assess parental as well as adolescent depressive symptoms, and for the assessment of critical situational events in the family, such as marital discord and violence.

In summarizing these studies on behavioral, cognitive, and affective problems among children of depressed parents, the common finding should be emphasized that there is no simple relationship between parental depression (maternal or paternal) and affective disorders in the offspring. Instead, studies are discovering a much more complicated pathway whereby children may become at a greater risk for a wide array of psychiatric problems when either or both parents suffers from depression. Based on the few studies conducted to date, differences in the behavior of children of unipolar versus bipolar depressed parents do not appear to be of clinical significance; rather, both subtypes appear to elevate the probability of receiving a psychiatric diagnosis during childhood or adolescence. Furthermore, the vast majority of studies to date have focused on maternal depression, and thus the role of paternal psychiatric illness is poorly understood.

We now turn to a closer look at the interactions between depressed parents and their children in order to see how their child-rearing methods and communications to their children may be responsible for developmental impairments.

Parent/Child Interactions in Families with a Depressed Parent

The characteristics of adult depression (i.e., feelings of helplessness, uselessness, being unable to function effectively, poor concentration, interpersonal disinterest), when combined with the responsibilities and demands of parenthood (e.g., feeding schedules, interrupted sleep, constant surveillance, disciplining the child) pose considerable odds against the likelihood of conflict-free, positive parent–child interactions. Furthermore, as noted by Weissman (1979), depression is more common in women, who also carry the bulk of the child-rearing responsibility in most families. Although the directionality issue cannot be easily resolved (i.e., do difficult infants bring about greater maternal depression, or do depressed mothers give rise to more difficult infants?), several important aspects of the daily interactions between depressed mothers and their infants or young children provide some clarity to the issue of how parental depression plays a pathogenic role in child development.

Weissman and her colleagues (1979; Weissman, Paykel, & Klerman, 1972; Weissman et al., 1987) concluded from their observations of interactions between depressed mothers and their offspring that these children were deprived of normal involvement with their parents. For example, during play these parents were unenthusiastic and provided little involvement or guidance for the child; as the children grew older, the parents continued this pattern by showing a lack of interest in the child's school activities, social events, or peers. Decreased involvement on the part of the parent took other forms as well, such as paying little attention to the child's physical health or appearance. The researchers further noted that the children were not as often encouraged to discuss their feelings or to discuss their daily activities, compared to comparison children from nondepressed families. Not only were the parent/child interactions marked by greater disinterest and less involvement, they observed that acutely depressed parents behaved in a more hostile fashion toward their children, a finding that has important implications as well for the child's development of a sense of self and self-mastery. Overall, these researchers interpreted their findings to highlight the four primary areas of parental dysfunction that can be identified in families with one or more depressed parents: involvement and disinterest, communication, affection, and hostility. All four of these areas (when phrased in positive terms) are deemed critical to healthy child development (Maccoby & Martin, 1983), and therefore the mechanisms by which parental depression plays a role in developmental psychopathology are becoming more apparent.

Additional studies have focused on the critical period of attachment between mother and infant during the first months of life, and have again revealed a pathogenic pattern among depressed parents of low involvement and responsivity toward their offspring. Cohn and Tronick (1983) used an experimental design to manipulate the presence or absence of maternal depressed mood while interacting with their 3-month-old infants (12 female and 12 male). Mothers in the study were instructed to interact normally or to interact with a simulated "depressed expression" with their infants. Results indicated that those mothers assigned to the "depressed" condition were significantly more undercontrolling and less elaborate compared to mothers in the normal condition. More importantly, condition effects revealed that infants in the "depressed" condition showed higher rates of wariness and protest (50% of the time), and less brief positive reactions. In contrast, in the normal condition, infants rarely exhibited protest or wary behavior and showed higher frequencies of brief positive displays. In commenting on these data, the researchers pointed out that "the sequencing of infant affect states is clearly related to the quality of maternal expression" (p. 190).

Radke-Yarrow, Cummings, Kuczynski, and Chapman (1985) also examined patterns of attachment, involving 2- and 3-year-old children and their mothers. Fourteen children had bipolar depressive mothers, 42 children had mothers diagnosed as major unipolar depression, 12 mothers were diagnosed as minor depression, and 31 were nondepressed. The results indicated that there was no difference between children of nondepressed mothers and children of mothers with minor depression in terms of the frequency of insecure attachments. However, there was a significantly greater incidence of insecure attachments in the major affective disorder group in comparison to normals. The researchers interpret these findings (in conjunction with additional findings not reviewed here) to suggest that maternal depression decreases the likelihood of secure attachment between the mother and child. Among the mothers with one of the forms of a major effective disorder, 55% were observed to have an insecure attachment with their child (this figure increased to 79% among mothers with a diagnosis of a bipolar depression, and was 47% and 29% among unipolar and nondepressed mothers, respectively). Once again, these results are quite clear in underscoring the limited range of affect among depressed mothers and the effects of such a pattern on the cognitive and emotional development of her child.

Changes in communication patterns under stressful and nonstressful conditions was the focus of attention in a study of 3-year-olds reported by Breznitz and Sherman (1987). These investigators studied 32 mother/child dyads in which the mother either suffered from periods of depression or had no psychiatric history or symptomatology. Not surprisingly, they found that the nondepressed mothers spoke significantly more often to their young children in comparison to depressed mothers during everyday, nonstressful circumstances. However, when placed in a stressful situation, depressed mothers increased the amount of speech they produced whereas nondepressed mothers had a slight decrease in their amount of speech. Both groups decreased their response latency during the stressful condition, but again the depressed mothers showed an even greater reduction in the amount of time it took for them to respond to their child. The investigators suggested on the basis of these findings that the two groups of mothers may handle stress quite differently. They interpreted the faster reaction time and increased speech productivity of the depressed mothers as an exaggerated or overreaction to the situation, which may convey anxiety or fear to the child. Consequently, maternal depression can be linked to developmental repercussions in the offspring that are due not only to the *content* of the interaction as discussed previously, but perhaps due as well to the patterning and delivery of such interactions.

The manner in which depressed mothers interact with and view the behavior of their older children has also been the focus of considerable inquiry in recent years. Investigating the reports of depressed ($N = 46$) and nondepressed ($N = 49$) mothers of the 3- to 8-year-old children, Webster-Stratton and Hammond (1988) found that depressed mothers rated their children significantly higher in the areas of externalizing, internalizing, and depression scales of the Child Behavior Checklist. Depressed mothers also reported greater stress in the parenting role as measured by the Parenting Stress Index, noting higher scores in such areas as attachment, depression, role restriction, low sense of competence, and socialization and health. Surprisingly, home observations of parent–child interaction did not reveal differences between the groups on five behavioral measures (although a trend for more critical statements among depressed mothers was noted). However, the results in total (including additional findings not reviewed herein) support the premise that the children of depressed mothers are *perceived* by the parent as being more disruptive and disturbed than they may be. This finding parallels the child abuse literature, in which abusive mothers have been found to perceive their children in a more negative light than do more objective observers (Wolfe, 1987), and is a reminder that the problems of children of disturbed parents cannot always be inferred or denied on the basis of parental report. As stated by Christensen, Phillips, Glasgow, and Johnson (1983), the perception of child behavior problems may be more related to marital discord and parental negative behavior rather than to the actual behavior of the child.

Further insights can be gained from our study of children of depressed parents by comparing these findings to those involving abusive parents. A logical connection exists between these two clinical populations, given the preponderance of negative interactions, low ratio of positive attention or reinforcement of the child, and reliance on critical commands (and punishment) to teach and control the child, found in both groups. However, as noted elsewhere (Wolfe, 1985), abusive parents are defined more specifically in terms of their singular behavior toward their children—extreme physical actions—rather than by the presence of a psychiatric condition or a syndrome of identifiable impairments, such as major affective disorder. Thus, child abuse is an event (more so than a psychiatric disorder) that is often associated with other prime examples of authoritarian parenting style, whereas depression can be more accurately described as the existence of a condition or cluster of symptoms that leads to impairments in the child-care role.

These distinctions notwithstanding, it is useful to compare the two populations of abusive and depressed parents to develop a consensus as to the similarities and differences in parent–child interactions. In an unusual study that involved subsamples of normal, abusive, and depressed mothers, Susman *et al.* (1985) found important differences in methods of child-rearing. Abusive mothers, in particular, were higher on self-reported ratings of authoritarianism, anxiety induction, guilt induction, and discipline inconsistency, and were lower on rationale guidance and enjoyment of the parenting role. Furthermore, abusive mothers were unlikely to encourage independence or openness to a new experience, tended to be very protective and to worry about the child, and to show less open expression of affect toward the child. Interestingly, this study revealed fewer deviations from the norm among the depressed mothers, with the exception of discipline inconsistency and need for control. However, depressed mothers were similar to the abusive mothers on 38% of the 21 child-rearing factors studied. Extrapolating from these findings, the authors suggested that the greater number and variety of child-rearing difficulties reported by the abusive mothers is indicative of their more specific deficits in the parenting domain, whereas the problems experienced by depressed mothers may interfere with child-rearing in a more general manner; that is, depending on mood or situational factors, depressed mothers may respond to their children in a more or less hostile and rejecting fashion (see also Lahey, Conger, Atkeson, & Treiber, 1984).

In general, the literature reviewed in this section on depressed parents underscores the relationship between parental affective disorder and developmental risk throughout the periods of infancy, childhood, and adolescence. Not only is there a direct association between the existence of a psychiatric diagnosis in the offspring and the presence of parental depression, but there is also evidence of the mechanisms by which parental depression interferes with the developing parent–child relationship. Depressed mothers, in particular, are observed to be less interactive and more critical of their children, a finding that mirrors to some extent the results of observational studies with abusive parents.

Moreover, studies have demonstrated that, in some depressed families, marital conflict accounts for more of the variance in child behavior problems than does the presence of parental depression. In turn, we also find that symptoms of maternal depression show a positive correlation with marital conflict, a finding that warrants greater attention if efforts at early detection and intervention of child behavior problems are to be maximally effective.

PARENTAL PSYCHOPATHOLOGY AND CHILD MALTREATMENT

When child maltreatment first began to receive the attention of researchers and practitioners over 25 years ago, it was considered to be a manifestation of severe parental psychopathology. Only psychiatrically disturbed individuals, it was reasoned, could show the lack of control and concern that was exhibited in documented cases of child abuse and neglect. Inspired by this early viewpoint, two decades of research studies have focused on developing an accurate understanding of the role that parental psychopathology might play in the expression of child abuse and neglect. Because the vast majority of parents are capable of dealing with difficult child behavior and stressful circumstances without resorting to physical violence or neglect, researchers have suspected that maltreating parents must lack some form of inner control, have experienced early trauma in their own families of origin, or suffer from a major thought disorder that limits their recognition of the consequences of their actions (see Green, 1978; Spinetta & Rigler, 1972). Although many of these disturbances have been identified among samples of maltreating parents, no *distinctive* psychological profile or pattern has been documented that supports the view that parental psychopathology is at the root of child maltreatment.

In order to understand the role of parental adjustment in the expression of abusive and neglectful behavior toward their offspring, it is necessary to clarify the context and nature of such behavior. In more recent studies, child maltreatment has been viewed as the product of an interaction between parental functioning and situational demands (rather than being limited primarily to parental psychopathology). Although the role of parental behavior still remains crucial in such a redefinition, the significance of parental disturbance has become less dramatic and less conspicuous than was originally assumed on the basis of their actions.

Early information on the behavior of abusive parents was derived primarily from clinical case studies, which provided a rich source of descriptive knowledge about the characteristics of such individuals. In the behavioral dimension, these case studies described abusive parents as chronically aggressive, isolated from family and friends, rigid and domineering, impulsive, and experiencing marital difficulties. Similarly, the cognitive-emotional functioning of these parents was reported to be marked by low frustration tolerance, emotional immaturity, role reversal, deficits in empathy and self-esteem, high expectations for their child's behavior, and problems in the expression and control of anger (see reviews by Parke & Collmer, 1975; Spinetta & Rigler, 1972; Wolfe, 1985, 1987).

These early clinical case studies became more sophisticated in the early 1970s, as more researchers entered the field and began to include matched control families to provide a basis for comparison on these psychological dimensions. The concept of an identifiable personality disorder or disturbance that could account for abusive behavior was contested by the social learning emphasis on person–situation interaction, which resulted in different methodological approaches to understanding this phenomenon. In contrast to personality dimensions, the emphasis shifted toward the daily interactions of family members (especially parent–child interactions) that might explain the escalation in intensity and severity that defines an abusive episode. In addition, self-report devices were developed that targeted the unrealistic expectations of some parents and the type and extent of physical and emotional symptoms experienced, which resulted in several significant contrasts between identified abusive parents and nonabusive parents.

The empirical findings that emerged from these more recent studies revealed many important similarities as well as differences in comparison to the earlier reports. In particular, several behavioral differences between abusers and nonabusers were reaffirmed, such as low frustration tolerance, social isolation, and impaired child-rearing skills. Moreover, several cognitive-emotional differences were supported, such as the tendency to demonstrate unrealistic expectations of their children, to report that their child's behavior is extremely stressful to them, and to describe themselves as being inadequate or incompetent in the parenting role (Wolfe, 1987).

A major description of abusive parents that was not confirmed or supported by these more recent studies had to do with personality disorders or psychopathology as the common element shared by abusive parents. Psychiatric descriptions, such as emotional immaturity, impulsivity, and low self-esteem have not received a great deal of consensus, perhaps because of the difficulty in defining and measuring these constructs. Thus, the notion of a distinctive personality profile or cluster of symptoms describing abusive parents can be modified to reflect the interactive nature of this phenomenon. Certain predispositional characteristics of some parents may place them at greater risk for abuse, because of such behavior patterns as inflexibility and maladaptive responses to certain situational contexts, especially those situations involving a difficult child, handling stressful situations, and solving family-related problems. Unfortunately, our knowledge of child neglect is far behind that of physical abuse. However, it appears from preliminary studies that neglect may involve an even greater degree of parental psychopathology than abuse which, coupled with situational events, leads to an *avoidance* response to stressful child behavior rather than to aggression (Wolfe, 1985). Whether these two forms of child maltreatment represent different manifestations of the same disorder or whether they are the two most identifiable patterns of parenting dysfunction (out of perhaps many more) remains to be investigated.

SUMMARY

We have reviewed a number of areas of parental psychopathology that have implications for child development. Because our attention was focused on the major psychosocial factors associated with parental disorders, we drew from the expanding literature on children of depressed parents to highlight the suspected processes involved in the transmission or transaction of developmental psychopathology in offspring. Despite the growing knowledge in this area of parental psychopathology, we again remind the reader that the studies covered in this review were limited primarily to situational and psychological variables. Interested readers will have to find elsewhere additional theoretical explanations, methodological procedures, and causal or correlational relationships associated with genetic, biological, and psychiatric fields of study.

Other important psychosocial variables that were not the focus of the present review merit some mention in closing. Parental alcoholism, for example, is known to interfere with normal child-rearing and the development of a healthy parent–child relationship. Consequently, it comes as no surprise that alcoholism in parents has been found to be associated with adjustment problems in children, especially males (Adler & Raphael, 1983; West & Prinz, 1987). Alcoholic parents appear to fit a pattern of inconsistent and unpredictable childcare that has been similarly discovered in many of the studies of parental disorders reviewed. In addition, we need to look more carefully at the cultural, familial, and social support factors that play a role in mediating the negative impact of poverty and disadvantage of children, because children from lower socioeconomic backgrounds tend to be more at risk for school problems (especially among minority children; Felner, Gillespie, & Smith, 1985).

The findings presented throughout this chapter support a social learning explanation of developmental psychopathology, which predicts a *disruption* or *alteration* in development as a function of significant factors affecting learning opportunities, of which parental depression is but one. Rather than assuming a one-to-one correspondence between parental psychopathology and developmental outcome, social learning theory suggests that events that have a significant influence on the child's learning environment can lead to changes or deviations in coping responses, expectations, problem-solving skills, and related developmental events. In this manner, parental depression represents one of the more visible and dramatic circumstances that can change the course of normal child development, much the same as do child abuse (Wolfe, 1987), parental divorce (Hetherington & Martin, 1986), wife battering (Wolfe *et al.*, 1985), and parental criminality (Lewis, Balsla, Shanok, & Snell, 1976), to name only a few. Consistency and predictability of child care may be the common threads that link many of these deviant forms of parenting practices to the wide variety of negative developmental outcomes (Wahler & Dumas, 1987).

Several methodological considerations emerge from the current literature in this area that justify further attention. Perhaps because of the inexact nature of our diagnostic systems, the criteria for determining and agreeing upon the type of problem(s) exhibited by some parents are often unclear. Furthermore, the choice of assessment instruments and procedures typically varies from study to study, and therefore it is difficult to draw comparative conclusions. One major direction that has been undertaken in this regard is a better understanding of the manner in which certain pathological conditions in parents affect their ratings of child behavior (see, for example, Jensen, Traylor, Xenakis, & Davis, 1988; Schaughency & Lahey, 1985). Most importantly, we need more longitudinal research on this topic in order to draw more firm conclusions about the long-term effects of parental psychopathology and the course and stability of such changes. Finally, we point to the growing recognition that a significant number of children survive without any detectable harm, even in very unhealthy environments (Beardslee & Podorefski, 1988), a reality that may offer assistance in understanding the plight of children of disturbed parents.

ACKNOWLEDGMENTS

Preparation of this chapter was supported in part by the Institute for the Prevention of Child Abuse (Toronto, Canada), and by a grant to David A. Wolfe from the Social Sciences and Humanities Research Council of Canada. We wish to thank the Charlestown Residential School, Adrienne Perry, Nancy Freeman, and Diane Factor for their assistance and support.

REFERENCES

Adler, R., & Raphael, B. (1983). Review: Children of alcoholics. *Australian and New Zealand Journal of Psychiatry, 17*, 3–8.
Anderson, C. (1987). Depression and families. *Journal of Psychotherapy and the Family, 3*, 33–48.
Barnett, P. A., & Gotlib, I. H. (1988). Psychosocial functioning and depression: Distinguishing among antecedents, concomitants, and consequences. *Psychological Bulletin, 104*, 97–126.
Baumrind, D. (1971). Current patterns of parental authority. *Developmental Psychology Monographs, 4* (1, pt. 2).
Beardslee, W. R., & Podorefsky, D. (1988). Resilient adolescents whose parents have serious affective and other psychiatric disorders: Importance of self-understanding and relationships. *American Journal of Psychiatry, 145*, 63–69.
Beardslee, W. R., Bemporad, J., Keller, M. B., & Klerman, G. L. (1983). Children of parents with major affective disorder: A review. *The American Journal of Psychiatry, 140*, 825–832.
Beardslee, W. R., Keller, M. B., & Klerman, G. L. (1985). Children of parents with affective disorder. *International Journal of Family Psychiatry, 6*, 283–299.
Bell, R. Q., & Harper, L. (1977). *Child effects on adults*. Hillsdale, NJ: Lawrence Erlbaum.
Blackford, K. A. (1988). The children of chronically ill parents. *Journal of Psychosocial Nursing, 26*, 33–36.
Breznitz, Z., & Sherman, T. (1987). Speech patterning of natural discourse of well and depressed mothers and their young children. *Child Development, 58*, 395–400.
Cantwell, D. P., & Baker, L. (1984). Parental mental illness and psychiatric disorders in "at risk" children. *Journal of Clinical Psychiatry, 45*, 503–507.
Christensen, A., Phillips, S., Glasgow, R. E., & Johnson, S. M. (1983). Parental characteristics and interactional dysfunction in families with child behavior problems: A preliminary investigation. *Journal of Abnormal Child Psychology, 11*, 153–166.
Cohn, J. F., & Tronick, E. Z. (1983). Three-month-old infants' reaction to simulated maternal depression. *Child Development, 54*, 185–193.
Cooper, S. F., Leach, C., Storer, D., Tonge, W. L. (1977). The children of psychiatric patients: Clinical findings. *British Journal of Psychiatry, 131*, 514–522.
Coyne, J. C., Kahn, J., Gotlib, I. H. (1987). Depression. In T. Jacob (Ed.), *Family interaction and psychopathology: Theories, methods, and findings* (pp. 509–533). New York: Plenum Press.

Emery, R. (1982). Interparental conflict and the children of discord and divorce. *Psychological Bulletin, 92,* 310–330.

Felner, R. D., Gillespie, J. F., & Smith, R. (1985). Risk and vulnerability in childhood: A reappraisal. *Journal of Clinical Child Psychology, 14,* 2–4.

Forehand, R., Brody, G., Slotkin, J., Fauber, R., McCombs, A., & Long, N. (1988). Young adolescent and maternal depression: Assessment, interrelations, and family predictors. *Journal of Consulting and Clinical Psychology, 56,* 422–426.

Goldstein, M. J. (1988). The family and psychopathology. *Annual Review of Psychology, 39,* 283–299.

Green, A. H. (1978). Child abuse. In B. B. Wolman, J. Egan, & A. Ross (Eds.), *Handbook of treatment of mental disorders in childhood and adolescence* (pp. 430–455). Englewood Cliffs, NJ: Prentice-Hall.

Hammen, C., Adrian, C., Gordon, D., Burge, D., Jaenicke, C., & Hiroto, D. (1987a). Children of depressed mothers: Maternal strain and symptom predictors of dysfunction. *Journal of Abnormal Psychology, 96,* 190–198.

Hammen, C., Gordon, D., Burge, D., Adrian, C., Jaenicke, C., & Hiroto, D. (1987b). Maternal affective disorders, illness, and stress: Risk for children's psychopathology. *American Journal of Psychiatry, 144,* 736–741.

Hetherington, E. M., & Martin, B. (1986). Family factors and psychopathology in children. In H. C. Quay, & J. S. Werry (Eds.), *Psychopathological disorders of childhood* (3rd ed., pp. 332–390). New York: John Wiley.

Jensen, P. S., Traylor, J., Xenakis, S. N., & Davis, H. (1988). Childhood psychopathology rating scales and interrater agreement: I. Parents' gender and psychiatric symptoms. *Journal of the American Academy of Child and Adolescent Psychiatry., 27,* 422–450.

Kandel, E., Mednick, S. A., Kirkegaard-Sorensen, L., Hutchings, B., Knop, J., Rosenberg, R., & Schulsinger, F. (1988). IQ as a protective factor for subjects at high risk for antisocial behavior. *Journal of Consulting and Clinical Psychology, 56,* 224–226.

Kashani, J. H., Burk, J. P., Horwitz, B., & Reid, J. C. (1985). Differential effect of subtype of parental major affective disorder on children. *Psychiatry Research, 15,* 195–204.

Klein, D. N., Clark, D. C., Dansky, L., & Margolis, E. T. (1988). Dysthymia in the offspring of parents with primary unipolar affective disorder. *Journal of Abnormal Psychology, 97,* 265–274.

Lahey, B. B., Conger, R. D., Atkeson, B. M., & Treiber, F. A. (1984). Parenting behavior and emotional status of physically abusive mothers. *Journal of Consulting and Clinical Psychology, 52,* 1062–1071.

Lee, C. M., & Gotlib, I. H. (1989). Clinical status and emotional adjustment of children of depressed mothers. *American Journal of Psychiatry, 146,* 478–483.

Lewis, D. O., Balla, D., Shanok, S., & Snell, L. (1976). Delinquency, parental psychopathology, and paternal criminality: Clinical and epidemiological findings. *Journal of the American Academy of Child Psychiatry, 15,* 665–678.

Maccoby, E. E., & Martin, J. A. (1983). Socialization in the context of the family: Parent-child interaction. In P. H. Mussen (Ed.), *Handbook of child psychology* (4th ed.). New York: Wiley.

Masten, A. S., & Garmezy, N. (1985). Risk, vulnerability, and protective factors in developmental psychopathology. In B. B. Lahey, & A. E. Kazdin (Eds.), *Advances in clinical child psychology* (Vol. 8, pp. 1–52). New York: Plenum Press.

Minuchin, S. (1974). *Families and family therapy.* Cambridge: Harvard University Press.

Minuchin, S., Rosman, B. L., & Baker, L. (1978). *Psychosomatic families.* Cambridge: Harvard University Press.

Olson, D. H., Sprenkle, D. H., & Russell, C. S. (1979). Circumplex model of marital and family systems: I. Cohesion and adaptability dimensions, family types, and clinical applications. *Family Process, 18,* 3–28.

Orvaschel, H. (1983). Maternal depression and child dysfunction: Children at risk. In B. B. Lahey, & A. E. Kazdin (Eds.), *Advances in clinical child psychology* (Vol. 6, pp. 169–197). New York: Plenum Press.

Orvaschel, H., Weissman, M. M., & Kidd, K. K. (1980). Children and depression. *Journal of Affective Disorders, 2,* 1–16.

Orvaschel, H., Walsh-Allis, G., & Ye, W. (1988). Psychopathology in children of parents with recurrent depression. *Journal of Abnormal Child Psychology, 16,* 17–28.

Parke, R. D., & Collmer, C. W. (1975). Child abuse: An interdisciplinary analysis. In E. M. Hetherington (Ed.), *Review of child development research* (Vol. 5, pp. 509–590). Chicago: University of Chicago Press.

Phipps-Yonas, S. (1980). Teenage pregnancy and motherhood: A review of the literature. *American Journal of Orthopsychiatry, 50,* 403–430.

Radke-Yarrow, M., Cummings, E. M., Kuczynski, L., & Chapman, M. (1985). Patterns of attachment in two- and three-year-olds in normal families and families with parental depression. *Child Development, 56,* 884–893.

Rutter, M. (1966). Children of sick parents: An environmental and psychiatric study. Institute of Psychiatry, Maudsley Monographs No 16. London: Oxford University Press.

Rutter, M. (1971). Parent-child separation: Psychological effects on the children. *Journal of Child Psychiatry, 12,* 233–260.

Rutter, M. (1979). Protective factors in children's response to stress and disadvantage. In M. W. Kent & J. E. Rolf (Eds.), *Primary prevention of psychopathology: Vol III. Social competence in children.* Hanover, NH: University Press of New England.

Sameroff, A. J., Seiffer, R., & Zax, M. (1982). Early development of children at risk for emotional disorder *Monographs of the Society for Research in Child Development, 47*(7 Serial No. 199).

Schaughency, E. A., & Lahey, B. B. (1985). Mothers' and fathers' perceptions of child deviance: Roles of child behavior, parental depression, and marital satisfaction. *Journal of Consulting and Clinical Psychology, 53,* 718–723.

Schore, E. L. (1988). Families, family roles and psychological diagnoses in primary care. *Developmental and Behavioral Pediatrics, 9,* 327–332.

Schwartz, B. A. (1979). Adolescent parents. In J. D. Nosphitz, I. N. Berling, & L. A. Stone (Eds.), *Basic handbook of child psychiatry: Prevention and current issues* (Vol. 4, pp. 360–363). New York: Basic Books.

Scott, K. G., Field, T., & Robertson, E. (1981). *Teenage parents and their offspring.* New York: Grune & Stratton.

Silverman, W. K., Cerny, J. A., Nelles, W. B., & Burke, A. E. (1988). Behavior problems in children of parents with anxiety disorders. *Journal of the American Academy of Child and Adolescent Psychiatry, 27,* 779–784.

Smets, A. C., & Hartup, W. W., (1988). Systems and symptoms: Family cohesion/ adaptability and childhood behavior problems. *Journal of Abnormal Child Psychology, 16,* 233–246.

Spinetta, J. J. & Rigler, D. (1972). The child abusing parent: A psychological review. *Psychological Bulletin. 77,* 296–304.

Susman, E. J., Trickett, P. K., Iannotti, R. I., Hollenback, B. E., & Zahn-Waxler, C. (1985). Child-rearing patterns in depressed, abusive, and normal mothers. *American Journal of Orthopsychiatry, 55,* 237–251.

Sylvester, C. E., Hyde, T. S., & Reichler, R. J. (1987). The diagnostic interview for children and personality inventory for children in studies of children at risk for anxiety disorders or depression. *Journal of the American Academy of Child and Adolescent Psychiatry, 26,* 668–675.

Turner, S. M., Beidel, D. C., & Costello, A. (1987). Psychopathology in the offspring of anxiety disorders patients. *Journal of Consulting and Clinical Psychology, 55,* 229–235.

Wahler, R. G., & Dumas, J. E. (1987). Family factors in childhood psychology: Towards a coercion-neglect model. In T. Jacob (Eds.), *Family interaction and psychopathology: Theories, methods, and findings* (pp. 581–627). New York: Plenum Press.

Webster-Stratton, C., & Hammond, M. (1988). Maternal depression and its relationship to life stress, perceptions of child behavior problems, parenting behaviors, and child conduct problems. *Journal of Abnormal Child Psychology, 16,* 299–315.

Weissman, M. M. (1979). Depressed parents and their children: Implications for prevention. In J. D. Noshpitz, I. N., Berlin, & L. A. Stone (Eds.), *Basic handbook of child psychiatry: Prevention and current issues* (Vol. 4, pp. 292–299). New York: Basic Books.

Weissman, M. M., Gammon G. D., John, K., Merikangas, K. R., Warner, V., Prusoff, B. A., & Sholomskas, D. (1987). Children of depressed parents. *Archives of General Psychiatry, 44* 847–853.

Weissman, M. M., Paykel, E. S., & Klerman, G. L. (1972). The depressed woman as a mother. *Social Psychiatry, 7,* 98–108.

Werner, E. E. (1989). High-risk children in young adulthood: A longitudinal study from birth to 32 years. *American Journal of Orthopsychiatry, 59,* 72–81.

West, M. O., & Prinz, R. J. (1987). Parental alcoholism and childhood psychopathology. *Psychological Bulletin, 102,* 204–218.

Wolfe, D. A. (1985). Child-abusive parents: An empirical review and analysis. *Psychological Bulletin, 97,* 462–482.

Wolfe, D. A. (1987). *Child abuse: Implications for child development and psychopathology.* Newbury Park, CA: Sage.

Wolfe, D. A., Jaffe, P. J., Wilson, S. K., & Zak, L. (1985). Children of battered women: The relation of child behavior to family violence and maternal stress. *Journal of Consulting and Clinical Psychology, 53,* 657–665.

Worland, J., Weeks, D. G., Janes, C. L., & Strock, B. D. (1984). Intelligence, classroom behavior, and academic achievement in children at high and low risk for psychopathology: A structural equation analysis. *Journal of Abnormal Child Psychology, 12,* 437–454.

Zahn-Waxler, C., Mayfield, A., Radke-Yarrow, M., McKnew, D. H., Cytryn, L., & Davenport, Y. B. (1988). A follow-up investigation of offspring of parents with bipolar disorder. *American Journal of Psychiatry, 145,* 506–509.

CHAPTER 8

PREDISPOSING CHILD FACTORS

ROBERT T. AMMERMAN

INTRODUCTION

Since the original description of the Battered Child Syndrome by Kempe and his colleagues (Kempe, Silverman, Steele, Droegemueller, & Silver, 1962), there has been a tremendous growth in professional and media interest in child abuse and neglect. Evidence of expanded awareness is found in the plethora of specialty journals (e.g., *Journal of Family Violence, Child Abuse and Neglect*) and books (MacFarlane, Waterman, Conerly, Damon, Durfee, & Long, 1986; Oates, 1982; Wolfe, 1987) devoted to this topic. This increased focus of attention is at least partly attributable to the dramatic rise in reported cases of child maltreatment in recent years. For example, there has been an 8% increase in reported cases of child abuse and neglect from 1985 to 1986 (American Association for Protecting Children, 1988). Although such an elevation in reports is partly related to greater professional awareness of child maltreatment, most experts agree that child abuse and neglect currently represent significant social problems (see Chapter 2 in this volume).

Because of the deleterious physical and psychological consequences associated with child maltreatment (see Ammerman, Cassisi, Hersen, & Van Hasselt, 1986; Friedrich & Einbender, 1983), recent investigators

ROBERT T. AMMERMAN • Western Pennsylvania School for Blind Children, Pittsburgh, Pennsylvania 15213.

have directed their efforts toward the prevention of abuse and neglect (e.g., Lutzker & Rice, 1984). An important component of such efforts is to identify children who are at high risk for maltreatment in an effort to curtail the processes leading to abuse or neglect (Parke & Collmer, 1975). At-risk populations have been targeted, using a variety of factors thought to be implicated in the etiology of abuse and neglect, including family demographics, socioeconomic status, parental psychopathology, parent history of abuse, and substance abuse disorders (see Starr, 1988). In addition, some theorists have suggested that certain child characteristics may play a role in the development and maintenance of abuse (deLissovoy, 1979). Thus, based upon this premise, it is possible that these child characteristics can be subsequently used in screening for potential child maltreatment or selecting at-risk populations for preventative interventions.

This chapter will review the evidence that child factors contribute to the etiology and maintenance of physical abuse and neglect. First, conceptual models that describe the process by which children can be involved in the development of maltreatment will be presented. Second, early childhood characteristics posited to be risk factors for abuse or neglect will be reviewed. Third, interactional studies describing the coercive relationship between abusive parents and their children will be discussed. These studies elucidate the ways in which child factors may contribute to the maintenance of abuse. Fourth, the role of child handicapping conditions in increasing risk for maltreatment will be considered. Finally, the utility of using child factors in assessing risk will be examined, and future directions that research might take are outlined. Child contributions to the etiology of sexual abuse will not be covered, and the reason for this is that it is widely acknowledged that the dynamics involved in sexual abuse differ greatly from those observed in physical abuse and neglect (see MacFarlane et al., 1986). Moreover, there is little support for the contention that children have any causative role in sexual abuse.

CONCEPTUAL MODELS OF CHILD ABUSE AND NEGLECT

Traditionally, three models have been used to explain the development and continuation of child abuse and neglect. These models emphasize parental psychopathology, sociological factors, and the social context of the parent–child relationship, respectively. The *Psychopathology Model* attributes child abuse and neglect to parental psychiatric disturbance or mental illness. According to this formulation, child abusers can be described as psychotic, impulsive, or sadistic. Also, physical abuse or neglect is seen as a manifestation of psychodynamic dysfunction or personality disturbance in the parent (Spinetta & Rigler, 1972). Although this model received early support in the literature, more recent investigations have failed to document severe psychopathology in child abusers (see Wolfe, 1985). Although parents who engage in maltreatment clearly exhibit maladjustment in a variety of areas of functioning (see Chapter 7 in this volume), their abusive behavior is rarely a direct product of specific psychiatric disorders.

The *Social-Cultural Model* of child maltreatment emphasizes social and cultural forces in the formation of child abuse and neglect. Within this framework, domestic violence is viewed as a response to stress engendered by unemployment, economic hardship, and educational disadvantage (Gelles, 1973). Moreover, cultural sanctioning of physical punishment to resolve family conflict further adds to the likelihood of abuse (Maurer, 1974). Empirical support for this model comes from multivariate studies that identify sociological and demographic factors as good predictors of maltreatment (Gaines, Sandgrund, Green, & Power, 1978; Garbarino, 1976). For example, Garbarino (1976) found that socioeconomic factors accounted for 36% of the variance in his sample of child abuse reports, whereas no other variable exhibited such explanatory power. Critics, however, have argued that social-cultural elements do not explain the *process* through which child maltreatment develops (Wolfe, 1987). Furthermore, the majority of socioeconomically disadvantaged parents do not abuse or neglect their children, thus demonstrating that this component alone does not fully account for the etiology of maltreatment (Egeland, Breitenbucher, & Rosenberg, 1980).

The *Social-Interactional Model* of child abuse and neglect focuses on the relationship between parent and child and the social context in which the maltreatment occurs (Parke & Collmer, 1975). This approach proposes that the unique characteristics of both the parent and the child interact to bring about maltreatment in particular conflict situations. For example, a parent with poor child-management skills, excessive expectations regarding child behavior, and a past history of being abused may be more likely to engage in physical abuse toward a difficult to manage, noncompliant child during times of stress (e.g., recent job loss, economic hardship). Therefore, the dynamic interchanges between parent and child in conjunction with situational variables are viewed as critical to the etiology and maintenance of abusive behavior. This model clearly suggests that child characteristics can contribute to the occurrence of abuse.

More recently, theorists have constructed comprehensive multi-casual models that attempt to combine the aforementioned conceptualizations and account for the complex interplay between etiological factors (Belsky, 1980; Burgess & Draper, 1988; Starr, 1988). Although these thorough models delineate the many levels of causative influence, they do not further our understanding of *how* such elements interact to bring about maltreatment. Wolfe (1987), on the other hand, has proposed a formulation that seeks to describe the ways in which individual and situational variables interact to inhibit or promote the likelihood of a family engaging in abuse. The *Transitional Model* views abuse as a product of the gradual escalation of power assertive parenting practices. Through the interaction of Destabilizing Factors (that increase the risk of abuse), and Compensatory Factors (that decrease the risk of abuse), parents pass through three stages reflecting increased likelihood of violence directed toward the child. The three stages are: (1) Reduced Tolerance for Stress and Disinhibition of Aggression, (2) Poor Management of Acute Crises and Provocation, and (3) Habitual Patterns of Arousal and Aggression with Family Members. Destabilizing factors within each stage include such variables as weak preparation for parenting (Stage 1), conditioned emotional arousal (Stage 2), and the child's increase in problem behavior (Stage 3). Compensatory factors consist of such elements as socioeconomic stability (Stage 1), improvement in child behavior (Stage 2), and use of community restraints and services (Stage 3). The important contributions of the Transitional Model are that it (1) describes child abuse as a gradually unfolding interactive process rather than an isolated phenomenon, (2) identifies both high-risk elements and protective factors critical to the occurrence of maltreatment, and (3) underscores the now widely accepted notion that a combination of risk factors, and not just those existing in isolation, are necessary for the development of abuse (see Ammerman, 1989; Starr, 1988). In addition, as with the Social-Situational Model, the Transitional Model clearly identifies child characteristics as a possible contributor to the development of child abuse. Further empirical study is required, however, to examine if, in fact, families do progress through these stages before engaging in maltreatment.

COMMENTS

The Social-Interactional Model and the Transitional Model of abuse elucidate the processes whereby child characteristics can contribute to the etiology of abuse. Specifically, children with severe behavior problems or those who are difficult to manage may add to the risk of maltreatment. However, it is important to emphasize that these characteristics alone are insufficient to bring about abuse. Rather, risk is heightened when child factors combine with preexisting elements (e.g., high levels of stress, poor coping skills, acceptance of physical punishment as a disciplinary technique) in the development of maltreatment.

EARLY CHILDHOOD RISK FACTORS

Initial formulations of the role of the child in the etiology of maltreatment focused on infant characteristics (see Friedrich & Boriskin, 1976). Specifically, these included such factors as prematurity, low birthweight, difficult infant temperament, or failure to develop secure mother–infant attachment. It was argued that the stress caused by the aforementioned conditions strained the parent–infant (especially the mother–infant) relationship that, in turn, led to abuse and neglect.

The impetus for implicating prematurity and low birthweight in the development of child maltreatment stemmed from the disproportionate occurrence of these conditions in abused and neglected samples. Based upon retrospective designs, numerous reports documented the over-representation of premature and low birthweight babies in maltreating families (Elmer & Gregg, 1967; Fontana, 1973; Klaus & Kennell, 1970; Klein & Stern, 1971). For example, Klein and Stern (1971) found that 23% of their sample of abused infants had low birthweight, whereas Elmer and Gregg (1967) noted that one third of their abused subjects received this diagnosis. There are two proposed mechanisms through which prematurity and low birthweight are posited to attribute to the development of maltreatment. First, frequent parent–infant separations secondary to complications associated with prematurity lead to an erosion of the attachment relationship or "bonding failure" between mother and infant (Klaus & Kennell, 1970). And second, the stress related to raising a difficult infant increases the overall risk of child maltreatment.

Preliminary studies of early separation as a contributor to maltreatment provided evidence for this association (Klaus & Kennell, 1970; Lynch, 1975; Lynch & Roberts, 1977). For example, Lynch (1975) reported that, in a study of 25 abused children and their siblings, maltreated children were more likely to have experienced birth complications or medical difficulties leading to postbirth hospitalizations than siblings. Likewise, Hawkins and Duncan (1985) reported a high incidence of chronic physical illnesses in a sample of substantiated child abuse cases. On the other hand, Sherrod, O'Connor, Vietze, and Altemeier (1984) failed to find differential patterns of early separation because of infant illness in abused, neglected, and non-maltreated children. Although abused children were found to experience more illnesses than their peers, these were most often attributed to the consequences of abuse.

Egeland and Vaughn (1981) rejected much of the research implicating the role of early separation in the etiology of maltreatment. They argued that (1) none of these investigations provides a *direct* measure of the strength of mother–infant attachment, and (2) that the retrospective design approaches utilized by these studies leaves numerous competing explanations for obtained findings (e.g., prenatal parental characteristics of the mother such as not obtaining proper medical care, poor nutrition, or substance abuse, may result in the birth complications and prematurity reported in these samples). In response to the methodological limitations of past investigations, Egeland and his colleagues (Egeland & Brunnquell, 1979; Egeland & Vaughn, 1981) conducted a prospective study of 267 mothers at high-risk for child maltreatment. Subjects were from low socioeconomic status (SES) backgrounds and were recruited during the last trimester of pregnancy. Of this sample, 32 infants were identified as receiving inadequate home care, whereas 33 were found to receive optimal care. Examination of birth complications and early separations revealed no differences between optimal and nonoptimal care groups (Egeland & Vaughn, 1981). Specifically, groups were statistically equivalent in terms of prematurity, birthweight, number of days spent in the hospital, delivery complications, and newborn medical problems. The authors emphasized the relative superiority of the prospective design when compared to a retrospective approach and they stated that "looking backward in time always provides a cause, but the inferred linearity is misleading. It may be the case . . . that a number of abused children are premature, but . . . the vast majority of premature children are not subsequently abused" (p 82).

Although there are conflicting data regarding the utility of using prematurity or low birthweight as a risk factor for child maltreatment, Frodi (1981) has elucidated the circumstances under which prematurity can contribute to maltreatment. She points out that premature infants display a variety of characteristics that are perceived as aversive and may precipitate an abusive response from caretakers. These consist of unattractive physical features (e.g., small size, developmentally retarded in growth) and a high-pitched, arhythmic cry.

Through a series of investigations, it has been demonstrated that many parents experience negative emotional and physiological arousal upon hearing the cry of a premature infant. For example, in one investigation (Frodi *et al.*, 1978) parents were shown videotapes of premature and full-term infants engaged in crying. Cries of the premature infant were dubbed onto the full-term baby's video tape, and vice versa, in order to control for the influence of physical characteristics on parental responding. Findings indicated increased emotional and physiological arousal in response to the premature baby's cry as contrasted with that of the full-term baby. Furthermore, parents reported less willingness to interact with the premature than with the full-term infant. Further examination revealed that parents react negatively to infants labeled as "premature" or "difficult" regardless of actual birth status (Frodi, Lamb, Leavitt, & Donovan, 1978). Frodi and Lamb (1980) extended their research on emotional and physiological responses to premature infants to child abusers. When compared to nonabusive parents, child abusers evidenced more pronounced increases in autonomic and emotional arousal when presented with the cries of a premature infant. In addition, abusive parents showed similar patterns of response to a smiling infant. Thus, abusive parents appear to view as aversive almost any social contact with a premature infant.

Although these studies describe the mechanisms through which prematurity may contribute to abuse, two methodological limitations prevent drawing firm conclusions from the data. First, the analogue nature of the aforementioned investigations do not demonstrate that such processes are found in the natural environment. And second, it is unclear from these findings that the negative behaviors displayed by premature infants precede and subsequently elicit abuse from caretakers. Rather, such aversive characteristics may develop as a function of abuse, although they also may serve to elicit further maltreatment in the future (Frodi, 1981).

Similar difficulty delineating cause and effect is encountered in the study of attachment formation in maltreated infants. Attachment is the affective and social bond between mother and infant formed via the unique contributions of parent and child (Ainsworth, Blehar, Waters, & Wall, 1978). Attachment is a qualitative construct that can be categorized as secure or insecure (Sroufe & Waters, 1977). Behavioral deficits in attachment-promoting behaviors exhibited by the mother and/or the infant can lead to insecure attachment. Ainsworth (1980), a pioneer in the empirical examination of attachment formation, has proposed that insecure attachment related to parental characteristics (e.g., unresponsiveness, inadequate caretaking) or aversive child behaviors (e.g., frequent crying, difficult to calm) can lead to maltreatment. However, no data are available showing that disruption in attachment leads to abuse or neglect, but numerous studies have shown disproportionate occurrence of insecure attachment in maltreated infants and their mothers (see Cicchetti, 1987), although it is most likely that such disruptions are a consequence rather than a cause of maltreatment (see Chapter 5 in this volume). Well-controlled prospective research is needed to examine more fully the possibility that insecure mother–infant attachment can lead directly to maltreatment.

Gaensbauer and Sands (1979) outlined the temperamental characteristics displayed by abused infants that may contribute to maltreatment. Based on observations of mother–infant interactions, they delineated the following disruptions in infant social and emotional responses that impede the formation of secure mother–infant attachment: affective withdrawal, lack of pleasure, inconsistency and unpredictability in affective communications, shallowness of affect communications, ambiguity or ambivalence in affective expression, and negative affect messages. The authors acknowledged the possibility that such infant behavioral disturbances may be a function of abusive caretaking rather than a cause, but point out the critical interdependence of the mother–infant relationship. They stated that

> disturbances in affective communication probably grow out of desynchronous, unsatisfying interactions with caretakers beginning very early in the child's life. Such desynchrony may result from constitutional factors in the child . . . or from inadequacies in the parents, or both . . . once established, such characteristics take on a life of their own and actively work upon the environment, including the caretakers who may have been instrumental in their initial development. (p. 248)

Crittenden (1985) empirically examined deviant infant behavior in abusive, neglecting, problematic, and adequate care mother–infant dyads. In general, maltreated infants were found to display behavior patterns that were more difficult to manage and more disagreeable than their non-maltreated counterparts. In a second experiment, Crittenden (1985) provided maltreating mothers with a program designed to enhance their sensitivity and responsivity to their infants. Results indicated that when these mothers showed gains in sensitivity, their infant's behavior subsequently improved as well. No changes in infant behavior were noted in families in which the abusive mother did not benefit from treatment. These findings provide compelling evidence for the relative primacy of mother behaviors over infant temperament in the relationship, and cast doubt on the infant's role in the development of maltreatment.

Egeland and Brunnquell (1979) provided the only prospective research data evaluating the role of child temperament in causing abuse. In their large-scale of high-risk mothers identified during pregnancy, Egeland and Brunnquell (1979) compared adequate care and inadequate care mothers and their infants using a variety of assessments, including measures of parenting attitudes, infant temperament, infant observations, and mother–infant observations. A discriminant analysis revealed that several infant characteristics distinguished adequate and inadequate care mothers. These consisted of infant orientation, irritability, and consolability. However, such other factors as maternal hostility and negative reactions to pregnancy, were more predictive of group classification than these infant behaviors. Thus, although infant variables' behaviors have some predictive power in distinguishing adequate from inadequate care mothers, other influences appear to be more salient in the development of maltreatment.

Relatively few empirical efforts have been directed toward the causative contribution of behavior problems in toddlers and preschool children to maltreatment. Despite its prominence in certain theoretical formulations, a paucity of data exists examining this relationship. There is no doubt that most maltreated children display extensive and varied behavior problems (see Ammerman *et al.*, 1986). But it is typically assumed that such psychopathologies are sequelae of abuse and neglect rather than causes of maltreatment. Also, it has been shown that child misbehavior can precipitate a specific abusive incident (Kadushin & Martin, 1981). Once again, this process is thought to take place in families already predisposed to abuse. Thus, although acting out, noncompliance, and oppositionality can be viewed as "abuse-provoking behaviors" (deLissovoy, 1979; Rusch, Hall, & Griffin, 1986), it is unclear to what extent such problems bring about an abusive relationship as opposed to maintaining or exacerbating previously extant maltreatment.

COMMENTS

Findings regarding the contribution of early childhood characteristics to maltreatment are equivocal. Retrospective studies underscore the high rate prematurity, low birthweight, early separations, and disrupted attachment in abused and neglected infants. Prospective studies, which offer a methodologically stronger experimental approach, provide little support for the hypothesis that difficult children are a major cause of abuse or neglect. The critical question is one of cause and effect: Are child characteristics contributors to or sequelae of maltreatment? Prospective designs are the only acceptable empirical approach to examining this issue and, to date, such studies have not indicated a major role for child characteristics in the etiology of abuse and neglect. However, it is documented that certain early childhood behavioral factors can be highly aversive, particularly to abusive parents (Frodi, 1981). According to the Transitional Model of maltreatment (Wolfe, 1987), childhood factors can lead to abuse *under specific conditions* related to the presence or absence of destabilizing and compensatory influences. Therefore, early childhood characteristics by themselves may be insufficient to elicit maltreatment, although within particular contexts (that have yet to be empirically identified) they might lead to abuse or neglect.

COERCIVE INTERACTIONS IN THE DEVELOPMENT AND MAINTENANCE OF ABUSE

Although findings linking child characteristics and maltreatment are equivocal, a growing body of literature indicates that children can contribute to an escalation of conflict that may lead to physical abuse. Indeed, recent theorists have identified interactions in the parent–child dyad as one of the most critical components in explaining the development and maintenance of abuse (Burgess & Draper, 1988). According to this framework, individual features of parent and child are less important than the interaction between the two. Thus, Wolfe (1987) rejected single-factor etiologic models of maltreatment and argued that "child abuse can best be explained as the *result of an interaction* between the parent and child within a system that seldom provides alternative solutions . . . or clear cut restraints . . ." (p. 51).

Numerous empirical efforts have been directed toward examining the nature of the interactions between maltreating parents and their children (see Wolfe & St. Pierre, 1989). These studies clearly document dysfunctional interaction patterns. In general, findings indicate that, although abusive parent–child dyads rarely exhibit higher levels of negative interactions, there is a paucity of reciprocal positive behaviors. Thus, parental responding is characterized by a lack of positive social interactions, low delivery of positive reinforcement, and restricted or negative affect. Likewise, abused children often are withdrawn, aggressive, and rarely initiate positive peer and adult contacts (Bousha & Twentyman, 1984; Schindler & Arkowitz, 1986).

Findings from the aforementioned studies, however, do not elucidate the coercive and interdependent processes of escalating conflict in maltreating parents and their children. Rather, it is possible that child misbehavior is a direct consequence of their parent's abusive and controlling management strategies. On the other hand, investigations employing sequential analytic techniques have documented the interactional nature of parent–child conflicts that leads to a mutual escalation of conflict and violence. For example, Oldershaw, Walters, and Hall (1986) compared the interactions of 10 abusive and 10 nonabusive mother–child pairs. Use of control strategies and child compliance were observed in a 40-min laboratory observational assessment during which mothers and their children simulated selected home activities. Results indicated that abusive mothers were more likely to use power assertive control strategies (e.g., threats, negative demand, disapproval) rather than more positively oriented approaches (e.g., reasoning, cooperation, approval) when contrasted with nonabusive mothers. In addition, abused children exhibited higher levels of disobedience and non-compliance than their nonabused peers. Sequential analyses further elucidated the tendency of abusive mothers to respond to child non-compliance with negative control strategies, thus worsening overall parent–child conflict.

In another study, Trickett and Kuczynski (1986) examined disciplinary practices in abusive and nonabusive mothers of children aged 4–10 years. Specifically, parents completed a Parent Daily Report of child transgressions and parental responses. Findings showed that abused children exhibited more behavior problems than nonabused children, and that abusive parents were more likely to use punitive disciplinary practices when compared to nonabusive parents. Moreover, abusive parents resorted to punitive strategies regardless of the severity of the child's misbehavior, whereas their nonabusive counterparts only employed punitive techniques for more serious misbehavior. These results underscore the coercive interaction that leads to the escalation of parent–child conflict in abusive families.

Stringer and LaGreca (1985) examined the relationship between coercive processes and child abuse in a hospital clinic sample of mothers. The authors hypothesized that, according to coercion theory (Patterson, 1981), potential for engaging in child abuse is related to an external locus of control and child behavior problems. Subjects were administered the Child Abuse Potential Inventory (CAP) (Milner, 1986), and measures of locus of control and child misbehavior. Findings revealed a positive relationship between elevated scores on the CAP and perceptions of control by others in mothers of male children. In addition, perceptions of control by others and CAP scores were associated with conduct and anxious-withdrawn behavior problems in children. Similar results were not noted in mothers of female children. However, this discrepancy is not surprising in that the coercive process appears to be more pronounced in families of male rather than female children. Although this investigation did not use mothers engaging in documented abuse or directly measure mother–child interactions, it does elucidate factors that contribute to the development of coercive dynamics in families.

Reid, Patterson, and Loeber (1982) provided one of the most comprehensive descriptions of coercive processes in abusive families. Reid *et al.* (1982) argued that the occurrence of child abuse is related to two factors: (1) the frequency of aversive interactions between parent and child that might lead to an abusive incident, and (2) the parent's ability to terminate quickly such parent–child confrontations. Observational studies have confirmed that abusive families engage in frequent and prolonged confrontations relative to nonabusive families. For example, Reid (1981, cited in Reid *et al.*, 1982) conducted home observations of distressed, distressed but not abusive, and abusive families. In general, there was a high positive correlation between rate of child oppositional/noncompliant behavior and parents engaging is threats or physically punitive behaviors across all groups. This association was most pronounced, however, in abusive families. Patterson (1981) further demonstrated that the child's acting out and parent's aversive behavior covary within families, as well. Finally, Reid, Taplin, and Loeber (1981) reported that nonabusive parents failed to terminate confrontations 14% of the time, whereas abusive parents were unsuccessful 35% of the time. Abusive mothers, in particular, demonstrated difficulty in discontinuing aversive interactions, failing to end them 53% of the time.

COMMENTS

There is compelling evidence that coercive parent–child interactions are a major component in the etiology and continuation of child abuse. Studies in this area are noteworthy because they (1) typically utilize well-controlled experimental designs, and (2) examine interactional and sequential elements of abusive family dynamics rather than using a more simplistic unidimensional formulation. The coercive approach to understanding child abuse clearly implicates the child as a contributor to abuse. However, findings in this area do not suggest that the child is necessarily an instigator of abuse. Rather, it is more likely that severe behavioral disturbance develops as a product of parental dysfunction. Once in place, however, the pattern of escalating conflict between parent and child assumes an independent existence, seemingly resistant to change from either family member. At this point, the child plays an active role in maintaining the abusive relationship, and outside intervention is required to break the maladaptive cycle.

HANDICAP AS A RISK FACTOR FOR MALTREATMENT

A number of recent reviews have suggested that handicapped children may be at heightened risk for abuse and neglect (Ammerman, Van Hasselt, & Hersen, 1988b; Jaudes & Diamond, 1985; White, Benedict, Wulff, & Kelley, 1987; Zirpoli, 1986). These authors proposed that, because many handicapped or disabled children exhibit characteristics implicated in maltreatment in nonhandicapped populations, they should be viewed as being particularly susceptible to maltreatment. In general, it is hypothesized that increased risk is manifested via three conditions: (1) disruptions in mother–infant attachment, (2) greater stress experienced by caretakers engendered by the behavior problems exhibited by many handicapped children, and (3) heightened vulnerability of children with disabilities to maltreatment.

There are six factors that may serve to disrupt the formation of mother–infant attachment in many children with disabling conditions (see Ammerman *et al.*, 1988b). First, there is evidence to suggest that some parents exhibit negative reactions upon the birth of a handicapped child (Gath, 1977; Waisbren, 1980). Typical responses include disbelief, shock, guilt, and disappointment (Emde & Brown, 1978). Although most parents adequately adjust to this occurrence (Drotar, Baskiewicz, Irvin, Kennell, & Klaus, 1975), some do not, and they may subsequently experience further disturbance in the development of the parent–child relationship. Second, some investigators have reported maternal loneliness, depression, and withdrawal following the birth of a handicapped infant (Emde & Brown, 1978; Lambert & West, 1980). The clinical significance of these symptoms, however, and their impact on parent–child functioning, is unclear. Third, there are reports in the clinical literature documenting hostile feelings directed by parents toward their handicapped children (Bauman & Yoder, 1966; Shaffer, 1964). Although empirical support for this factor is lacking, it is possible that such hostility can lead to maltreatment in handicapped children.

Fourth, several investigations have reported disruptions in the formation of secure mother–infant attachment in handicapped populations (Cicchetti & Serafica, 1981; Emde & Brown, 1978; Fox, 1988; Stone & Chesney, 1978; Wasserman, 1986; Wasserman, Lennon, Allen, & Shilansky, 1987). Such disturbances are partly a function of the behavioral deficits (e.g., hypo or hypertonicity, unresponsiveness, lack of eye contact) displayed by many disabled children, particularly those with severe impairments. Moreover, mothers may misinterpret these behavioral deficits and lack of responsiveness as "disinterest" on the part of the infant. In turn, this may result in a reciprocal decrease in attachment-promoting behaviors exhibited by the mother, thus further eroding the attachment bond (Wasserman, Allen, & Solomon, 1985). A fifth negative influence on the parent–child relationship often found in handicapped populations is the frequent early separations between the child and his or her family because of hospitalizations secondary to medical complications at birth. Because of several retrospective studies indicating a relationship between early separation and maltreatment (e.g., Lynch, 1975), this might be an additional risk factor for handicapped children. Finally, a sixth aspect affecting the parent–child relationship in handicapped populations are unrealistic and inaccurate expectations held by some parents regarding their disabled child's development and abilities. Excessive expectations and parental denial (Warren, 1977) may result in profound disappointment and frustration as the child repeatedly fails to meet anticipated goals (Scott, 1969). This may, in turn, increase the probability of abusive behavior.

Numerous investigators have documented the role of stress, and particularly the lack of adequate coping skills, in the development of maltreatment (Browne, 1986; Egeland et al., 1980; Straus, 1980). Specifically, it is proposed that stress leads to increased frustration that can lead to physical abuse. In particular, prolonged exposure to stress appears to be more related to abuse than isolated stressful incident (Rohner & Rohner, 1978). This issue is particularly critical for families with a handicapped child. Indeed, the introduction of a handicapped child into the home raises parental stress levels because of increased care requirements, greater financial obligations, and difficult-to-manage behavior problems (see Gallagher, Beckman, & Cross, 1983). In fact, the behavior problems evinced by many handicapped children, and especially those with multiple handicapping conditions (Van Hasselt, Ammerman, & Sisson, in press), can be very aversive and difficult to manage. Some examples of these include: rocking, eye poking, hand flapping, disruptiveness, aggression, and screaming. These problems often require consistent application of behavior management techniques in order to bring them under control. Moreover, most parents require specific training to use these techniques in an effective manner (Sisson, Van Hasselt, Hersen, & Aurand, 1988). Thus, the chronicity and pervasiveness of the more severely handicapped children's dysfunctions would seem to place them at high risk for abuse (Ammerman, Lubetsky, Hersen, & Van Hasselt, 1988a).

The final risk factor associated with maltreatment in the handicapped is vulnerability. Infants are often overrepresented in child abuse reports partly because they are more vulnerable to abuse (Gelles, 1978). This fact may be an artifact, however, in that infants also are more likely to be injured by maltreatment when contrasted with older children, and therefore are more likely to come to the attention of authorities. Handicapped children, particularly those with severe disabilities, also can be categorized as vulnerable. Depending upon the extent and severity of their handicap, these children may be unable to defend themselves (Morgan, 1987). Furthermore, children with cognitive or language deficits may be "easy targets" given their inability to report incidents of maltreatment. Detection of abuse and neglect in severely handicapped children may be further confounded by the occurrence of bruises and abrasions resulting from accidents related to their impairment (e.g., falling down, bumping into objects). At times, distinguishing between accidental and abuse-related injury may be difficult. Also, many disabled children are more prone to neglect because of their increased care requirements and medical needs (Ammerman *et al.*, 1988b).

INCIDENCE OF MALTREATMENT IN
HANDICAPPED POPULATIONS

Although several investigations have reported a disproportionate number of handicapped children in abused and neglected samples, findings vary considerably. A wide range of incidence levels (4% to 70%) has been found (Birrell & Birrell, 1968, Crittenden, 1985; Gil, 1970; Hawkins & Duncan, 1985; E. C. Herrenkohl & R. C. Herrenkohl, 1979; Iowa Department of Social Services, 1977; Johnson & Morse, 1968; Lightcap, Kurland, & Burgess, 1982; Sandgrund, Gaines, & Green, 1974; Starr, 1982). Discrepancies in results are related to differences in criteria for what constitutes a handicap, and difficulties in identifying abuse and neglect in handicapped children. Many of the studies employ unclear and incomplete definitions of disabling conditions, whereas others provide no such information. Thus, samples include children with minor physical anomalies as well as those with more severely handicapping sensory and orthopedic handicaps. Another impediment to accurate epidemiological investigation of the occurrence of maltreatment in these populations is the problem of recognizing and substantiating assault. As previously mentioned, many more severely handicapped children are unable to understand or report the occurrence of physical and/or sexual abuse. In addition, some physically handicapped children suffer contusions and abrasions related to their handicap rather than abuse *per se*.

Although a large body of research has accrued suggesting greater risk for abuse and neglect in handicapped children, a few investigators have questioned the relationship between having a handicapping condition and subsequent maltreatment. At issue, in general, is the child's role in the etiology of maltreatment (Egeland & Vaughn, 1981), and, in particular, the increased risk for abuse in handicapped children (Starr, Dietrich, Fischhoff, Ceresnie, & Zweier, 1984). Paradoxically, it has been suggested that the more severely disabled child is at *decreased* risk for assault (Martin & Beezley, 1974; Steele, 1980). Starr *et al.* (1984) and Steele (1980) base their conclusions on the methodological weaknesses (i.e., retrospective designs) of studies linking certain child characteristics (e.g., prematurity) with maltreatment. Also, Martin and Beezley (1974) cite their clinical experience that handicapped children are not likely targets for maltreatment. They propose that, for the parent, a handicapped child's misbehavior is clearly related to his or her impairment, and not intent. This understanding, in turn, mitigates the frustration that may lead to abuse. Children with conditions that are less evident to the parent (e.g., Attention Deficit Hyperactivity Disorder), it is hypothosized, are more likely to be at risk for maltreatment (Martin & Beezley, 1974). However, perceptions of intent appear to have little relation to the occurrence of abusive incidents (Rosenberg & Reppucci, 1983). Rather, abusive parents are more likely to respond negatively to child problem behaviors that are resistant to intervention regardless of intentionality (e.g., crying). In addition, although incidence rates of abuse are higher in hyperactive children relative to the general population (Heffron, Martin, Welsh, Perry, & Moore, 1987), they are not significantly different from other clinic-referred or psychiatrically disturbed children.

There are several methodological and conceptual problems with the aforementioned positions. First, very few of the studies on child characteristics and their causal role in abuse include handicapped children in their samples. Second, investigations that do involve handicapped children primarily examine those with more minor physical anomalies (e.g., extra digits, cleft palate) rather than those with more severely debilitating handicapping conditions. Third, almost no multihandicapped children are represented in these efforts. Because it is hypothesized that the form and magnitude of behavior problems exhibited by many multihandicapped children (e.g., aggression, stereotypic behaviors) play an important role in the development of maltreatment, it is of paramount importance that such children be carefully evaluated before conclusions about their risk for abuse and neglect are reached (Ammerman *et al.*, 1988a).

Some investigations, however, have assessed the incidence of maltreatment in samples of handicapped children. In a retrospective analysis, Diamond and Jaudes (1983) reviewed medical charts of 86 children and adolescents with cerebral palsy. Their results indicated that 9% had been maltreated following the diagnosis of cerebral palsy, and an additional 14% were labeled as "at risk" for maltreatment using numerous criteria thought to be related to maltreatment risk. In a more recent effort, Ammerman, Hersen, Van Hasselt, McGonigle, and Lubetsky (1989) examined abuse and neglect in psychiatrically hospitalized multihandicapped children. These children were selected for study because of their extensive handicaps and, in most cases, severe behavioral dysfunction, that would place them at especially high-risk for abuse and neglect. A retrospective analysis of 150 charts revealed that 39% had been victims or warranted high suspicion of past and/or current maltreatment. Physical abuse was the most common form, occurring in 69% of the subgroup that was maltreated. This was followed by neglect (45%) and sexual abuse (36%). Of particular significance was the severity of maltreatment. For example, 66% of the sexual abuse cases involved penetration. Also, 40% of the sexually abused children were assaulted by multiple perpetrators. Finally, 52% of the subgroup of maltreated children experienced more than one form of maltreatment (e.g., abuse *and* neglect), many of them concurrently.

COMMENTS

The role of the handicapped child in the etiology of maltreatment is, at best, unclear. Researchers are equally divided in their confidence that disability is (Morgan, 1987) or is not (Starr *et al.*, 1984) a risk factor for abuse and neglect. Unfortunately, this area has not received the research attention required to resolve this issue. An overreliance on retrospective designs prevents the examination of a causal relationship between handicapping conditions and maltreatment. In addition, much of the prospective research fails to examine more severely handicapped and multihandicapped children. Thus, inferences drawn from these data may be inapplicable to multihandicapped populations. As with the association between other child characteristics and maltreatment, it is unlikely that handicaps in isolation cause abuse and neglect (Ammerman *et al.*, 1988b). Rather, presence of a handicap *in combination with other factors* raises the overall risk for maltreatment.

SUMMARY

This chapter began with the premise that child characteristics can contribute to the etiology of physical abuse and neglect. The framework for this hypothesis is drawn from recent theoretical formulations (the

Social-Interactional Model and the Transitional Model) that describe the processes through which certain child factors increase maltreatment risk. The impetus for research in this area comes from the pressing need to identify populations at risk for abuse and neglect so that they can receive preventive interventions before maltreatment ultimately develops.

Current findings do not provide strong support for the role of the child in abuse and neglect. Prospective studies have identified several behavioral characteristics that can contribute to maltreatment (Egeland & Brunnquell, 1979), but the explanatory power of these variables is minor relative to other causative factors. However, a variety of well-controlled studies have documented that child noncompliance and oppositionality can serve to maintain a preexisting abusive relationship (Reid et al., 1982). In this instance, the child may have little to do with the development of abuse, although he or she may contribute to the occurrence of subsequent abusive incidents. Finally, several authors have proposed that presence of a severe handicap can uniquely increase the overall likelihood of maltreatment (Ammerman et al., 1986; Morgan, 1987). Although preliminary studies document high rates of abuse and neglect in these populations (Ammerman et al., 1989; Diamond & Jaudes, 1983), few direct empirical investigations have been conducted in this area.

A major problem afflicting the study of child characteristics is that child maltreatment is a multidetermined phenomenon that defies unitary causal explanation. By its very nature, child abuse grows out of an interaction between two individuals: the perpetrator and the child. The most promising area of future research is to identify characteristics of the interaction or parent–child relationship rather than individual factors as predictors of maltreatment. The important question then becomes under what conditions do which child characteristics lead to maltreatment? What combination of variables (related to the child, perpetrator, or situation) heighten risk for abuse? Such a multivariate empirical approach is critical at this juncture in the search for childhood risk factors.

ACKNOWLEDGMENTS

Preparation of this chapter was facilitated in part by grant No. G008720109 from the National Institute on Disabilities and Rehabilitation Research, U.S. Department of Education, and a grant from the Vira I. Heinz Endowment. However, the opinions reflected herein do not necessarily reflect the position of policy of the U.S. Department of Education or the Vira I. Heinz Endowment and no official endorsement should be inferred. The author wishes to thank Mary Jo Horgan for her assistance in preparation of the manuscript.

REFERENCES

Ainsworth, M. D. (1980). Attachment and child abuse. In G. Gerber, C. Ross, & E. Zigler (Eds.), *Child abuse: An agenda for action* (pp. 35–47). New York: Oxford University Press.

Ainsworth, M. D. S., Blehar, M. C., Waters, E., & Wall, S. (1978). *Patterns of attachment: A psychological study of the strange situation.* Hillsdale, NJ: Lawrence Erlbaum.

American Association for Protecting Children. (1988). *Highlights of official child neglect and abuse reporting 1986.* Denver: American Humane Association.

Ammerman, R. T. (1989). Child abuse and neglect. In M. Hersen (Ed.), *Innovations in child behavior therapy* (pp. 353–394). New York: Springer.

Ammerman, R. T., Cassisi, J. E., Hersen, M., & Van Hasselt, V. B. (1986). Consequences of physical abuse and neglect in children. *Clinical Psychology Review, 6,* 291–310.

Ammerman, R. T., Lubetsky, M. J., Hersen, M., & Van Hasselt, V. B. (1988a). Maltreatment of children and adolescents with multiple handicaps: Five case examples. *Journal of the Multihandicapped Person, 1,* 129–139.

Ammerman, R. T., Van Hasselt, V. B., & Hersen, M. (1988b). Maltreatment of handicapped children: A critical review. *Journal of Family Violence, 3,* 53–72.

Ammerman, R. T., Hersen, M., Van Hasselt, V. B., McGonigle, J. J., & Lubetsky, M. J. (1989). Abuse and neglect in psychiatrically hospitalized multihandicapped children. *Child Abuse and Neglect, 13,* 335–343.

Bauman, M. K., & Yoder, N. M. (1966). *Adjustment to blindness—Reviewed.* Springfield, IL: Charles C Thomas.

Belsky, J. (1980). Child maltreatment: An ecological integration. *American Psychologist, 35,* 320–335.

Birrell, R., & Birrell, J. (1968). The maltreatment syndrome in children: A hospital survey. *Medical Journal of Australia, 2,* 1023–1029.

Bousha, D. M., & Twentyman, C. T. (1984). Mother-child interactional style in abuse, neglect, and control groups: Naturalistic observations in the home. *Child Development, 93,* 106–114.

Browne, D. H. (1986). The role of stress in the commission of subsequent acts of child abuse and neglect. *Journal of Family Violence, 1,* 289–297.

Burgess, R. L., & Draper, P. (1988). A biosocial theory of family violence: The role of natural selection, ecological instability, and coercive interpersonal contingencies. In L. Ohlin & M. H. Tonry (Eds.), *Criminal and justice—An annual review of research: Family violence.* Chicago: University of Chicago Press.

Cicchetti, D. (1987). Developmental psychopathology in infancy: Illustration from the study of maltreated youngsters. *Journal of Consulting and Clinical Psychology, 55,* 837–845.

Cicchetti, D., & Serafica, F. C. (1981). Interplay among behavioral systems: Illustrations from the study of attachment, affiliation, and wariness in young children with Down's Syndrome, *Developmental Psychology, 17,* 36–49.

Crittenden, P. M. (1985). Maltreated infants: Vulnerability and resilience. *Journal of Child Psychology and Psychiatry, 26,* 85–96.

deLissovoy, V. (1979). Toward the definition of "abuse provoking child." *Child Abuse and Neglect, 3,* 341–350.

Diamond, L. J., & Jaudes, P. K. (1983). Child abuse in a cerebral-palsied population. *Developmental Medicine and Child Neurology, 25,* 169–174.

Drotar, D., Baskiewicz, A., Irvin, N., Kennell, J., & Klaus, M. (1975). The adaptation of parents to the birth of an infant with congenital malformation: A hypothetical model, *Pediatrics, 56,* 710–717.

Egeland, B., & Brunnquell, D. (1979). An at-risk approach to the study of child abuse. *Journal of the American Academy of Child Psychiatry, 18,* 219–236.

Egeland, B., & Vaughn, B. (1981). Failure of "bond formation" as a cause of abuse, neglect, and maltreatment. *American Journal of Orthopsychiatry, 51,* 78–84.

Egeland, B., Breitenbucher, M., & Rosenberg, D. (1980). Prospective study of significance of etiology of child abuse. *Journal of Consulting and Clinical Psychology, 48,* 195–205.

Elmer, E., & Gregg, G. S. (1967). Developmental characteristics of abused children. *Pediatrics, 40,* 596–602.

Emde, R. N., & Brown, C. (1978). Adaptation to the birth of a Down's Syndrome infant. Grieving and maternal attachment. *Journal of the American Academy of Child Psychiatry, 17,* 299–323.

Fontana, V. J. (1973). The diagnosis of the maltreatment syndrome in children. *Pediatrics, 51,* 780–782.

Fox, N. A. (1988). The effect of prematurity and postnatal illness on the mother-infant interaction: A study of a high-risk dyad. In E. J. Anthony & C. Chiland (Eds.), *The child in his family: Perilous development: Child raising and identity formation under stress* (pp. 211–222). New York: Wiley.

Friedrich, W. N., & Boriskin, J. A. (1976). The role of the child in abuse: A review of the literature. *American Journal of Orthopsychiatry, 46,* 580–590.

Friedrich, W. N., & Einbender, A. J. (1983). The abused child: A psychological review. *Journal of Clinical Child Psychology, 12,* 244–256.

Frodi, A. M. (1981). Contribution of infant characteristics to child abuse. *American Journal of Mental Deficiency, 85,* 341–349.

Frodi, A. M., & Lamb, M. E. (1980). Child abusers' responses to infant smiles and cries. *Child Development, 51,* 238–241.

Frodi, A. M., Lamb, M. E., Leavitt, L., & Donovan, W. (1978). Fathers' and mothers' responses to infant smiles and cries. *Infant Behavior and Development, 1,* 187–198.

Frodi, A. M., Lamb, M., Leavitt, L., Donovan, W., Neff, C., & Sherry, D. (1978). Fathers' and mothers' responses to the appearance and cries of premature and normal infants. *Developmental Psychology, 14,* 490–498.

Gaensbauer, T. J., & Sands, K. (1979). Distorted affective communications in abused/neglected infants and their potential impact on caretakers. *Journal and the American Academy of Child Psychiatry, 18,* 236–250.

Gaines, R., Sandgrund, A., Green, A. H., & Power, E. (1978). Etiological factors in child maltreatment: A multivariate study of abusing, neglecting, and normal mothers. *Journal of Abnormal Psychology, 87,* 531–540.

Gallagher, J. J., Beckman, P., & Cross, A. H. (1983). Families of handicapped children: Sources of stress and its amelioration. *Exceptional Children, 50,* 10–19.

Garbarino, J. (1976). A preliminary study of some ecological correlates of child abuse: The impact of socioeconomic stress on mothers. *Child Development, 47,* 178–185.

Gath, A. (1977). The impact of an abnormal child upon the parents. *British Journal of Psychiatry, 130,* 405–410.

Gelles, R. J. (1973). Child abuse as psychopathology: A sociological critique and reformulation. *American Journal of Orthopsychiatry, 43,* 611–621.

Gelles, R. J. (1978). Violence toward children in the United States. *American Journal of Orthopsychiatry, 48,* 580–592.

Gil, D. (1970). *Violence against children: Physical child abuse.* Cambridge: Harvard University Press.

Hawkins, W. E., & Duncan, D. F. (1985). Children's illnesses as risk factors for child abuse. *Psychological Reports, 56,* 638.

Heffron, W. M., Martin, C. A., Welsh, R. J., Perry, P., & Moore, C. K. (1987). Hyperactivity and child abuse. *Canadian Journal of Psychiatry, 32,* 384–386.

Herrenkohl, E. C., & Herrenkohl, R. C. (1979). A comparison of abused children and their nonabused siblings. *Journal of the American Academy of Child and Adolescent Psychiatry, 18,* 260–269.

Iowa Department of Social Services. (1977). *Statistical data on child abuse cases.* Report Series A-4.

Jaudes, P. K., & Diamond, L. J. (1985). The handicapped child and child abuse. *Child Abuse and Neglect, 9,* 341–347.

Johnson, B., & Morse, H. (1968). Injured children and their parents. *Children, 15,* 147–152.

Kadushin, A., & Martin, J. A. (1981). *Child abuse: An interactional event.* New York: Columbia University Press.

Kempe, C. H., Silverman, F. N., Steele, B. F., Droegemueller, W., & Silver, H. K. (1962). The battered child syndrome. *Journal of American Model Association, 181,* 105–112.

Klaus, M., & Kennell, J. (1970). Mothers separated from their newborn infants. *Pediatric Clinics of North America, 17,* 1015–1037.

Klein, M., & Stern, L. (1971). Low birth weight and the battered child syndrome. *American Journal of Diseases in Childhood, 122,* 15–18.

Lambert, R., & West, M. (1980). Parenting styles and the depressive syndrome in congenitally blind individuals. *Journal of Visual Impairment and Blindness, 74,* 333–337.

Lightcap, J. L., Kurland, J. A., & Burgess, R. L. (1982). Child abuse: A test of some predictions from evolutionary theory. *Ethology and Sociobiology, 3,* 61–67.

Lutzker, J. R., & Rice, J. M. (1984). Project 12-Ways: Measuring outcome of a large in-home service for treatment and prevention of child abuse and neglect. *Child Abuse and Neglect, 8,* 519–524.

Lynch, M. A. (1975). Ill-health and child abuse. *Lancet, 2,* 317–319.

Lynch, M. A., & Roberts, J. (1977). Predicting child abuse: Signs of bonding failure in the maternity hospital. *British Medical Journal, 1,* 624–626.

MacFarlane, K., Waterman, J., Conerly, S., Damon, L., Durfee, M., & Long, S. (Eds.). (1986). *Sexual abuse of young children.* New York: Guilford Press.

Martin, H. P., Beezley, P. (1974). Prevention and the consequences of child abuse. *Journal of Operational Psychiatry, 6,* 68–77.

Maurer, A. (1974). Corporal punishment. *American Psychologist, 29,* 614–626.

Milner, J. S. (1986). The child abuse potential inventory manual (2nd ed.). Webster, NC: Psytec.

Morgan, S. R. (1987). *Abuse and neglect of handicapped children.* Boston: Little, Brown.

Oates, K. (Ed.). (1982). *Child abuse: A community concern.* New York: Brunner/Mazel.

Oldershaw, L., Walters, G. C., & Hall, D. K. (1986). Control strategies and noncompliance in abusive mother-child dyads: An observational study. *Child Development, 57,* 722–732.

Parke, R. D., & Collmer, C. W. (1975). Child abuse: An interdisciplinary analysis: In E. M.

Hetherington (Ed.), *Review of child development research* (Vol. 5, pp. 509–590). Chicago: University of Chicago Press.

Patterson, G. R. (1981). *Families of antisocial children: An interactional approach.* Eugene, OR: Castalia Publishing.

Reid, J. B., Taplin, P., & Loeber, R. (1981). A social interactional approach to the treatment of abusive families. In R. B. Stuart (Ed.), *Violent behavior: Social learning approaches to prediction, management, and treatment* (pp. 83–101). New York: Brunner/Mazel.

Reid, J. B., Patterson, G. R., & Loeber, R. (1982). The abused child: Victim, instigator, or innocent bystander? *Nebraska Symposium on Motivation, 29,* 47–68.

Rohner, R. P., & Rohner, E. C. (1978). *A multivariate model for the study of parental acceptance-rejection and child abuse.* Storrs, CT: University of Connecticut.

Rosenberg, M. S., & Reppucci, N. D. (1983). Abusive mothers: Perceptions of their own and their children's behavior. *Journal of Consulting and Clinical Psychology, 51,* 674–682.

Rusch, R. G., Hall, J. C., & Griffin, H. C. (1986). Abuse-provoking characteristics of institutionalized mentally retarded individuals. *American Journal of Mental Deficiency, 90,* 618–624.

Sandgrund, A., Gaines, R., & Green, A. H. (1974). Child abuse and mental retardation: A problem of cause and effect. *American Journal of Mental Deficiency, 79,* 327–330.

Schindler, F., & Arkowitz, H. (1986). The assessment of mother-child interactions in physically abusive and nonabusive families. *Journal of Family Violence, 1,* 247–258.

Scott, R. A. (1969). The socialization of blind children. In D. Goslin (Ed.), *Handbook of socialization theory and research.* Chicago: Rand McNally.

Shaffer, H. R. (1964). The "too-cohesive" family: A form of group pathology. *International Journal of Social Psychiatry, 10,* 266–275.

Sherrod, K. B., O'Connor, S., Vietze, P. M., & Altemeier, W. A. (1984). Child health and maltreatment. *Child Development, 55,* 1174–1183.

Sisson, L. A., Van Hasselt, V. B., Hersen, M., & Avrand, J. (1988). Tripartite behavioral intervention to reduce stereotypic and disruptive behaviors in young multihandicapped children. *Behavior Therapy, 19,* 503–526.

Spinetta, J. J., & Rigler, D. (1972). The child abusing parent: A psychological review. *Psychological Bulletin, 77,* 296–304.

Sroufe, L. A., & Waters, E. (1977). Attachment as an organizational construct. *Child Development, 48,* 1184–1199.

Starr, R. H., Jr., (1982). A research-based approach to the prediction of child abuse. In R. H. Starr, Jr. (Ed.), *Child abuse prediction: Policy implications.* Cambridge, MA: Ballinger.

Starr, R. H., Jr. (1988). Physical abuse of children. In V. B. Van Hasselt, R. L. Morrison, A. S. Bellack, & M. Hersen (Eds.), *Handbook of family violence* (pp. 119–155). New York: Plenum Press.

Starr, R. H., Jr., Dietrich, K. N., Fischhoff, J., Ceresnie, S., & Zweier, D. (1984). The contribution of handicapping conditions to child abuse. *Topics in Early Childhood Special Education, 4,* 55–69.

Steele, B. (1980). Psychodynamic factors in child abuse. In C. H. Kempe & R. E. Helfer (Eds.), *The battered child* (3rd ed., pp. 49–85). Chicago: University of Chicago.

Stone, N. W., & Chesney, B. H. (1978). Attachment behaviors in handicapped infants. *Mental Retardation, 16,* 8–12.

Straus, M. A. (1980). Stress and child abuse. In C. H. Kempe and R. E. Helfer (Eds.), *The battered child* (3rd ed., pp. 86–102). Chicago: University of Chicago Press.

Stringer, S. A., & LaGreca, A. M. (1985). Correlates of child abuse potential. *Journal of Abnormal Child Psychology, 13,* 217–226.

Trickett, P. K., & Kuczynski, L. (1986). Children's misbehaviors and parental discipline strategies in abusive and nonabusive families. *Developmental Psychology, 22,* 115–123.

Van Hasselt, V. B., Ammerman, R. T., & Sisson, L. (in press). Physical disability. In A. S. Bellack, M. Hersen, & A. E. Kazdin (Eds.), *International handbook of behavior modification and therapy* (2nd ed.). New York: Plenum Press.

Waisbren, S. E. (1980). Parents' reactions after the birth of a developmentally disabled child. *American Journal of Mental Deficiency, 84,* 345–351.

Warren, D. A. (1977). *Blindness and early childhood development.* New York: American Foundation for the Blind.

Wasserman, G. A. (1986). Affective expression in normal and physically handicapped infants: Situational and developmental effects. *Journal of the American Academy of Child Psychiatry, 25,* 393–399.

Wasserman, G. A., Allen, R., & Solomon, C. R. (1985). At-risk toddlers and their mothers: The special case of physical handicaps. *Child Development, 56,* 73–83.

Wasserman, G. A., Lennon, M. C., Allen, R. & Shilansky, M. (1987). Contributors to attachment in normal and physically handicapped infants. *Journal of the American Academy of Child and Adolescent Psychiatry, 26,* 9–15.

White, R., Benedict, M. I., Wulff, L., & Kelley, M. (1987). Physical disabilities as risk factors for child maltreatment: A selected review. *American Journal of Orthopsychiatry, 57,* 93–101.

Wolfe, D. A. (1985). Child abusive parents: An empirical review and analysis. *Psychological Bulletin, 97,* 462–482.

Wolfe, D. A. (1987). *Child abuse: Implications for child development and psychopathology.* Newbury Park, CA: Sage.

Wolfe, D. A., & St. Pierre, J. (1989). Child abuse and neglect. In T. H. Ollendick & M. Hersen (Eds.), *Handbook of child psychopathology,* (2nd ed., pp. 377–398). New York: Plenum Press.

Zirpoli, T. J. (1986). Child abuse and children with handicaps. *Remedial and Special Education, 7,* 39–48.

Part IV

PREVENTION AND TREATMENT

CHAPTER 9

PREVENTION PROGRAMS

MAXINE R. NEWMAN AND JOHN R. LUTZKER

INTRODUCTION

A discussion of the prevention of child abuse or neglect, as any discussion of prevention, requires definition. In a seminal book *Principles of Preventive Psychiatry* (1964), Caplan defined three types of prevention, some of which were already in use by psychiatrists and psychologists as early as the mid-1960s: primary prevention, secondary prevention, and tertiary prevention. In this chapter, we will discuss these three levels of prevention generically, give a brief historical overview of past efforts to identify and prevent child abuse or neglect, define prevention in the area of child abuse or neglect, specifically when the intervention is intended to: prevent further abuse or prevent first abuse, consider some programs designed to prevent further abuse and others which focus on intervening before abuse occurs, and provide some recommendations for future prevention programs.

MAXINE R. NEWMAN AND JOHN R. LUTZKER • Department of Psychology, University of Judaism, Los Angeles, California 90077.

PREVENTION LEVELS

TERTIARY PREVENTION

Tertiary prevention has been described as a process that has the community-at-large as a client (Rappaport, 1977). The aim of tertiary prevention is to lower the rate of emotional or behavioral dysfunction in a given community. This label, then, would cover large-scale community programs directed toward the rehabilitation of individuals already diagnosed as suffering from a mental, emotional, or behavioral problem. The goals of tertiary programs are to reduce the severity and duration of these disorders. Caplan (1964) argued that the terms *rehabilitation* and *tertiary prevention* are not synonymous. For Caplan, the term rehabilitation refers to work that is done with an individual client, whereas tertiary prevention implies programs that intervene in an entire community. Thus, Caplan's definition covers large-scale service programs that effectively reach the total population of identified mental patients within a community. For example, the Joint Commission on Mental Health and Illness (1961) and the Joint Commission on Mental Health of Children (1970) were involved in tertiary prevention when they recommended removing as few patients as possible from their homes and their communities (Rappaport, 1977). The purpose of these decisions was to stop the process that Cumming and Cumming (1957) had labeled "closing the ranks," that is, the process whereby individuals living in a system, in which a member is removed, "close ranks" and another individual takes the identified patient's role in the system. The longer the duration of removal, the more difficult it is for the identified patient to resume a role within the system because it has been filled. Therefore, tertiary prevention deals with a policy of creating local community facilities for day-and-night care, including hospitals in which the duration of removal from the home or community is minimal in the belief that the shorter the removal, the less likely the chance of long-term problems. These tertiary prevention programs include an assumption that there will be a reduction in such problems across the community as a result of the intervention stance.

Further, tertiary prevention has implications for the quality of hospital or institutional care, should such care be necessary. Following the goals of tertiary prevention, an institution would provide much more than custodial care. When the stated or unstated goal is to get the patient back into the community as soon as possible, then rehabilitation programs, "milieu" or socioenvironmental treatment, token economies designed to teach adequate social functioning, use of "significant others" as volunteers, use of nonprofessional mental health workers in hospital and in the community, halfway houses, and vocational training programs are offered, all of which are examples of tertiary prevention (Rappaport, 1977).

SECONDARY PREVENTION

Although tertiary prevention is directed at large-scale community- or institution-based programs geared toward keeping diagnosed patients within their homes or communities and providing the necessary care and training to accomplish this end, secondary prevention has as its goal the early identification of and intervention into problems *before* they become major mental illnesses. In this context, Rappaport (1977) defined secondary prevention programs as those that are intended to reduce the rate of a given disorder by lowering its prevalence in an identified high-risk population. Thus, in secondary prevention the emphasis is on early identification of the problem and the risk factors in the life cycle of an individual. For example, secondary prevention programs are often aimed at children in order to provide an "enhanced opportunity to cope with developmental tasks" (Rappaport, 1977, p. 64). The goal of such programs is to prevent problems that may develop and thereby reduce the incidence and the prevalence of mental dysfunction. Although secondary prevention is most often geared toward the detection of risk factors in children, it can also mean such detection in adults who are at risk before their problems develop into severe disorders.

Caplan (1964) suggested that sharpening diagnostic tools and encouraging early referral are strategies that can be effective in early detection of risk factors. For example, Rappaport (1977) noted that during World War II the United States Army used the Minnesota Multiphasic Personality Inventory (MMPI) as a prescreening device to detect possible problems in inductees before they were sent to training or combat situations. Although he emphasized the shortcomings of such large-scale testing and the sacrifices in accuracy that may occur, he, nevertheless, recommended them to maximize efficiency and to get a global identification of problem groups. Cowen, Dorr, Clarfield, Kreling, McWilliams, Pokracki, Pratt, Terrell, and Wilson (1973) developed a brief 11-item scale that is designed so that teachers can record the symptom frequency of dysfunctional classroom behaviors among elementary school children that is another example of sharpening diagnostic tools to detect risk factors before problems actually develop. An example of encouraging early referral to treatment if a problem is suspected is the use of public education through the mass media (Rappaport, 1977). Rappaport (1977) further suggested consultation with physicians, psychologists, teachers, and clergy, and recommended that so-called walk-in clinics should be part of every hospital's services. Next, he prescribed gearing the diagnosis to specific treatment steps rather than separating diagnosis from treatment planning. Caplan (1964) urged that no diagnosis or labeling be done unless there is prompt and effective treatment available. He pointed out that labeling maladaptive behaviors may, in and of itself, create problems for the individual who is thus labeled. Finally, Rappaport (1977) cautioned professionals to withhold diagnosis and intervention in those types of cases in which "spontaneous recovery" is likely. Encouraging the collection of such data is a way of making community mental health facilities more accountable (Rappaport, 1977).

Primary Prevention

Caplan (1964) referred to primary prevention as a "community concept"; that is, it does not have as its goal the reduction of risk to any given individual. Rather, primary prevention programs seek to reduce the rate of new cases of disorders in a population over time by counteracting adverse influences before they have a chance to produce dysfunction. Primary prevention programs seek to lower the risk for a whole population. In this situation, some members of the population may become ill, but their numbers will be reduced in the population as a whole.

Such a definition per se involves mental health professionals in areas outside their customary practice. For example, to meet primary prevention goals a professional might become involved in political or social action. Further, the professional, in this instance, is encouraged to look at those factors that lead to health as well as those that lead to illness. And illness, in the context of primary prevention, is viewed as having a much wider scope than is usual, thereby inspiring professionals to intervene in areas that include societal problems or problems of living that might not, in the usual course of their work, fall into their province (Caplan, 1964). Rappaport (1977) concluded that primary prevention programs must focus on identifying environmental factors that influence a community. Some of these factors may be harmful and may therefore decrease a community's ability to cope with the stresses of life; others may be helpful and increase the coping ability of the community. Therefore, the goals of primary prevention programs are to produce optimum outcomes for a community, to discover what negatively influences a community, and provide treatment and/or social-political action to lower negative circumstances, to increase positive forces, and to reduce the incidence and prevalence of dysfunction in a community.

HISTORICAL OVERVIEW

CHILD ABUSE BEFORE THE BATTERED CHILD SYNDROME

During the Hellenistic period, the Greek, Soranus, advocated infanticide based upon a list of factors similar to the now-known risk factors for child abuse and neglect. In A.D. 900, Rhazes, a Persian, speculated that in cases of "prominence of the umbilicus" and "hernia of children," the child may have been intentionally injured. Writings from seventeenth and eighteenth century sources indicate knowledge of willful abuse of children by teachers and family members (Lynch, 1985). During the nineteenth century, experts were divided between two positions in cases of child maltreatment; some pleaded eloquently for medical recognition of the problem and included calls to action in their writings, whereas others, describing injuries and/or the results of neglect, were content to attribute such phenomena to unknown causes. It was during this same period that some physicians were instrumental in founding the English Society for the Prevention of Cruelty to Children, which brought to public and judicial attention 762 cases of child abuse and succeeded in obtaining 120 convictions. During this period the link between alcoholism and child abuse was openly discussed (Lynch, 1985). In the United States, the American Society for the Prevention of Cruelty to Animals gave rise to the New York Society for the Prevention of Cruelty to Children (Carstens, 1921). Schultz (1968) suggested that because the child protective movement grew out of the animal protective movement, the initial concern was with physical abuse, and the goal was to remove the child from the abusive environment. At the turn of the century, a new view of child protection was articulated. Fostered primarily by the Massachusetts Society for the Prevention of Cruelty to Children, the emphasis turned from removal and punishment, which were chiefly the province of the police, to interventions designed to reduce environmental causes of abuse and neglect and to promote improved conditions of family life, which were the province of humane societies (Schultz, 1968). Carstens (1911–1912), the general secretary of the Massachusetts Society for the Prevention of Cruelty to Children, looked to social workers to provide programs dealing with infant mortality, birth registration, child labor, pauperism, dependency, and venereal infection—that is, a "complete social program." Along with the Massachusetts society, other groups joined in the call for social programs to reduce poverty, disease, and dependency. After World War I, the New York Society for the Prevention of Cruelty to Children joined its more liberal colleagues by including the concepts of rehabilitation of perpetrators and reconstruction of family life into its program (Carstens, 1921). During the Great Depression and the years of social programming that followed, professionals involved in the protection of children no longer focused on law enforcement, but rather on rehabilitative interventions combined with a commitment to extensive social action.

After World War II, Caffey (1946) wrote of the continued reluctance of physicians to draw the "obvious conclusion" from the association of subdural hematomas and fractures in children. Although many authors writing from the 1930s through the 1950s still did not connect the characteristic X-ray appearances of injuries in very young children as being caused by parental abuse (Bakwin, 1956; Barmayer, Alderson, & Cox, 1951; Silverman, 1952; Snedecor, Knapp, & Wilson, 1935), others began to discuss the possibility of children being willfully mistreated by parents (Fisher, 1958), criminally neglected by parents (Kempe & Silver, 1959), and murdered by parents or caretakers (Adelson, 1969). By calling attention to the resistance of physicians and social workers to acknowledge the diagnosis (Elmer, 1960) and by describing a project in which legal authorities and hospital staff cooperated as advocates to protect children (Boardman, 1961), researchers in child abuse further set the stage for Kempe's seminal paper in 1961.

THE BATTERED CHILD SYNDROME

In 1961, at the meeting of the American Academy of Pediatrics, C. Henry Kempe and his associates at the Denver Medical Center first proposed the diagnosis of child abuse and neglect in a symposium entitled, "The Battered Child Syndrome" (Kempe, Silverman, Steele, Droegemuller, & Silver, 1962). Kempe and his colleagues clearly stated that

> the radiologic manifestations of trauma are specific and the metaphysical lesions in particular occur in no other disease of which we are aware. (p. 23)

Although physicians had previously relied on such diagnoses as scurvy, syphillis, osteogenisis imperfecta, infantile cortical hyperostosis, paraplegia, and congenital indifference to pain, after Kempe *et al.* (1962) it became difficult to avoid the obvious distinctions between the pathogenic manifestations of these conditions and the traumas inflicted in cases of child abuse and neglect (Lutzker & Newman, 1986). In this historic presentation, Kempe and his colleagues further suggested management strategies, including the controversial issue of reporting such cases to authorities. They further recommended strategies to communicate therapeutically with perpetrators. Finally, they urged physicians who had been disinclined to believe that parents could ever inflict such pain on their children, to reevaluate the evidence, and accept their duty to protect the child under their care.

AFTER KEMPE

Although it had become clear that the reporting of child abuse and/or neglect was crucial before any treatment or intervention could occur, there were differences between the Children's Bureau, the American Medical Association, and the American Humane Association over who should report (physicians only, or others who came in professional contact with children), to whom reports should be made (the police or a protective agency), and what kinds of abuse and neglect were to be reported (physical only or neglect and other forms of abuse) (Paulsen, 1968). However, by 1967, all 50 states had enacted some form of reporting law, and by 1973, a mandatory reporting law that required reports in all cases of suspected abuse and that protected the mandated reporter from reprisal for any action was in place in every state in the United States (Lucht, 1975).

Over the years, the medical model of child abuse and neglect has grown in acceptance, and child abuse and neglect have even been described as an "infectious disease" (Child Protection Report, 1976). This emphasis tends to neglect the social and environmental stressors that were recognized in earlier years as contributing factors in child abuse and neglect (Carstens, 1911–1912; Carstens, 1921; Schultz, 1968). Only recently have health professionals begun to integrate the two points-of-view and to recognize that child abuse and neglect are ecobehavioral problems influenced by parent characteristics, child characteristics, and socioenvironmental factors (Lutzker & Newman, 1986).

PREVENTION IN CHILD ABUSE AND NEGLECT

In the area of child abuse and/or neglect, prevention efforts may focus on reducing or eliminating further abuse in families already identified as abusive or neglectful, or actually preventing abuse or neglect before the problem occurs. In the first instance, prevention is likely to be tertiary or secondary; in the second, it will be primary or secondary. An emphasis was found in the literature on prevention programs that focus on sexual abuse of adolescents or programs dealing with either physical or emotional abuse.

A five-part tertiary prevention strategy emerged from a working conference on "Preventing Child Sexual Abuse: A Focus on the Potential Perpetrator" (Cohn, 1986). The following 10 points comprise the rationale for such a strategy: (1) child sexual abuse is a complex problem requiring multiple prevention strategies; (2) knowledge about abuse and prevention is not generally based on empirical findings; (3) because there is no data-based profile of the sexual abuser, consequently, prevention efforts cannot be geared to a specific group of potential perpetrators; (4) since sexual abuse does not only occur after age 21, adolescents and even younger children should also be targeted; (5) sexual abuse is not only an issue of power, thus such areas as sexual ideas, beliefs, misconceptions, and preferences must also be addressed; (6) there are no strongly voiced taboos in our society against molesting children, and often the values and messages transmitted through the media may even appear to condone behaviors that might lead to sexual abuse; (7) children do not know how to resist abuse; (8) children are sometimes placed in nonprotective environments; (9) there is no single law and no single profession that can handle a problem so deeply embedded in our societal values as sexual abuse; and (10) it is essential to increase public understanding of the problem and get public support for prevention programs. Given these assumptions, Cohn (1986) reported five prevention methods recommended by the conference: (1) quality sex education programs for teens and preteens; (2) training professionals and others who work with children how to identify and help abused children; (3) providing education to parents on attachment, bonding, appropriate and inappropriate touching, how to identify inappropriate behaviors in mates or others, how to identify abuse and help their children; (4) ensuring that all institutions and programs that serve children offer children training in self-awareness and self-protection; and (5) changing media messages for adults and adolescents to say: "Child sexual abuse is a crime; there is help out there; abuse is a chronic problem unless you get help; children get hurt when you sexually abuse them; children cannot consent to this kind of behavior." The message to children should say: "It's okay to say no; it's not your fault; reach out for help should this begin to happen to you; help is available out there for you."

As we previously mentioned, goals of secondary prevention efforts include the early identification of high-risk individuals or groups *before* abuse occurs, the reduction of the rate of abuse in high-risk populations, and the identification of risk factors for abuse and/or neglect. For example, Hagenhoff, Lowe, Hovell, and Rugg (1987) recommended a social learning theory approach to the prevention of teenage pregnancy. Hagenhoff and her colleagues (1987) suggested that Bandura's (1977) self-efficacy model may be useful in addressing this growing societal problem. They noted the following factors that govern the use of contraceptives by teens: (1) accessibility; (2) social/cultural factors; (3) family factors; (4) social skills and peer influence; (5) life career goals; (6) knowledge; and (7) expectations of personal mastery. Because such programs would be directed to a high-risk population, they would be considered secondary prevention interventions.

Another secondary prevention approach was described by Englert, Marneffe, Soumenkoff, and Hubinont (1985) regarding the use of tubal sterilization in a population at risk for abusing or neglecting their children. In their study, Englert et al. (1985) noted the following preconditions for tubal sterilization of regular maternity patients at the prenatal clinic at Saint-Pierre Hospital in Brussels: (1) the woman must be at least 30 years old; (2) there must be two living children; (3) there must be a stable communal background of at least 5 years; and (4) the couple must give written consent. In a comparison of 19 sterilized high-risk women and 18 regular maternity patients, Englert et al. (1985) found that the high-risk women differed from the regular maternity population: (1) they tended to be younger; (2) they tended not to be in a stable communal relationship; and (3) their children, if alive, were often either abandoned or in foster homes. Englert et al. (1985) concluded that there may be some institutional abuse in such a secondary prevention policy. Tubal sterilization is, "an aggressive act upon a woman's reproductive system." However, a physician has an ethical dilemma when serving the mother and the unborn child. If the physician's ultimate goal is "family health," then such ethical conflicts must be confronted.

Azar, Barnes, and Twentyman (1988) discussed secondary prevention with a focus on the characteristics of the abused child, assessment of the physically abused child, and treatment approaches for the abused child. They noted that the physically abused child appears to show problems in five areas: (1) neurological; (2) cognitive; (3) social skills; (4) peer interaction; and (5) behavioral dysfunction. Azar et al. (1988) suggested that little data-based literature currently exists regarding the assessment of such children and recommend such strategies as (1) a review of social service and school records to establish patterns. For example, abuse occurring at the end of the month may indicate financial difficulties in the child's family; abuse occurring after pay day may point to some form of parental substance abuse. (2) Thorough medical and neurological examinations, including such areas as speech, language, and articulation problems. (3) Careful cognitive testing done in a manner that is sensitive to the particular population. For example, an abused child may become anxious with an adult psychologist in a closed room; with the door open and extra time spent on establishing rapport and a safe environment, results may change. (4) Collection of behavioral data by asking parents or caregivers to complete standardized problem checklists. With the exception of foster care placement, treatment has seldom been focused directly on the abused child. Although Azar and her colleagues (1988) suggested that multiple interventions, such as day care, individual and group counseling, and parent training, may be employed, there has not, to date, been extensive, empirical study of the impact of behavioral interventions with abused and/or neglected children. Studies that have been done include one that compared the effectiveness of peer and teacher prompts on the socially withdrawn behavior of 36 maltreated preschool children (Fantuzzo, Azar, & Twentyman, 1985) and another that examined the effectiveness of bibliotherapy (Pardek & Pardek, 1984).

Browne (1986) discussed the role of stress in the commission of subsequent acts of child abuse and/or neglect. She found that stressful situations, along with the seriousness of the first abuse, significantly influenced the explanation of the commission of further abuse.

Family violence is another descriptor that has been found to be associated with individuals who are at high-risk for abuse and neglect (White, Snyder, Bourne, & Newberger, 1987). White and her colleagues (1987) asserted that, although the focus in the child abuse and neglect literature is often on the maltreatment of children, it may be more accurate to conceptualize domestic violence as a family problem. For example, children may be victimized by watching other family members being attacked rather than being attacked themselves. They also pointed out the difference between factors that may have clinical significance as opposed to factors that may have research significance. As an example, they suggested that researchers may argue that parental alcohol abuse occurs only in a small percentage of child abuse and neglect cases, whereas the clinician may see families in which parental alcohol abuse may be a highly significant factor in the maltreatment of their children. White, et al. (1987) also pointed out the differences between the rosy picture of family life painted by the media and the possibility that family members may actually cause harm to each other. They cited the seminal work by Straus, Gelles, and Steinmetz (1980) in their book, *Behind Closed Doors*, which brought the incidence of family violence out of the societal

closet. They noted the Bittner and Newberger (1981) model for understanding child abuse in which predisposing factors to family violence
were described as (1) child-produced stresses (handicapped, retarded,
difficult, hyperactive, foster child); (2) family stresses (poverty, unemployment, isolation, poor housing, relationship difficulties, parent–
child problems, inappropriate child-rearing style); and (3) parent-pro-
duced stresses (low self-esteem, abused as a child, depression, substance abuse, psychiatric disorder, ignorance of child-rearing, unrealistic
expectations). These factors are then influenced by a triggering situation, such as a discipline problem, substance abuse, an argument or
family conflict, or some acute environmental problem, followed by maltreatment by one family member toward another.

Identifying a similar population, Meredith, Abbott, and Adams
(1986) found that, as the use of physical violence among family members
increased, there were significant decreases in the family perception of
family strengths, marital satisfaction, and parental satisfaction. This
highlights the high risk for abuse or neglect in families who practice
physical violence toward each other.

Primary prevention methods, similar to tertiary prevention measures, have a community focus. Although as we have noted, tertiary
prevention is geared toward the already diagnosed situations of child
abuse and neglect, primary prevention has a broader goal: To reduce the
rate of new cases in a population over time by counterbalancing adverse
influences, and to reduce the risk of child abuse and neglect for the
entire community. Thus, primary prevention programs for child abuse
and neglect would include political/social action, examination of factors
that produce healthy family behaviors, as well as examination of factors
that lead to family dysfunction, exploration of problems of living, and,
the study of environmental factors that impact family life.

Paisley (1987) discussed legislative actions to prevent child abuse
and neglect enacted by states and, in particular, the legislation efforts in
North Carolina. She described the role of the school counselor and
noted that primary prevention programs should be geared toward reducing the parent's unrealistic expectations of child and adolescent behaviors, caretaker responsibilities, long-term costs of inappropriate parent skills, and family isolation. She recommended programs that enhance parent–child bonding, emotional ties, and improved communication skills. She further suggested programs that would help parents
increase coping skills, especially when under stress. Peer support, access to social services and medical/health resources, and parental home-
management/child-management skills are also recommended.

Hodson and Skeen (1987) reviewed the research and theories of child sexual abuse and found that family life education could make a significant contribution to the prevention and treatment of sexual abuse. Thus, family life educators and other professionals who routinely work with children and their families must be supplied with information on the prevention and detection of childhood sexual abuse, including such issues as (1) the theoretical explanations of childhood sexual abuse, (2) the characteristics of abusers, (3) the characteristics of victims, (4) the means of detecting abuse, and (5) the prevention and response interventions.

In his presidential address for the International Society for Prevention of Child Abuse and Neglect, Ferrier (1986) suggested that, even though the need for tertiary prevention exists because "accidents always occur," he urged that professionals agree that cases of abuse and neglect should only be accidents and "rare ones at that (p. 280)." He noted the difficulty in secondary prevention because though the identifying of high-risk groups is attractive it may be, "fraught with the danger of self-fulfilling prophecy (p. 281)." Ferrier (1986) stated that his "personal bias is primary prevention." He recommended using education of the general public to create a change in current attitudes, values, and beliefs about the use of violence as an acceptable method of child-rearing as well as heightening societal awareness of the "devastating effect of rejection or verbal abuse." He supported the position of the American Academy of Pediatrics in its condemnation of the lack of censorship in television to ban the most "viciously realistic forms of violence" presented for home viewing. Finally, he suggested that the further study of those children who survive abuse or neglect and overcome their circumstances compared with those children who are unable to overcome the abuse or neglect, would "boost our morale and lift our spirits."

Nelson (1984) analyzed four arenas of political action on behalf of children: the U.S. Children's Bureau, the media, state legislators, and Congress. She found that child abuse is a "consensual issue"; that is, everyone agrees that child abuse is a problem. It also appears to be relatively high on the agenda of those who make policy decisions. However, she noted that such decisions are often made from the heart rather than on the basis of empirical information or data-based studies. Thus, although made with the best of intentions, state response often unwittingly offers the least effective response.

School sexual abuse prevention programs may produce some unintended consequences and dilemmas (Trudell & Whatley, 1988). This primary prevention strategy often involves the use of classroom teachers and other elementary school personnel as instructors or guides for students. Although child sexual abuse is a complex issue that is likely to be

affected by the decrease of traditional societal controls over sexual behavior, varying sexual expectations, family isolation, an increase in divorce rates, an increase in the number of families joined by remarriage,
differences in the way male and females are socialized, media and por-
nographic depictions of children as sexual objects, changing norms of
child obedience to adults, and low rates of identification, prosecution,
and conviction of perpetrators, school prevention programs frequently
focus on the prospective perpetrator's access to the child and neglect to
address such issues as the adult's attraction to a child, his or her lack of
internal controls, and the lack of external controls. Trudell and Whatley
(1988) argued that, because of the complexity of the problem and the
necessary oversimplification of a wide-based primary prevention program, simply offering a prevention program in every classroom would
not lead to a significant decrease in child sexual abuse. Furthermore, the
emphasis on the child's behavior may encourage blaming the victim. In
such programs, parents have been informed that in 80% of the cases, the
victim could have stopped the assault by just saying no. Implied within
this message is that the child is powerful enough to stop the victimization and therefore responsible for the consequences. Trudell and Whatley (1988) also pointed out several dilemmas for classroom teachers in
this prevention approach: (1) the increased use of predeveloped curricu-
lar materials may lead to deskillling teachers; (2) these materials are
often designed to be brief interventions because packages that involve a
minimum of extra teacher and student time are more marketable; and (3)
such programs are designed to avoid controversy, and since one of the
most controversial issues in the area of childhood sexual abuse is ex-
plicitness, these programs are often vague rather than clear. Also, many
teachers are reluctant to use such programs because of the mandatory
reporting laws, which, as some critics argue, obscure the ethical nature
of teacher decisions; assume that reporting will, necessarily, produce
positive outcomes; and, neglect the educational context of the classroom
in order to encourage the openness and trust necessary for child-to-
teacher disclosure. Trudell and Whatley (1988) concluded that broad-
based school programs to prevent childhood sexual abuse may not solve
the problem. Rather, they suggested the primary prevention strategy of
social action to make "fundamental changes in a society that allows and
even encourages child sexual abuse" (p. 111).

    Rosenberg and Reppucci (1985) examined three categories of pri-
mary prevention in child abuse: (1) programs that helped families become more competent; (2) programs geared toward the prevention of
first-time abuse; and (3) programs that focused on high-risk populations. They pointed out three methodological problems that appeared to

cut across all such programs: (1) there were not enough appropriate comparison groups; (2) outcome measures were poorly chosen; and (3) there was a "failure to measure proximal programmatic objectives and distal prevention goals." They concluded that although the programs studied offered some exciting possibilities in the area of primary prevention of child abuse and neglect, many have not proved that they could actually accomplish this goal.

PREVENTION PROGRAMS

Tertiary prevention programs are directed toward an already diagnosed population and have, as their goals, the rehabilitation of the perpetrator, keeping the family intact, and the prevention of further abuse.

Wolfe, Kaufman, Aragona, and Sandler (1981) developed an intervention model for child abusers that consists of a series of step-by-step procedures to teach abusive parents the skills required in managing their children's activities, problem-solving and conflict resolution, anger and impulse control, and building and maintaining positive social relationships outside the home. Wolfe and his colleagues (1981) presented a treatment and assessment program and a series of evaluative studies.

The Kansas Child Abuse Prevention Trust Fund Program, which was founded in 1980 (Poertner, 1987), offers programs to abusive parents that include parenting education, public awareness (a primary prevention program), home visits, and special programs for latchkey children and children from homes in which spousal abuse has been reported.

Secondary prevention programs target an at-risk population and have as their goals the prevention of first-time abuse or the prevention of further abuse.

Wolfe, Edwards, Manion, and Koverola (1988) evaluated an early intervention program for parents who were at-risk of abusing or neglecting their children. The subjects were women, aged 16–25, who were living on welfare, with young children aged 9–60 months. Even though many of the women had male friends who visited them for different lengths of time, only three were married or involved in permanent relationships. These women and their children were assigned to one of two intervention groups: an information-only program offered by the child protection agency, or a behavioral parent-training program in addition to the other program. Although both groups showed improvement in their child-rearing environments and child behaviors, only the women who received the behavioral parent-training package showed significant improvements in parenting risk and child-behaviors problems at posttest and at a 3-month follow-up. Further, at a 1-year follow-up case-workers rated these women as having lower risks of maltreatment and higher abilities to manage their children.

The Children's Hospital Program on Family Violence (White *et al.*, 1987) in Boston was developed to provide an interdisciplinary team-treatment approach to the problem of child abuse and neglect. The program adopted the term "Trauma X," rather than use what was then referred to as the "battered child syndrome," as an expression of general emphasis on violence and neglect directed to problems of family systems rather than attributes attributable to pathological parents. The clinical work of the Trauma X team led to the creation of a family violence research center—The Family Development Center. The Children's Hospital also provides a clinical training program and inservice teaching. Funded by federal grants, this model hospital-based training program on family violence provides an ongoing Family Violence Seminar and a fellowship program for pediatricians and behavioral and social scientists.

Project 12-Ways, supported by Title XX federal funds operates out of the Southern Illinois University at Carbondale and evolved out of the logic of ecologically oriented research. An ecobehavioral approach to the treatment of child abuse and neglect (Lutzker, 1984; Lutzker, Frame, & Rice, 1982; Lutzker & Rice, 1984; Lutzker, Wesch, & Rice, 1984; Lutzker & Newman, 1986), Project 12-Ways focuses on the remediation of several of the known risk factors contributing to the problem, including premature birth and birth complications, mental retardation, physical handicaps and developmental difficulties, behavioral problems, such as whining, crying, hyperactivity, and other negative behaviors, unemployment, large family, unstable marriage, stress-producing events, single-parenting, and poverty. Project 12-Ways provides such services as parent training, using contingency management and activity training programs (Dachman, Halasz, Bickett, & Lutzker, 1984; Lutzker, Megson, Webb, & Dachman, 1985); stress reduction, using progressive muscle relaxation, biofeedback, or behavioral relaxation training (Campbell, O'Brien, Bickett, Newman, & Lutzker, in press); self-control training, such as weight or anger control; social support and basic skills for children, such as personal hygiene (Lutzker, Campbell, & Watson-Perczel, 1984); activity training for parents and children, such as health maintenance and nutrition, home cleanliness, and nutritious meal planning and serving (Rosenfield-Schlichter, Sarber, Bueno, Greene, & Lutzker, 1983; Sarber, Halasz, Messmer, Bickett, & Lutzker, 1983; home safety (Barone, Greene, & Lutzker, 1986; Tertinger, Greene, & Lutzker, 1984); and job-finding, problem-solving, money management, and prenatal/postnatal care for single parents (Lutzker, Lutzker, Braunling-McMorrow, & Eddelman, 1987).

Project Ecosystems which is based in southern California, is a replication of Project 12-Ways and is directed at families with developmentally disabled children who are at-risk for abuse or neglect. Lutzker, Campbell, Newman, and Harrold, (1990) described the multiple in-home services provided by Project Ecosystems in the first 6 months of its existence. Goals include keeping the child at home wherever possible, preventing incidents of child abuse or neglect, improving adaptive functioning within families, and providing training and research opportunities to students in applied behavior analysis and human services. Project Ecosystems maintains a caseload of 30–50 families within any given fiscal year. Its objectives are that, in any fiscal year, no more than three children being served will be placed in a more restrictive setting. A further objective is that no more than three parents will be indicted for abuse or neglect. Project Ecosystems provides the same kind of multi-faceted interventions described in Project 12-Ways, including basic skill training, problem-solving; job-finding; money management; nutrition, behavioral pediatrics; hygiene; and, home-safety. Assessment is accomplished with parent self-report measures and child-observation measures. Clinical evaluation, single-case experiments, and program evaluation are the three methods used to evaluate services.

Primary prevention programs are broad-based, with the community at-large as their target. These programs are designed to prevent first-ever abuse in the general population. The programs often use the public media to communicate their message although not always.

A special comic book issue of *Spiderman*, which dealt with sexual abuse, was presented to 73 2nd, 3rd, and 4th-grade children (Garbarino, 1987). This low-cost, primary prevention approach was effective in teaching children and their parents how to report sexual abuse. Garbarino recommended enhancing the power of the comic book by presenting it in the framework of an ongoing and comprehensive program geared not only to children but to parents as well.

The *Red Flag/Green Flag People* coloring book and a film, *Better Safe than Sorry II*, was given to 289 3rd and 4th-graders, 276 parents, and 13 teachers from two schools (Kolko, Moses, Litz, & Hughs, 1987), along with a discussion of imaginary and actual scenarios involving inappropriate touching. Kolko and his colleagues (1987) evaluated this program to promote awareness and prevent child sexual victimization by comparing it to a group of 41 3rd and 4th-graders, 41 parents, and 2 teachers from a control school. Children in the experimental group learned more about the differences between appropriate and inappropriate touching, were more likely to report abuse, and were more able to use learned skills than those in the control group. The program was also effective in increasing parents' knowledge about the program and in enhancing communication about abuse at home.

Wurtelle, Marrs, and Miller-Perrin (1987) compared a sexual abuse prevention program that included participant modeling with a similar program using symbolic modeling. Wurtele and her colleagues (1987) found that the participant modeling program that taught self-protective skills through modeling and active rehearsal provided superior efficacy than the symbolic modeling program that taught the same skills, but that involved observation of the experimenter rather than hands-on practice.

Similarly, Stillwell, Lutzker, and Greene (1990) evaluated the Sexual Abuse Prevention Program for Preschoolers (SAPPP), which added such components as behavioral training, rehearsal, and evaluation to the format of a popular prevention program. Children participated in six SAPPP lessons that included the topic introduction (for example, different types of touch, how to say no and how to tell others), stories related to the topic, behavioral rehearsal of a target behavior, and finally class discussion. Stillwell and her colleagues (1990) found that all of the children improved their scores on correct verbal responses from pretest to posttest. However, none of the children showed improvement on behavioral demonstration. Stillwell et al. (1990) concluded that an important goal of future prevention programs should be to train children to demonstrate optimum prevention *behaviors*.

Conte, Rosen, Saperstein, and Shermack (1985) evaluated a 3-hour program that taught common sexual abuse prevention concepts, such as the difference between OK and not-OK touching. Using a repeated measures multivariate analysis of variance, they found that children in a prevention training group significantly increased their knowledge of prevention concept, as opposed to children in a control group who did not. Furthermore, older children learned more than younger children, and both groups had difficulty with concepts presented in the abstract rather than in the concrete.

As noted, Rosenberg and Reppucci (1985) reviewed primary prevention programs in the area of child abuse and neglect. They found programs that addressed three major areas: competency enhancement, preventing the onset of abusive behavior, and targetting high-risk groups. Competency enhancement programs included the use of theater and television to increase parenting skills (Inter-Act: Street Theater for Parents); a large-scale comprehensive program to decrease the prevalence of child abuse and improve children's school performance (Project C.A.N. Prevent); and parent education groups to enhance parents' abilities to cope with child-rearing problems resulting from cultural differences (Pan Asian Parent Education Project). Programs to prevent the onset of abusive behavior included media campaigns, information, crisis, and referral networks, and projects designed to empower social groups to provide support to families. Some projects that were reviewed included a comprehensive community education and referral campaign designed to strengthen formal and informal helping networks (Project Network, Atlanta University); a multifaceted public awareness project for rural counties (Primary Prevention Partnership); and telephone hotlines (Parents Anonymous, Michigan's Warm Line, Connecticut's Care-Line). In their review of primary prevention projects, Rosenberg and Reppucci (1985) included programs that targetted high-risk groups. We would consider these interventions secondary prevention; however, in this instance we will include them here. Those reviewed are a service for prospective mothers expecting a first child with emphasis on young, single, and women of lower socioeconomic status (Prenatal/Early Infancy Project), and another multileveled program, discussed earlier, with an emphasis on home safety (Project 12-Ways).

RECOMMENDATIONS

The traditional mental health concept of prevention, as we have shown, includes three seemingly distinct levels of interventions. However, Rosenberg and Reppucci (1985) argued that tertiary level programs that have as their target population individuals whose disorders are already identified are not, in the strictest sense, prevention programs at all. On the other hand, we suggest that prevention of *further* abuse is a valid perspective.

In searching the literature, we found very few large-scale community programs that had as their goal the rehabilitation of *all* members of the diagnosed population. We included Project 12-Ways (Lutzker & Newman, 1986) in our section on secondary prevention because it addresses many of the risk factors in child abuse and neglect; however, it is an example of how a tertiary prevention program might succeed. For example, Project 12-Ways is community-based; it provides in-home, *in-situ* services with the goal of keeping the family intact, where feasible, increasing the parenting and living skills of caregivers, decreasing dysfunctional child behaviors, and decreasing abuse and/or neglect.

Programs must also be cost effective. Lutzker and Newman (1986) pointed out that Project 12-Ways provided services at approximately one half the cost that would have been incurred if similar services had been provided under the auspices of a mental health facility. Program evaluation and empirical examination must support claims of success by any prevention program. Project 12-Ways has an ongoing research, assessment, and evaluation arm that provides consistent feedback about interventions (Lutzker & Newman, 1986).

In the area of secondary prevention, we note the many risk-factors that impact on families and that may lead to abuse or neglect. There are parent characteristics, child characteristics, and environmental characteristics, which, when triggered by an event, may lead to abusive or neglectful environments (White et al., 1987). Project 12-Ways (Lutzker & Newman, 1986) and Project Ecosystems (Lutzker, Campbell, Newman & Harrold, 1990) provide multilevel services directed at these three aspects of the problem. We recommend "ecologically orientated" interventions and research; that is, we suggest that future secondary prevention programs examine and address the many complex factors that seem necessary and sufficient to produce child abuse and neglect.

At the same time, primary prevention is the simplest and the most complex issue of our time. There appears to be money and enthusiasm for large-scale, media-based campaigns to "just say no." However, in the attempt to reach everyone, the message becomes vague rather than concrete. Often, with the best will in the world, programs are watered down to be palatable to the largest common denominator to the point of being ineffective and possibly harmful. For example, if children are taught that they have only to say no, then we are blaming the victims for their victimization (Trudell & Whatley, 1988). Social action is another aspect of primary prevention. For example, Zuravin (1986) found a connection between residential density and urban child maltreatment. In this instance, it is incumbent upon health care professionals to publish such findings, not only for each other in professional journals, but to make such research known to the general public. Hermalin, Melendez, Kamarck, Kievans, Ballen, and Gordon (1979) noted the usefulness of self-help groups as support networks for more formal health care delivery systems in enhancing primary prevention. Thus, it is the responsibility of the health care professional to provide an environment supportive of the growth of self-help groups. Finally, our society has values and a culture that supports such axioms as "spare the rod and spoil the child"; we even admire such lone killers as *Rambo*, and we laugh at such lines as Noel Coward's quip "women should be beaten regularly, like a gong." In this atmosphere, which is hostile to nurturance, it is necessary for the health care professional to become an activist, to publically boy-cott films, music, and books that promote violence to women and chil-dren, and to protest policies that keep a major segment of our popula-tion in despair.

SUMMARY

There are three levels of child abuse or neglect prevention: tertiary, secondary, and primary. Tertiary prevention in the area of child abuse and neglect refers to large-scale community programs, often institution-based, whose goal is to prevent further abuse or neglect in already cited families. Secondary prevention in the area of child abuse and neglect is concerned with reaching those groups or individuals who appear to be at risk for abuse and/or neglect, either because of parental charac-teristics, child characteristics, or environmental characteristics. The goal of such programs is to prevent further abuse or first-time abuse. Primary prevention in the area of child abuse and neglect considers the entire population as its target. Media campaigns, bibliotherapy, school-based programs, films, and social and political action are components of these interventions. Although much work has been done that has proven of value in the area of prevention programs for child abuse and neglect, there is still much more to be accomplished in the future.

REFERENCES

Adelson, L. (1969). Slaughter of the innocents. *New England Journal of Medicine, 264*, 1345–1349.

American Humane Association. (1963). Child abuse: Preview of a nationwide survey. Denver, CO: Author.

Azar, S. T., Barnes, K. T., & Twentyman, C. T. (1988). Developmental outcome in phys-ically abused children: Consequences of parental abuse on the effects of a more gener-al breakdown in caregiving behaviors. *The Behavior Therapist, 11*, 27–32.

Bakwin, H. (1956). Multiple skeletal lesions in young children due to trauma. *American Journal of Pediatrics, 49*, 7–15.

Bandura, A. (1977). *Social learning theory.* Englewood Cliffs, NJ: Prentice Hall.

Barmayer, G. H., Alderson, L. R., & Cox, W. R. (1951). Traumatic periostitis in young children. *American Journal of Pediatrics, 38*, 184–190.

Barone, U. J., Greene, B. F., & Lutzker, J. R. (1986). Home safety with families being treated for child abuse and neglect. *Behavior Modification, 10*, 93–114.

Bittner, S., & Newberger, E. H. (1981). Pediatric understanding of child abuse and neglect. *Pediatrics in Review, 2*, 197.

Boardman, H. E. (1961). A project to rescue children from inflicted injuries. *Social Work* (Am. Ed.) *1*, 43–51.

Browne, D. H. (1986). The role of stress in the commission of subsequent acts of child abuse and neglect. *Journal of Family Violence, 1*, 289–297.

Caffey, J. (1946). Multiple fractures in the long bones of infants suffering from chronic subdural hematoma. *American Journal of Roentgendogy Radium Therapy and Nuclear Medicine, 56*, 163–174.

Campbell, R. V., Twardosz, S., Lutzker, J. R., & Cuvo, A. J. (1983, May). *Comparison study of affectionate behavior across status of abuse neglect and non-abuse neglect.* Paper presented at the annual convention of the Association for Behavior Analysis, Milwaukee, Wisconsin.

Campbell, R. V., O'Brien, S., Bickett, A. D., Newman, M. R., & Lutzker, J. R. (in press). Migraine headaches and marriage and family happiness: An ecobehavioral approach. In S. Diamond & M. Maliszewski (Eds.), *Sexuality and headache: A medical-behavioral overview.* New York: International Universities Press.

Caplan, G. (1964). *Principles of preventive psychiatry.* New York: Basic Books.

Carstens, C. C. (1911–1912). The prevention of cruelty to children. *Proceedings of the Academy of Political Science, 2*, 616–617.

Carstens, C. C. (1921). The development of social work for child protection. *Annals of the American Academy of Political and Social Science, 98*, 137–141.

Child Protection Report. Vol. 2, January 14, 1976.

Cohn, A. A. (1986). Preventing adults from becoming sexual molesters. *Child Abuse and Neglect, 10*, 559–562.

Conte, J. R., Rosen, C., Saperstein, L., & Shermack, R. (1985). An evaluation of a program to prevent the sexual victimization of young children. *Child Abuse and Neglect, 9*, 319–328.

Cowen, E. L., Dorr, D., Clarfield, S., Kreling, B., McWilliams, S. A., Pokracki, D., Pratt, M., Terrell, D., & Wilson, A. (1973). The AML: A quick screening device for early identification of school maladaption. *American Journal of Community Psychology, 1*, 12–35.

Cumming, J., & Cumming, E. (1957). *Closed ranks.* Cambridge: Harvard University Press.

Dachman, R. S., Halasz, M. M., Bickett, A. D., & Lutzker, J. R. (1984). A home-based ecobehavioral parent-training and generalization package with a neglectful mother. *Education and Treatment of Children, 7*, 183–202.

Elmer, E. (1960). Abused young children seen in hospitals. *Social Work, 5*, 98–102.

Englert, Y., Marneffe, C., Soumenkoff, G., & Hubinont, P. O. (1985). Institutional abuse: Tubal sterilization in a population at risk of ill-treating their children. *Child Abuse and Neglect, 9*, 31–35.

Fantuzzo, J., Azar, S. T., & Twentyman, C. T. (1985, November). *Child abuse and psychotherapy research: Merging social concerns and empirical investigation.* Paper presented at the annual convention of the Association for Advancement of Behavior Therapy, Philadelphia, Pennsylvania.

Ferrier, P. E. (1986). Presidential address: The International Society for Prevention of Child Abuse and Neglect. *Child Abuse and Neglect, 10*, 279–281.

Fisher, S. H. (1958). Skeletal manifestations of parent induced trauma in infants and children. *Southern Medical Journal, 51*, 956–960.

Gambrill, E. D. (1983). Behavioral intervention with child abuse and neglect. In M. Hersen, R. M. Eisler, & P. M. Miller (Eds.), *Progress in behavior modification: Vol. 15* (pp. 1–56). Orlando, FL: Academic Press

Garbarino, J. (1987). Children's response to a sexual abuse prevention program: A study of the *Spiderman* comic. *Child Abuse and Neglect, 11*, 143–148.

Hagenhoff, C., Lowe, A., Hovell, M. F., & Rugg, D. (1987). Prevention of the teenage pregnancy epidemic: A social learning theory approach. *Education and Treatment of Children, 10,* 67–83.

Helfer, R. B. (1982). A review of literature on the prevention of child abuse and neglect. *Child Abuse and Neglect, 6,* 251–261.

Hermalin, J., Melendez, L., Kamarck, T., Kievans, F., Ballen, E., & Gordon, M. (1979). Enhancing primary prevention: The marriage of self-help groups and formal health care delivery systems. *Journal of Clinical Child Psychology, 8,* 125–129.

Hodson, D., & Skeen, P. (1987). Child sexual abuse: A review of research and theory with implications for family life educations. *Family Relations: Journal of Applied Family and Child Studies, 36,* 215–221.

Joint Commission on Mental Health and Illness. (1961). *Action for Mental Health.* New York: Wiley.

Joint Commission on Mental Health of Children. (1970). *Crisis in child mental health: Challenge for the 1970's.* New York: Harper & Row.

Kempe, C. H., & Silver, H. K. (1959). Problem of parental criminal neglect and severe physical abuse of children. *American Journal of Diseases of Children, 98,* 529.

Kempe, C. H., Silverman, F. N., Steele, B. F., Droegemueller, W., & Silver, H. K. (1962). The battered-child syndrome. *Journal of the American Medical Association, 181,* 105–112.

Kolko, D. J., Moses, J. T., Litz, J., & Hughs, J. (1987). Promoting awareness and prevention of child sexual victimization using the Red Flag/Green Flag Program: An evaluation with follow-up. *Journal of Family Violence, 2,* 11–35.

Lucht, C. (1975). Providing a legislative base for reporting child abuse. *Fourth National Symposium on Child Abuse.* Denver, CO: American Humane Association.

Lutzker, J. R. (1984). Project 12-Ways: Treating child abuse and neglect from an ecobehavioral perspective. In R. F. Dangel & R. A. Poloten (Eds.), *Parent training: Formulations of research and practice* (pp. 260–291). New York: Guilford Press.

Lutzker, J. R., & Newman, M. R. (1986). Child abuse and neglect: Community problem, community solutions. *Education and Treatment of Children, 9,* 344–354.

Lutzker, J. R., & Rice, J. M. (1984). Project 12-Ways: Measuring outcome of a large in-home service for treatment and prevention of child abuse and neglect. *Child Abuse and Neglect, 8,* 519–524.

Lutzker, J. R., Campbell, R. V., & Watson-Perczel, M. (1984). Utility of the case study method in treatment of several problems of a neglected family. *Education and Treatment of Children, 7,* pp. 315–353.

Lutzker, J. R., Frame, R. E., & Rice, J. M. (1982). Project 12-Ways: An ecobehavioral approach to treatment and prevention of child abuse and neglect. *Education and Treatment of Children, 5,* 141–155.

Lutzker, J. R., Wesch, D., & Rice, J. M. (1984). A review of Project 12-Ways: An ecobehavioral approach to treatment and prevention of child abuse and neglect. *Advances in Behaviour Research and Therapy, 6,* 63–73.

Lutzker, J. R., Campbell, R., Newman, M. R., & Harrold, M. (1989). Ecobehavioral intervention for abusive, neglectful, and high-risk families: Project 12-Ways and Project Ecosystems. In G. H. S. Singer & L. K. Irvin (Eds.), *Family support services: Emerging pertnerships between families with severely handicapped individuals and communities* (pp. 313–326). Baltimore, MD: Paul H. Brookes.

Lutzker, J. R., Megson, D. A., Webb, M. E., & Dachman, R. S. (1985). Validating and training adult-child interaction skills to professionals and to parents indicated for child abuse and neglect. *Journal of Child and Adolescent Psychotherapy, 2,* 91–104.

Lutzker, S. Z., Lutzker, J. R., Braunling-McMorrow, D., & Eddelman, J. (1987). Promoting to increase mother-baby stimulation with single mothers. *Journal of Child and Adolescent Psychotherapy, 4,* 3–12.

Lynch, M. A. (1985). Child abuse before Kempe: An historical review. *Child Abuse and Neglect, 9,* 7–15.

Meredith, W. H., Abbott, D. A., & Adams, S. L. (1986). Family violence: Its relation to marital and parental satisfaction and family strengths. *Journal of Family Violence, 1,* 299–309.

Nelson, B. J. (1985). *Making an issue of child abuse: Political agenda setting for social problems.* Chicago: University of Chicago Press.

Paisley, P. O. (1987). Prevention of child abuse and neglect: Legislative response. *School Counselor, 34,* 226–228.

Pardek, J. T., & Pardek, J. A. (1984). Treating abused children through bibliotherapy. *Early Child Development and Care, 16,* 195–205.

Paulsen, M. (1968). The law and abused children. In R. Helfer & C. H. Dempe (Eds.), *The battered child.* Chicago: University of Chicago Press.

Poertner, J. (1987). The Kansas family and child trust fund: Five year report. *Child Welfare, 66,* 3–12.

Rappaport, J. (1977). *Community psychology: Values, research, and action.* New York: Holt, Rinehart, & Winston.

Rosenberg, M. S., & Reppucci, N. D. (1985). Primary prevention of child abuse. *Journal of Consulting and Clinical Psychology, 55,* 576–585.

Rosenfield-Schlichter, M. D., Sarber, R. E., Bueno, G., Greene, B. F., & Lutzker, J. R. (1983). Maintaining accountability for ecobehavioral treatment of one aspect of child neglect: Personal cleanliness. *Education and Treatment of Children, 6,* 152–164.

Sarber, R. E., Halasz, M., Messmer, M. C., Bickett, A. D., & Lutzker, J. R. (1983). Teaching menu planning and grocer shopping skills to a mentally retarded mother. *Mental Retardation, 21,* 101–106.

Schultz, W. J. (1968). *The humane movement in the United States, 1910–1922.* New York: AMS Press.

Silverman, F. N. (1952). The roentgen manifestation of unrecognized skeletal trauma in infants. *American Journal of Roentgenology, Radium Therapy, and Nuclear Medicine, 69,* 413–427.

Snedecor, S. T., Knapp, R. E., & Wilson, H. B. (1935). Traumatic ossifying periostitis of the newborn. *Surgery, Gynecology, and Obstetrics, 61,* 385–387.

Stillwell, S. L., Lutzker, J. R., & Greene, B. F. (1988). Evaluation of a sexual abuse prevention program for preschoolers. *Journal of Family Violence, 3,* 269–280.

Straus, M. A., Gelles, R. S., & Steinmetz, S. (1980). *Behind closed doors: Violence in the American family.* Garden City, NY: Doubleday.

Tertinger, D. A., Greene, B. F., & Lutzker, J. R. (1984). Home safety: Development and validation of one component of an ecobehavioral treatment program for abused and neglected children. *Journal of Applied Behavior Analysis, 17,* 159–177.

Trudell, B., & Whatley, M. H. (1988). School sexual abuse prevention: Assessing consequences and dilemas. *Child Abuse and Neglect, 12,* 103–113.

United States Department of Health, Education, and Welfare. (1963). *The abused child: Principles and suggested language for legislation on reporting of the physically abused child.* Washington, DC: U.S. Government Printing Office.

Vasta, R. (1982). Physical child abuse: A dual-component analysis. *Developmental Review, 2,* 125–149.

White, K. M., Snyder, J., Bourne, R., & Newberger, E. H. (1987). *Treating family violence in a*

Pediatric Hospital: A program of training, research, and service. U.S. Department of Health and Human Services. Rockville, MD: Public Health Service, Alcohol, Drug Abuse, and Mental Health Administration, National Institute of Mental Health.

Willems, E. P. (1974). Behavioral technology and behavioral ecology. *Journal of Applied Behavior Analysis, 7,* 151–165.

Wolfe, D. A., Edwards, B., Manion, C., & Koverola, C. (1988). Early intervention for parents at risk of child abuse and neglect: A preliminary investigation. *Journal of Consulting and Clinical Psychology, 56,* 40–47.

Wolfe, D., Kaufman, K., Aragona, J., & Sandler, J. (1981). *The child management program for abusive parents: Procedures for developing a child abuse intervention program.* Florida: Anna Publishing.

Wurtelle, S. K., Marrs, S. R., & Miller-Perrin, C. L. (1987). Practice makes perfect? The role of participant modeling in sexual abuse prevention programs. *Journal of Consulting and Clinical Psychology,* 599–602.

Zuravin, S. J. (1986). Residential density and urban child maltreatment: An aggregate analysis. *Journal of Family Violence, 1,* 307–314 .

CHAPTER 10

TREATING THE ABUSED CHILD

ANTHONY P. MANNARINO AND JUDITH A. COHEN

INTRODUCTION

In most clinical settings, treatment for child abuse rarely focuses solely
on the victim, which is inherently sensible since the perpetrator of abuse
must also be treated if the risk for re-abuse is to be significantly reduced.
Particularly in the area of physical abuse, treatment has largely focused
on abusive parents, whereas little has been written about the treatment
of child victims. (For a discussion of treatment of the child abuser, see
Chapter 11 in this volume.) More recently, however, our understanding
of how to treat abused children has increased as data have begun to
accumulate regarding the impact of abuse on victims.

This chapter will address a number of issues related to the treatment of abused children. First, we will present a discussion of definitional issues, and methodological concerns that have impeded our
efforts to develop appropriate and effective treatment modalities followed by discussions of treatment methods and clinical themes relevant
to physically and sexually abused children. We will not address the
concept of emotional abuse in this chapter because we believe that this
type of abuse is so unspecified and ill-defined that a section on treatment devoted to it is simply not possible.

ANTHONY P. MANNARINO AND JUDITH A. COHEN • Department of Psychiatry, Western
Psychiatric Institute and Clinic, University of Pittsburgh School of Medicine, Pittsburgh,
Pennsylvania 15213.

Furthermore, we contend that for a number of legitimate clinical reasons, a discussion of the treatments applicable to sexually and physically abused children should be separated. First, whereas physical abuse is largely perpetrated by parents, sexual abuse can be intra- or extrafamilial. In addition, although physical abuse is clearly an act of aggression toward a child, it is uncommon for sexual abuse to be accompanied by violence. Finally, little empirical evidence exists pertaining to familial factors that contribute to physical or sexual abuse. Current data do not suggest that family dynamics and related factors are necessarily similar for these two types of abuse (Walker, Bonner, & Kaufmann, 1988). For these reasons, we will provide separate treatment of victims of physical and sexual abuse. If the discussion of one type of abuse has relevance to the other, there will be an attempt to highlight the areas of overlap.

DEFINITIONAL AND METHODOLOGICAL ISSUES

DEFINITIONAL PROBLEMS

In order to develop and provide effective treatment, the problem to be addressed needs to be clearly specified. This has not been the case in the area of child abuse. Various types of abuse (e.g., physical, sexual, emotional) are frequently lumped together and handled as if they are one entity (Blythe, 1983). In some treatment studies, the nature of the abuse is not even documented (Isaacs, 1982).

Even when attempts are made to separate physical from sexual abuse, definitional problems persist. For example, what exactly constitutes physical abuse? Must there be physical evidence of an injury? Or, in the area of sexual abuse, how are these cases investigated and what criteria are used in determining credibility? We readily acknowledge that these are complex issues that are not easily resolved. However, more serious efforts should be made by researchers studying the kinds of treatments potentially useful to abused children to specify clearly how abuse is defined and what criteria are utilized in making this determination.

In addition to definitional issues, characteristics of the treated populations have been infrequently specified in studies of child abuse (Smith, Rachman, & Yule, 1984). It is very surprising that sometimes not even the age range or sex of the abused group is mentioned. There are other sample characteristics as well, such as race, socioeconomic level, and intellectual status that rarely are addressed. All of these factors can have a profound impact on the course of treatment and its outcome. Failure to specify these variables has been a major limiting factor in treatment studies involving abused children.

Methodological Problems

The study of potentially effective treatments for abused children has also been beset by other types of severe methodological difficulties. For example, control groups or alternative treatments have rarely been employed (Smith *et al.*, 1984). In addition, the specific nature of the treatment program often is unclear (Blythe, 1983). Details of the intervention are so seldom given that it is sometimes difficult to discern if treatment is being provided to the victim, the alleged perpetrator, or to both.

The kind of outcome data collected in studies of child abuse are typically subjective and unsystematic (Isaacs, 1982). Subjective ratings by the treating clinician are the norm. It is uncommon for empirically validated questionnaires, rating scales, or semistructured interviews to be used. Moreover, the lack of adequate follow-up has been another methodological shortcoming.

These definitional problems and methodological issues have been major stumbling blocks to progress in the general area of child abuse and in the specific area of treatment for this population. Fortunately, these issues are beginning to be addressed adequately by a number of researchers. Particularly in the area of sexual abuse, more recent studies (Cohen & Mannarino, 1988; Conte & Schuerman, 1987; Friedrich, Urquiza, & Beilke, 1986) have been methodologically more sophisticated and precise. It is hoped that this trend will continue in order to build a foundation of solid data and outcome studies in this field.

TREATING THE PHYSICALLY ABUSED CHILD

In the area of child physical abuse, the focus of treatment has largely been on the abusive parent. In a thorough review of the existing literature, the authors found that in the vast majority of studies, there was either no treatment provided for children or it was clearly secondary to that being given to parents (Gabinet, 1983a,b; Green, Power, Stonebrook, & Gaines, 1981; Lutzker & Rice, 1984; Pelcovitz, Kaplan, Samit, Krieger, & Cornelius, 1984; Shelton, 1982; Trowell & Castle, 1981).

It is difficult to assess why child victims of physical abuse have so frequently been ignored in the development of interventions. Typically, elimination of further abuse has been the major treatment goal. Accordingly, there has been a natural tendency to gear treatment toward parents who perpetrate abuse against their children—an approach that has been somewhat short-sighted, though, because it fails to recognize that children may continue to suffer from emotional problems caused by earlier abuse.

Other reasons may exist why treatment has not focused on child victims. As Williams (1980) pointed out, child physical abuse has commonly been perceived to be in the professional domain of the physician and not the mental health practitioner. Accordingly, there has been a major concern about physical injuries and not necessarily the emotional trauma caused by the abuse. Moreover, from a societal-legal perspective, some pressure has been focussed on abusive parents who are perceived as needing treatment or punishment.

Recently, an increased emphasis was seen in the emotional and behavioral difficulties that children experience as a result of having been physically abused. Several studies have pointed to anxiety, aggression, and social skills deficits, as being significantly correlated with physical abuse in children (Mask, Johnson, & Kovitz, 1983; Reid, Taplin, & Loeber, 1981; Wolfe & Mosk, 1983). With this added focus on the problems experienced by victims, a more serious interest has developed in the kinds of interventions that would be most appropriate and effective for this population.

Although assessment is not the focus of this chapter, it is important to underscore that any potentially effective treatment for physically abused children must be based on careful assessment. Walker *et al.* (1988) have stressed the significance of a thorough evaluation in order to develop a method of intervention that is tailored to the individual needs of each child. This issue cannot be overemphasized. Appropriate clinical decisions should be made only after each case has been comprehensively evaluated. More informed judgments can then be formed regarding what kinds of treatment would potentially be most effective for the child, parent, or family.

REVIEW OF TREATMENT STUDIES OF CHILD VICTIMS

Few published studies are available that have specifically implemented treatment programs for child physical abuse victims. The studies that do exist are not linked in any empirical or theoretical way and will be reviewed briefly to provide the reader with some sense of what has transpired in the field.

One of the earliest attempts to investigate the impact of treatment with abuse victims was part of a national demonstration project (Cohn, 1979). In this study, treatment was provided to 70 abused children, aged 2–7 years, in three different centers. These children manifested a wide array of behavioral problems. Based on the subjective reports of treating clinicians, it was determined that victims made gains in receiving affection, interacting with adults, and in the area of self-image. Unfortunately, the nature of the treatment provided to these children was unclear. In addition, the use of subjective, nonblind clinician ratings to assess treatment progress was a serious methodological shortcoming. Despite these criticisms, Cohn's study was the first attempt to examine whether treatment of victims and not only of abusive parents may be potentially efficacious.

Other treatment programs designed for child physical abuse victims have been extremely diverse. Myers, Brandner, and Templin (1985) assessed developmental gains in 53 preschoolers who participated in a therapeutic preschool and whose parents were actively involved in a parenting group. Results demonstrated that most children made modest developmental progress. As with the Cohn (1979) investigation, the nature of the intervention provided to the children in this study was unspecified. Also there was no control group used or alternate treatment employed.

A methodologically more sophisticated project was designed by Heide and Richardson (1987) in which one half of a group of neglected but not necessarily abused children (mean age = 3) was placed in a day treatment program while the other half comprised waiting list controls. Children remained in day treatment for an average of nearly 8 months. The authors reported that treated children made significantly greater gains than did controls in five areas of functioning: perceptual-motor, cognition, gross motor, social/emotional, and language. The design and results of this study are very encouraging. However, it is again quite frustrating that the nature of the treatment provided was only minimally reported.

Other types of treatment for physically abused children have been described in the literature but not empirically evaluated. Huebner (1984) discussed the potential usefulness of group counseling for middle school abused and neglected children. The group intervention consisted of techniques to improve problem-solving skills and self-esteem. In a contrasting model, Frazier and Levine (1983) suggested "reattachment therapy" for young abuse victims. Critical elements in this approach are helping children to become attached to a therapist and then assisting them to learn to elicit attachment behavior from their caretaker. An enlightened concept advanced by these authors is that certain child behaviors can provoke a parent into more abusive behaviors. Accordingly, helping the child to change these behaviors can break down the typical abuse cycle. Although this model has yet to be evaluated, it offers an innovative, theoretically based approach to the treatment of abuse victims. More details will be discussed in the next section of this chapter regarding the notion of "provocative child behaviors" and how they might serve as the focus of treatment of abused children.

This brief review has demonstrated that there are few published studies of potentially effective treatments for physically abused children. Moreover, most of the studies presented have not been guided by a particular theoretical or conceptual framework and have typically been characterized by serious methodological shortcomings.

NEW DIRECTIONS IN THE CLINICAL TREATMENT OF ABUSE VICTIMS

Treatment for Abuse-Related Symptoms or Problems

One way to conceptualize physical abuse is as a traumatic event in the life of a child that may have a wide range of outcomes, many of which are deleterious. Unfortunately, our current knowledge of the impact of physical abuse on children is quite limited. Recent studies (Mask et al., 1983; Reid et al., 1981; Wolfe & Mosk, 1983) have suggested that abused children experience significantly greater levels of anxiety, aggression, social skills deficits, and other behavioral problems when contrasted with nonabused children. It is clearly premature to assume, however, that all abused children will manifest similar difficulties. There is little doubt that the effects of physical abuse will be a function of the child's preabuse characteristics, including developmental status, relationship with the abusive parent, and other family factors, and that there will be a range of outcomes. All abused children must have a comprehensive assessment to determine what symptoms or problems they present in response to the abuse and how these problems can be treated most effectively.

There are a number of clinical interventions that have been demonstrated to be effective with children with specific emotional or behavioral difficulties. Regrettably, this chapter does not have sufficient space to review all of these techniques and, moreover, they have not been developed specifically for abused children. Nonetheless, a few that may have special relevance for abused children will be briefly mentioned.

Problem-solving strategies have been found to be useful in treating a variety of problems, including hyperactivity, aggressiveness, and impulsivity (Kendall & Braswell, 1985). This model could be employed with abused children who display any of these types of "externalizing" problems in response to physical abuse (see Spivack, Platt, & Shure, 1976, and Meichenbaum, 1977, for specific clinical instructions on how to use problem-solving techniques with children). In a similar light, systematic desensitization and other relaxation techniques with documented effectiveness could be used to treat anxiety and fears in children who have been abused or neglected (Walker *et al.*, 1988). Finally, social skills training (Michelson, Sugai, Wood, & Kazdin, 1983; Mannarino, Christy, Durlak, & Magnussen, 1982) could be the treatment of choice for abused children with interpersonal deficits.

None of the aforementioned clinical interventions have been systematically evaluated as to their potential utility with abused children. Furthermore, empirical studies need to be conducted that examine how the effectiveness of these clinical procedures is affected by the child's developmental status, family situation, or other variables. Nonetheless, the important point that we are trying to make is that clinical child psychology and child psychiatry have a number of treatment techniques (primarily behavioral or cognitive-behavioral) with documented clinical efficacy and that clinicians working with abused children should not hesitate to utilize these interventions as part of their overall treatment strategy.

Treatment of "Provocative Child Behaviors"

Another perspective in the treatment of physically abused children is more specifically abuse-related. It is well known among therapists who treat abusive families that the children who are at highest risk for abuse may engage in a number of "provocative" behaviors that increase parental frustrations and aggressiveness, including inattentiveness, restlessness, noncompliance, and temper outbursts. These behaviors can contribute to an interactive pattern in which the child's behaviors raise parental frustrations and elicit greater aggressiveness which, in turn, reinforce the child's provocative behaviors. A self-perpetuating cycle is thus created that increases the probability of physical abuse.

A potentially useful model to deal with the kind of interactive pattern mentioned above is to help the abused or at-risk child change these provocative behaviors. As discussed earlier, Frazier and Levine (1983) focused on assisting the victim to eliminate "child produced stressors" that contribute to the total abuse cycle. A number of useful interventions have also been outlined by Walker *et al.* (1988), who suggested that anger management techniques can be used to help abused children reduce the level of aversive behaviors displayed toward parents. If the child can learn to reduce the number and intensity of angry outbursts and to exhibit increased self-control, this may have a positive impact in the form of a decreased likelihood of future abuse.

There are other ways in which children at risk for abuse can change the behaviors that perpetuate this abusive pattern. For example, children can learn how to obey commands promptly and how to earn rewards for adaptive behaviors (Walker *et al.*, 1988). Moreover, self-instructional training (Kendall & Braswell, 1985) and other cognitive-behavioral strategies can be employed to reduce inattentiveness, restlessness, and impulsivity.

It is important to state that this discussion in no way implies that abused children bear any responsibility for having been physically assaulted. The authors recognize fully that abusive parents must take complete responsibility for their assaultive behaviors. Nonetheless, if children at-risk for abuse can be helped to alter some of the behaviors that contribute to the abusive cycle discussed earlier, then perhaps the likelihood of subsequent physical maltreatment can be lowered.

None of the strategies to alter provocative behaviors in abused children have been empirically investigated. It is certainly possible that some will prove to be fruitful whereas others will not. Perhaps the greatest advantage of this perspective is that it is inherently preventive in nature. Specifically, it addresses one subset of variables (i.e., child provocative behaviors) that contribute to a pattern of abuse in families. If interventions can be implemented that reduce these provocative behaviors, then future abuse can perhaps be prevented or at least the risk significantly reduced.

This section on the treatment of physical abuse has focused almost exclusively on clinical interventions with individual victims. Space does not permit a discussion of other potentially useful techniques such as family treatment (which is sometimes suggested as an appropriate intervention for physically abusive families). Moreover, a thorough discussion of parent training and other clinical procedures with physically abusive parents can be found in Chapter 11 of this volume.

TREATING THE SEXUALLY ABUSED CHILD

GENERAL CONSIDERATIONS

There is a growing body of literature addressing techniques for treating sexually abused children. As is the case with treatment studies of child physical abuse, almost all of these are based on clinical rather than empirical information. It is important to recognize that no study exists to date that examines empirically the efficacy of any of these therapeutic interventions in a methodologically sound manner. Thus, although many of the clinical approaches to sexually abused children seem inherently logical, there is no objective evidence that they are indeed effective. This should be born in mind throughout the following discussion.

In designing treatment programs, it would seem essential to define what precisely is to be treated. One of the most important issues in the field of child sexual abuse has been determining just what kind of problems these children experience. For many years, no one examined this question empirically, because it was assumed that, based on clinical experience, psychodynamic theory, or methodologically weak retrospective studies, sexually abused children had such problems as depression, anxiety, poor self-esteem, dysfunctional families, impaired ability to trust others, and poor assertiveness skills. Although these ideas often seemed to fit with theoretical concepts of child sexual abuse and represented the best information available at the time, recent empirical studies have challenged some of those assumptions.

Researchers have demonstrated almost uniformly that sexually abused children do not necessarily display significant symptoms of depression, anxiety, or low self-esteem as measured by standardized self-report measures (Cohen & Mannarino, 1988; Tufts New England Medical Center, 1984; Einbender & Friedrich, 1989). No studies have empirically examined such issues as trust or assertiveness in these children, no doubt in part because such variables are difficult to measure objectively. Empirical studies of family functioning of sexually abused children are also lacking. Even studies that have demonstrated significant psychopathology in sexually abused children (as measured by parental ratings on standardized instruments), have noted that about one half of the abused subjects were not rated as having any significant pathology (Friedrich, Urquiza, & Beilke, 1986; Tufts New England Medical Center, 1984). Thus, it is not always obvious what problems need to be treated in children who have been sexually abused. Also there seems to be great variability in the type and severity of symptoms experienced.

This is not surprising if sexual abuse is conceptualized as a life event (or series of events) rather than as a discrete psychiatric syndrome. In this way, it is similar to experiencing a divorce or a death, and its impact can vary enormously depending on many factors, some of which have yet to be determined. Sexual abuse is a very diverse phenomenon. It may be intra- or extrafamilial, vary in type of abuse, frequency, and level of force used. The context in which it occurs may greatly affect the impact it has on a child. Abuse may occur in the context of a supportive cohesive family who believe the child, or in a chaotic dysfunctional family who either blame the child for the abuse or disbelieve him or her altogether. It may happen to a well-adjusted socially skilled child, or to a child who exhibited multiple behavioral, developmental, or emotional problems prior to the abuse. Some children may be removed from the home and go through criminal court proceedings, whereas others will have no involvement in the criminal or child protective systems. Certain aspects of the child's temperament, such as general adaptability to stress and cognitive style, may influence the impact of abuse as well.

Because of the above factors, it stands to reason that child sexual abuse would have variable effects on children. Thus, in planning treatment it is not helpful to conceptualize sexual abuse as a unitary clinical syndrome with certain constant behavioral and emotional features. Each child and family must be evaluated carefully and individually to determine what issues are relevant and what problems need to be addressed in therapy, rather than categorizing the child as a "sexual abuse victim" and planning treatment around that label.

REVIEW OF TREATMENT STUDIES OF CHILD VICTIMS

In the last ten years, increasing numbers of treatment models for sexually abused children have appeared in the literature. Virtually all of these have come from clinical programs, whose primary focus is treatment rather than research. This is one reason why these models have lacked systematic empirical data regarding their utility. These methodological shortcomings do not necessarily imply that these treatment models are ineffective. Rather they highlight the fact that research in this field is in its infancy, and that more controlled outcome studies are needed.

Individual Psychotherapy

The case histories of sexually abused children, which have appeared in the psychoanalytic literature for over half a century, have been of theoretical interest and may have provided insight into the dynamic issues of some of these children. Unfortunately, because of their focus on the analytic process, the general applicability of such studies has been limited.

With the advent of the women's movement in the late 1960s, rape crisis centers and women's shelters provided an alternative resource for abused women and children. Many of the innovative individual and group therapy techniques for sexually abused children were started in these centers. As many of the staff in these settings were not professional child therapists, but rather former victims or feminist activists, their treatment approaches were not rooted in any particular theoretical framework. The increasing numbers of sexual abuse victims coming to treatment, however, enabled individual therapists to identify issues that had been overlooked by the traditional analytic model. Porter, Bleck, and Sgroi (1982) summarized these newly recognized treatment issues: the "damaged goods" syndrome (where victims feel irreversibly physically or otherwise damaged as a result of the abuse), guilt, fear, depression, low self-esteem, repressed anger, impaired ability to trust, blurred intrafamilial role boundaries, pseudomaturity, and impaired self-mastery and control. Although recent empirical data have challenged the idea that these problems typify most sexually abused children, recognition of these as potential issues to be explored was a major advance at that time.

Many therapists have relied on play therapy to treat young victims based on the assumption that emotionally laden experiences are easier for children to express symbolically through play than to talk about directly. One study (Mitchum, 1987) described the use of developmental play therapy with five 4-year-old children over the course of 10 weeks. Although Mitchum stressed the importance of developing a new trusting relationship with an adult partner, details of the therapeutic interventions used were vague. In large part this is due to the nature of nondirective play therapy, which is generally unstructured and difficult to describe.

Although there is a wealth of anecdotal information written about individual therapy in sexually abused children, systematic descriptions of these therapeutic intervention techniques are lacking.

Group Therapy

Many therapists have described group treatment approaches for child sexual abuse victims. The idea of group therapy has been appealing not only for its relatively high cost-effectiveness, but also because of the observation that many of these victims feel different from other children after having been abused; consequently, group treatment allows them to meet and interact with other abuse victims and feel more "normal." None of the following descriptive studies included outcome measures, but they have expanded the kinds of approaches that could be attempted with this population of children.

Lubell and Soong (1982) described group therapy with sexually abused children who had been placed in foster care (presumably because the perpetrator remained at home). They noted the importance of addressing the feelings of loss that these children experienced as a result of removal from the parental home. They also focused on the sense of isolation the children felt because abuse had made them feel "different" from peers. Another issue addressed in this model was the children's anger toward the perpetrator, their families, and the system. They stressed the utility of having co-therapists lead these groups, not only for the additional sense of support it provided the clients but also to give support to the therapists.

Berliner and Ernst (1984) described a group program that highlighted issues of self-protection, victims' acknowledgment that abuse had occurred, and appropriate attribution of responsibility to the perpetrator. They used a variety of therapeutic activities, including art projects, educational exercises, and focusing on appropriate intragroup interactions.

Sturkie (1983) provided a structured 8-week therapy group for latency-aged children who had been sexually abused. In this format, one major treatment theme was addressed during each session, including believability (i.e, the importance of telling the truth about abuse until someone believes you), guilt and responsibility, body integrity and protection, secrecy and sharing, anger, powerlessness, other life crises and tasks, and court attendance. They stressed the value of using role playing to model and practice appropriate behaviors and expression of feelings.

Damon and Waterman (1986) designed a parallel group treatment model for treating abused children (aged 8 and younger) and their mothers in concurrent groups. They provided a clear and detailed description of their therapeutic interventions. Thirteen modules were presented to the children and parents, carefully coordinated, so that the mothers would be sensitive to and prepared for what the children had addressed each week in therapy. Some of the issues focused on included the right to say no, the emphasis that private parts are private, whom to tell if abuse occurs, fault and responsibility, anger and punishment, and sex education. These authors offered a unique wealth of clinical materials, such as stories and activities, that are particularly useful with younger children, as well as many practical suggestions. In sum, Damon and Waterman have provided an excellent descriptive account of an innovative group therapy model for sexually abused children.

Family Therapy

Much of the writing in the field of child sexual abuse exclusively addresses intrafamilial abuse. For many years, there was a widespread assumption that most sexual abuse was incestuous, and that in these cases the mother was collusive with the abuse. Recent demographic studies have challenged both of these assumptions, because most reported abuse has been found to occur outside of the nuclear family (Finkelhor, 1979; Mannarino & Cohen, 1986). Furthermore, studies have noted that the majority of mothers of incest victims report the abuse to authorities, as soon as it is disclosed to them (Mannarino & Cohen, 1986), and choose to reject their mate in order to protect their children (Myer, 1985). This challenges the theory that intrafamilial abuse is largely a function of problematic mother–child relationships or that mothers of abused children know about and tolerate the abuse.

On the other hand, there are clearly some cases where the mother knows about and colludes with ongoing abuse. In addition, often family members are in need of therapeutic interventions even in cases of extrafamilial abuse. Thus, it is once again essential to assess each child and family, to clarify which members need treatment, and what issues are pertinent in their particular situation.

Sgroi (1982) suggested a format for evaluating the type and degree of family treatment required in child sexual abuse cases. She stated that in all cases, five factors should be examined: (1) poor supervision of the children, (2) poor choice of surrogate caretakers, (3) inappropriate sleeping arrangements, (4) blurred role boundaries, and (5) sexual abuse by a family member. She discussed varying treatment approaches to the family depending on which of these factors is problematic. She also pointed out the need for more family treatment programs and studies of treatment outcome.

Furniss-Tilman (1983) proposed a treatment approach for incestuous families, specifically those cases involving father–daughter incest. The program is based on the author's clinical experience with 27 of these families. In this program, the initial step is work on intergenerational boundaries in the family system, including defining and strengthening appropriate generational bonds and boundaries. Then the problems in the mother–daughter dyad are addressed, including issues of competition and the mother's responsibility to protect the child. After those problems are resolved, the relationship between the mother and father is the focus of attention. When this relationship becomes more appropriate, the father–daughter relationship is examined.

A treatment program described by Giarretto (1982) has received a great deal of attention, largely because of its very low (1%) reported recidivism rate. This project primarily treats father–daughter incest cases, and is based on work with over 4,000 such families. Treatment consists of a joint effort involving professionals in the mental health, criminal justice, and child protective service systems. There are self-help components (Parents United, Daughters and Sons United) that provide support and other ancillary services. Therapy focuses on mother–daughter counseling to overcome their mutual alienation. A variety of services are provided, including group, family, and individual therapy. Giarretto's study is unusual in that it provides follow-up data. Ninety percent of the victims were reunited with their families, and the reported recidivism rate was less than 1%, a result that is very promising, but it must be noted that these statistics do not necessarily reflect healthy outcomes. Children returned home were not necessarily free of psychopathology. Also, the lack of reported reabuse does not necessarily imply that it did not recur. It is possible that many victims or families, after having gone through extensive interventions, including the child's removal from the home, may have been more hesitant to report abuse a second time.

The major limitation of this study, however, is that 90% of the offenders in this program took full responsibility for the sexual abuse. This fact is unrepresentative of sexual abuse cases in general, where the overwhelming majority of perpetrators deny either responsibility for the abuse or that it happened at all. This suggests that Giaretto's program treats a highly selected population, and raises questions of how applicable it would be to the majority of incestuous families. Nevertheless, it is an impressive program for many reasons, including the high level of cooperation among agencies.

Zimmerman, Wolbert, Burgess, and Hartman (1987) described a modified family group treatment method, used in cases in which multiple children are abused by the same offender. This model makes use of artwork within a group of intrafamilial peers, with a great deal of attention paid to the attributions the children form about the abuse. Specifically, the authors used attributional questions to examine the victims' causal beliefs about the abuse. This model also used peer/family support to prepare the children for court appearances.

In many families in which the nonabusive members respond promptly and appropriately, the main issues may be in dealing with the stress of the disclosure, possible feelings of guilt regarding the abuse, the loss of the perpetrator from the family, and the subsequent legal proceedings that occur with regard to custody, visitation, and criminal charges. Porter et al. (1982) pointed out that ambivalent feelings are very common in this situation, and that these need to be addressed in therapy with the family members who are affected. There is a lack of studies addressing family treatment in cases of extrafamilial abuse. However, it is generally accepted among therapists that family members experience stress regarding sexual abuse and disclosure and may need education and support concurrent with the victim's involvement in therapy.

Educational Interventions

Many programs have included victim and family education as part of the treatment, including such interventions as teaching self-protective skills, assertiveness training and the right to say no to intrusive behavior (Berliner & Ernst, 1984; Damon & Waterman, 1986; Sturkie, 1983), differentiating between appropriate and inappropriate touching (Damon & Waterman, 1986; Sturkie, 1983), what to do if abuse occurs again (Damon & Waterman, 1986), and education about legal procedures and going to court (Sturkie, 1983; Zimmerman et al., 1987). Parents as well as victims often need information about the complex criminal justice system and support with regard to court appearances. The kinds of educational tools available have increased greatly. Coloring books about recognizing and reporting sexual abuse, card and board games teaching how to avoid potentially abusive situations, and children's books and videotapes about going to court are now commonplace in centers that treat sexually abused children. Some of these are also used in sexual abuse prevention programs. Although the efficacy of such interventions has yet to be demonstrated, clinicians have frequently found these aids very helpful.

But because of the complex systems involvement in many sexual abuse cases, often the therapist is obliged to take on the task of coordinating the various services available, including making a referral for a physical examination (to rule out or treat possible sexually transmitted diseases or traumatic genital injuries), educating the family about, and possibly accompanying the child to, various legal proceedings (juvenile or criminal court hearings for charges pressed against the perpetrator, family court hearings to resolve custody and visitation issues), and remaining in close contact with child protective services workers to keep mutually informed about progress and recommendations regarding the child's situation. Many victims' centers provide advocates who assume some of these responsibilities, allowing the therapist to concentrate on treatment. However, any therapist working with sexually abused children should have a thorough understanding of the systems involved and be prepared to spend considerable time on case management and liaison activities. Often it seems that providing these services is as helpful to the child and family as is the actual therapy.

New Directions in the Treatment of Sexually Abused Children

Attribution Theory

Zimmerman *et al.* (1987) devoted a great deal of time in treatment to the attributions children make about sexual abuse. Attributional style has received increased attention recently among researchers. It appears that this may be one of the important mediating factors in determining how symptomatic a child may become following sexual abuse. At the present time, however, there is no empirical evidence to support or challenge this idea.

Theoretically, two related attributional factors may be involved. The first pertains specifically to the abuse: To what does the child attribute the abuse? Some children place full responsibility on the perpetrator, whereas other victims feel the abuse was entirely their own fault. Many children fall somewhere in between, believing that the abuse was basically the perpetrator's fault, but that some facets of the victim (such as being handsome or pretty, being friendly, or being too weak to fight back) also contributed in some degree to the abuse. The second factor is the child's general attributional style: To what does the child attribute typical life experiences, such as failing an exam or making a new friend? Is the child's style to attribute such occurrences to aspects of himself or herself, or to aspects of the outside world, or to some combination?

Future studies could focus on whether either of these attributional factors affect significantly the development or avoidance of psychopathology, and whether there is an attributional style that is optimal for recovery from the abuse. If so, cognitive therapy approaches could be utilized to alter the child's attributions in a way that could positively affect outcome. Clearly, more research is needed before conclusions can be drawn about the role of attributional style; however, it is a promising area for future treatment designs.

Traumagenic Dynamics

Other possible directions for treatment have been suggested by Finkelhor and Browne (1985) who discuss four concepts that are potential foci for therapy: traumatic sexualization, stigmatization, betrayal, and powerlessness. They described these concepts as "traumagenic dy-

namics" that alter the child's cognitive and emotional orientation to the
world, and distort the child's self-concept, world view, or affective abilities. This conceptualization suggests that possible intervention strategies could be designed to correct these cognitive and emotional distor-
tions.

Behavior Therapy

Berliner and Wheeler (1988) proposed a conceptualization that child
sexual abuse results in conditioned anxiety and socially learned maladaptive responses. They suggested that effective therapy may involve
the use of established modalities, such as systematic desensitization,
relaxation training, and problem-solving training.

Finally, behavior modification programs may be useful in controlling many of the problematic symptoms displayed by some sexually
abused children. Aggressive behavior, sexually provocative or overt sexual behavior, and enuresis are all potentially responsive to behavioral
interventions that could be implemented concurrently with other therapeutic strategies. Although this approach has been used by some clinicians, it seems to be dismissed by many others who believe that focusing
on behavioral symptoms will obscure the underlying psychological issues. It is not suggested that these psychological, abuse-related issues
are less important to address. However, it does seem critical to reduce
these types of maladaptive behaviors quickly, in order to prevent secondary problems, such as loss of peers through aggressive behavior, or
ostracism or re-abuse because of inappropriate sexual behavior.

The future direction of treatment for sexually abused children depends to a large degree on the availability of empirical information. In
order to choose effective treatment approaches, there must be more
systematic data gathered with regard to the impact of abuse, and the
effect and outcome of well-defined treatment modalities.

SUMMARY

This chapter has attempted to accomplish a number of tasks. First,
the methodological issues and problems in conducting treatment outcome research with abused children were addressed. Next, in separate
sections, existing treatment studies for physically and sexually abused
children were reviewed and a clinically oriented discussion of potentially useful therapeutic techniques with each group was presented.
Emphasis throughout this chapter has been that there is little empirical

documentation of the effectiveness of treatment modalities with abused children and that further research is clearly needed to fill this void.

REFERENCES

Berliner, L., & Ernst, E. (1984). Group work with preadolescent sexual assault victims. In I. R. Stuart & J. G. Greer (Eds.), *Victims of sexual aggression: Treatment of children, women and men* (pp. 105–124). New York: Van Nostrand Reinhold.

Berliner, L., & Wheeler, J. R. (1988). Treating the effects of child sexual abuse on children. *Journal of Interpersonal Violence, 2,* 415–434.

Blythe, B. J. (1983). A critique of outcome evaluation in child abuse treatment. *Child Welfare, 62,* 325–335.

Cohen, J. A., & Mannarino, A. P. (1988). Psychological symptoms in sexually abused girls. *Child Abuse and Neglect, 12,* 571–577.

Cohn, A. H. (1979). An evaluation of three demonstration child abuse and neglect treatment programs. *Journal of the American Academy of Child Psychiatry, 18,* 283–291.

Conte, J., & Schuerman, J. R. (1987). The effects of sexual abuse on children: A multidimensional view. *Journal of Interpersonal Violence, 2,* 380–390.

Damon, L., & Waterman, J. (1986). Parallel group treatment of children and their mothers. In K. MacFarlane & J. Waterman (Eds.), *Sexual abuse of young children: Evaluation and treatment* (pp. 244–298). New York: Guilford Press.

Einbender, A. J., & Friedrich, W. N. (1989). The psychological functioning and behavior of sexually abused girls. *Journal of Consulting and Clinical Psychology, 57,* 155–157.

Finkelhor, D. (1979). *Sexually victimized children.* New York: Free Press.

Finkelhor, D., & Browne, A. (1985). The traumatic impact of child sexual abuse: A conceptualization. *American Journal of Orthopsychiatry, 55,* 530–541.

Frazier, D., & Levine, E. (1983). Reattachment therapy: Intervention with the very young abused child. *Psychotherapy: Theory, research and practice, 20,* 90–100.

Friedrich, W. N., Urquiza, A. J., & Beilke, R. (1986). Behavior problems in sexually abused young children. *Journal of Pediatric Psychology, 11,* 47–57.

Furniss-Tillman, T. (1983). Family process in the treatment of intrafamilial child sexual abuse. *Journal of Family Therapy, 5,* 263–278.

Gabinet, L. (1983a). Child abuse treatment failures reveal need for redefinition of the problem. *Child Abuse and Neglect, 7,* 395–402.

Gabinet, L. (1983b). Shared parenting: A new paradigm for the treatment of child abuse. *Child Abuse and Neglect, 7,* 403–411.

Giarretto, H. (1982). A comprehensive sexual abuse treatment program. *Child Abuse and Neglect, 6,* 263–279.

Green, A. H., Power, E., Stonebrook, B., & Gaines, R. (1981). Factors associated with successful and unsuccessful intervention with child abuse in families. *Child Abuse and Neglect, 5,* 45–52.

Heide, J., & Richardson, M. T. (1987). Maltreated children's developmental scores: Treatment versus nontreatment. *Child Abuse and Neglect, 11,* 29–34.

Huebner, E. S. (1984). A group treatment approach for abused middle school students. *Techniques, 1,* 139–143.

Isaacs, C. D. (1982). Treatment of child abuse: A review of the behavioral interventions. *Journal of Applied Behavioral Analysis, 15,* 273–294.

Kendall, P., & Braswell, L. (1985). *Cognitive-behavioral therapy for impulsive children.* New York: Guilford Press.

Lubell, D., & Soong, W. (1982). Group therapy with sexually abused adolescents. *Canadian Journal of Psychiatry, 27,* 311–315.

Lutzker, J. R., & Rice, J. M. (1984). Project 12-Ways: Measuring outcome of a large in-home service for treatment and prevention of child abuse and neglect. *Child Abuse and Neglect, 8,* 519–524.

Mannarino, A. P., Christy, M., Durlak, J. A., & Magnussen, M. G. (1982). Evaluation of social competence training in the schools. *Journal of School Psychology, 20,* 11–19.

Mannarino, A. P., & Cohen, J. A. (1986). A clinical-demographic study of sexually abused children. *Child Abuse and Neglect, 10,* 17–28.

Mask, E., Johnson, C., & Kovitz, K. (1983). A comparison of the mother-child interactions of physically abused and non-abused children during play and task situations. *Journal of Clinical Child Psychology, 12,* 337–346.

Meichenbaum, D. (1977). *Cognitive-behavior modification: An integrative approach.* New York: Plenum Press.

Michelson, L., Sugai, D. P., Wood, R. P., & Kazdin, A. E. (1983). *Social skills assessment and training with children: An empirically based handbook.* New York: Plenum Press.

Mitchum, N. T. (1987). Developmental play therapy: A treatment approach for child victims of sexual molestation. *Journal of Counseling and Development, 65,* 320–321.

Myer, M. H. (1985). A new look at mothers of incest victims. *Journal of Social Work and Human Sexuality, 3,* 47–58.

Myers, P. A., Brandner, A., & Templin, K. (1985). Developmental milestones in abused children and their improvement with a family-oriented approach to the treatment of child abuse. *Child Abuse and Neglect, 9,* 245–250.

Pelcovitz, D., Kaplan, S., Samit, C., Krieger, R., & Cornelius, D. (1984). Adolescent abuse: Family structure and implications for treatment. *Journal of the American Academy of Child Psychiatry, 23,* 85–90.

Porter, F. S., Bleck, L. C., & Sgroi, S. M. (1982). Treatment of the sexually abused child. In S. M. Sgroi (Ed.), *Handbook of clinical intervention in child sexual abuse* (pp. 113–148). Lexington, MA: Lexington Books.

Reid, J. B., Taplin, P. S., & Loeber, R. (1981). A social interactional approach to the treatment of abusive families. In R. B. Stuart (Ed.), *Violent behavior: Social learning approaches to prediction, management, and treatment* (pp. 83–101). New York: Brunner/Mazel.

Sgroi, S. M. (1982). Family treatment of child sexual abuse. *Journal of Social Work and Human Sexuality, 1,* 109–128.

Shelton, P. R. (1982). Separation and treatment of child-abusing families. *Family Therapy, 9,* 53–60.

Smith, J. E., Rachman, S. J., & Yule, B. (1984). Non-accidental injury to children-III. *Behaviour Research and Therapy, 22,* 367–383.

Spivack, G., Platt, J. J., & Shure, M. B. (1976). *The problem-solving approach to adjustment.* San Francisco: Jossey-Bass.

Sturkie, K. (1983). Structured group treatment for sexually abused children. *Health and Social Work, 8,* 299–308.

Trowell, J., & Castle, R. L. (1981). Treating abused children. *Child Abuse and Neglect, 5,* 187–192.

Tufts New England Medical Center, Division of Child Psychiatry (1984). *Sexually exploited children: Service and research project.* Final report for the Office of Juvenile Justice and Delinquency Prevention. Washington, DC: U.S. Department of Justice.

Walker, C. E., Bonner, B. L., & Kaufman, K. L. (1988). *The physically and sexually abused child: Evaluation and treatment*. New York: Pergamon Press.

Williams, G. J. (1980). Management and treatment of parental abusive and neglect of children. In G. J. Williams & J. Money (Eds.), *Traumatic abuse and neglect of children at home* (pp. 483–487). Baltimore: Johns Hopkins University Press.

Wolfe, D., & Mosk, M. (1983). Behavioral comparisons of children from abusive and distressed families. *Journal of Consulting and Clinical Psychology, 51*, 702–708.

Zimmerman, M. L., Wolbert, W. A., Burgess, A. W., & Hartman, C. R. (1987). Art and group work: Interventions for multiple victims of child molestation (Part II). *Archives of Psychiatric Nursing, 1*, 40–46.

TREATING THE CHILD ABUSER

JEFFREY A. KELLY

INTRODUCTION

Scientific, empirically based approaches to the treatment of any problem depend upon the adequacy of theoretical models concerning the cause of the problem. As discussed in other chapters, for many years there was a paucity of sound empirical data that could be used either to account for the presence of child abusive patterns or to guide the development of effective interventions for child abusers. Prior to the mid-1970s, most models of child abuse were unifactorial in nature and attempted to predict the occurrence of child maltreatment in families from single etiological causes, such as parent psychopathology or sociological disadvantage (see reviews by Belsky, 1980; Burgess, 1979; Parke & Collmer, 1975). Treatment interventions based on such models also tended to be unifactorial, usually emphasizing treatment of a parent's postulated underlying psychiatric disorder or the alleviation of socioeconomic distress. However, most of these therapeutic interventions were unevaluated or investigated only with uncontrolled and anecdotal outcome reports.

Over the past 10 years, theories of child abuse have become more ecological and multifactorial, stressing the functional interplay between a variety of child characteristics; parent characteristics, cognitive-behavioral skills, and coping strategies; and environmental influences on the

JEFFREY A. KELLY • Division of Psychology, University of Mississippi Medical Center, Jackson, Mississippi 39216.

family (Burgess, 1979; Burgess & Richardson, 1984; Kelly, 1983; Parke & Collmer, 1975; Wolfe, 1985). The emergence of these more complex social-interactional conceptual models of child abuse has given rise to new approaches to the treatment of child abusive parents. Because outcomes of therapy for child maltreating parents have been studied scientifically for only a short period of time, this field is still in its earliest stages, and many questions remain uninvestigated. However, sufficient information has already been gained to guide the development of clinical research and intervention for child abusive parents. Thus, this chapter will briefly discuss conceptual and practical issues related to treatment for child abusers, review empirical research on therapy outcomes for this population, and consider topics important for further treatment research.

MULTIFACTORIAL MODELS OF CHILD ABUSE: IMPLICATIONS FOR TREATMENT

If the occurrence of child maltreatment is deemed to be a consequence of what potentially are multiple parent, child, and environmental factors (and the reciprocal influences between them), it is apparent that there also are many different potential targets or objectives for treatment intervention. For example, it has now been well-established that child abusive parents relative to their nonabusive counterparts exhibit deficits in child management skills (Burgess, 1979; Burgess & Conger, 1978), emotional overreactivity to aversive cues of child behavior (Disbrow, Doerr, & Caulfield, 1977; Frodi & Lamb, 1980; Wolfe, Fairbank, Kelly, & Bradlyn, 1983), higher levels of conflict and violence with family members other than the abused child (Burgess & Conger, 1978; Lahey, Conger, Atkeson, & Treiber, 1984; Reid, Taplin, & Lorber, 1981), greater mislabeling and misattributions concerning child behavior (Mash, Johnston, & Kovitz, 1983), higher behavioral impulsiveness (Rohrbeck & Twentyman, 1986), and deficient social problem-solving skills (Azar, Robinson, Hekinans, & Twentyman, 1984). Such findings indicate that treatment for child abusive parents might include parent training, anger control and stress management training, marital and family therapy, cognitive and reattributional therapy, and problem-solving training. Furthermore, although psychiatric and sociological "single-factor" theories of child abuse are criticized as overly narrow and simplistic, between 5% and 10% of abusive parents do exhibit demonstrable and severe psychopathology (Bell, 1973; Kempe, 1973; Kempe & Kempe, 1978), and socioeconomic stress is implicated in a significant proportion of reported abuse cases (Garbarino, 1976; Garbarino & Sherman, 1980; Giovannoni

& Billingsley, 1970). Multifactorial models of child abuse create multiple potential targets for therapeutic intervention although it is not necessarily the case that all abusive families have all these problems. A question of practical clinical and research importance is that of determining *which* factors contribute functionally to child maltreatment in a given family so that parent treatment can address the most relevant problem areas for that family (Kelly, 1983).

In addition to multiple problem areas related to abuse that can be targeted in treatment, the term *child abuse* itself is very broad and subsumes a number of different patterns of child maltreatment. Extreme physical violence directed by an adult toward a child is the form of maltreatment most often considered abuse and is the problem most often studied in the child abuse literature. However, child maltreatment because of neglect may occur even more often than cases of physically violent abuse (Mayhall & Norgard, 1983), and recent studies suggest that sexual abuse occurs at a rate and with psychological consequences more widespread than previously believed (Finkelhor & Hotaling, 1984; Kolko, 1987; Mrazek, 1983). Although physically abusive and neglectful parents share similar patterns in certain treatment-relevant areas, such as child management skill deficits (Burgess & Conger, 1978) and physiological arousal to cues of child behavior (Disbrow *et al.*, 1977), there is little *à priori* evidence that physical abuse, sexual abuse, and child neglect share the same causes or will respond to identical therapeutic interventions. Treatment that is effective for certain child maltreating parents may prove less effective or be ineffective for parents who maltreat their children in different ways and for different reasons.

If multifactorial and ecological perspectives have produced more complex models of child abuse and family violence, they also set the stage for more innovative and well-controlled studies of treatment outcome. Prior to the mid-1970s, there was little, if any, empirical research on the efficacy of treatment for child abusers. Since that time, uncontrolled descriptive and anecdotal reports have gradually given rise to more scientifically sound evaluations. We will next turn our attention to treatment interventions for abusive parents.

INTERVENTIONS TO IMPROVE PARENTING SKILLS

The rationale of child management training for abusive parents is that violent parenting acts, which can result in child injury, may develop because of the parent's failure to manage child behavior in a more appropriate, nonviolent manner. From this perspective, a parent's overreliance on ineffective child control strategies and high rates of corporal punishment increase child aversive behavior, escalate the intensity and frequency of aversive interchanges between the parent and child, and establish an ongoing "coercive cycle" between them (cf. Patterson, 1977; Patterson, Reid, Jones, & Conger, 1975). Use of physical punishment is maintained probably because it can produce temporary suppression of child's misbehavior, although organisms adapt to the intensity of frequently administered punishment (Azrin, Holz, & Hake, 1963; Reynolds, 1975) and, over time, escalating levels of punishment are needed to produce the same degree of behavioral suppression. Ultimately, parents who rely excessively on physically punitive controls may in fact injure their children. This formulation is consistent with a substantial body of observational research that has demonstrated the occurrence of fewer positive parental behaviors, more frequent negative and aversive behaviors, and lower levels of attentiveness to the child by abusive parents than control parents, even during routine parent–child interactions (Bousha & Twentyman, 1984; Burgess, 1979; Burgess & Conger, 1978). For these reasons, a number of investigators have employed parent-training methods to alter the disciplinary style and parent–child interaction patterns of abusive parents.

Parenting Skills Interventions with Individual Clinical Cases

Mastria, Mastria, and Harkins (1979) conducted one of the earlier case study parent-training interventions with a mother who physically abused her 7-year-old child. Treatment in the study consisted of videotaping parent–child interactions that took place in a clinic playroom and providing video feedback, therapist modeling of appropriate means to handle child misbehavior, and homework assignments to practice the same skills *in vivo*. Parent behaviors targeted for intervention included the use of positive verbal reinforcement, ignoring inappropriate child behavior, and problem-solving skills to identify nonviolent methods to handle child misbehavior. Mastria *et al.* (1979) reported increases in observed appropriate parenting skill behavior after treatment and at a 3-month followup. Moreover, these changes were corroborated by parent, child, and therapist reports of improved adjustment and coping by the parent and her child. However, this early study did not employ experimental controls and presented limited data on the specific nature of change observed in parent–child interactions.

Sandler, Van Dercar, and Milhoan (1978) also conducted an early investigation of parent-training effectiveness, but provided intervention and conducted observational assessments within the homes of two abusive families rather than in a clinic setting. In both cases, the abusive parents were single mothers who were reported to have beaten their children. Observations were conducted over seven to nine occasions at mealtimes to establish pretreatment baselines for the occurrence of 29 different categories of parent and child behavior using the coding system developed by Patterson, Ray, Shaw, and Cobb (1969). The parents initially exhibited low rates of positive verbal and positive physical behavior, frequent negative commands, and minimal conversational talk with their children. Intervention in this project consisted of child management technique reading assignments, therapist modeling of appropriate parenting skills, and tangible reinforcement for parent compliance in the training. Treatment produced substantial increases in positive verbal and positive physical parent behavior, increased conversational talk between parent and child, decreased use of negative commands, and more frequent affectionate laughter. Most changes were well maintained at 4-month follow-up, although the Sandler et al. (1978) study did not employ an experimental design.

A similar intervention was also conducted by Wolfe and Sandler (1981). In this study, each of three physically abusive parents received training to improve interactions with their children, including the handling of child misbehavior. As in the Sandler et al. (1978) investigation, both parent-training and family observations took place in family homes, and the parent-training intervention included child-management reading assignments, therapist modeling of appropriate skills, role-playing of problem situations, and feedback to the parent following behavior rehearsal. Over the course of the 10-session intervention, substantial decreases were observed in aversive child behavior (such as crying, noncompliance, and verbal or physical negativity) and aversive parent behavior (including negative commands and yelling). Increases in the proportion of child compliance to parental commands were also associated with treatment, and all effects were maintained at long-term follow-up. Treatment conditions in the Wolfe and Sandler (1981) study were manipulated to determine whether contingency contracting with the parent to utilize one new child-management technique at home each week would produce greater skill change. Although the investigators reported that this additional homework contracting was useful clinically, it was not associated with improvement beyond that produced by in-the-home parent training alone.

A somewhat different parent-training approach was employed in a case reported by Wolfe, St. Lawrence, Graves, Brehony, Bradlyn, and

Kelly (1982), with treatment conducted in a clinic playroom setting and its impact assessed by observations of parent–child interaction behavior made during "staged" tasks in both clinic playroom and home settings. The staged tasks involved situations that were intended to elicit child noncompliance (picking up and sorting a large number of toys) as well as positive parent–child behavior (playing a game together). The parent who received treatment in this case demonstration was a 29-year-old single mother of two mentally retarded 9-year-old twin boys; welfare authorities reported the children were difficult to control and that the mother injured them during frequent spankings and whippings. Following baseline playroom observations, the therapists providing treatment coached and modeled appropriate means to handle child behavior, including the use of verbal and physical touch reinforcement, selective ignoring of minor misbehavior, and time out for more serious misconduct. During practice parent–child interaction in each session, the mother was prompted and herself reinforced by the observing therapists via a "bug-in-the-ear" remote receiver that she wore for using trained skills. Experimental control in the study was achieved by means of a multiple baseline introduction of treatment attention first targeting the mother's hostile physical and verbal behavior and then improving her positive interaction skills. Reductions in hostile behavior and increases in positive reinforcing skills during clinic and at-home observations were found and were maintained 2 months following intervention. There were no further reports of child maltreatment by welfare caseworkers after the completion of treatment. A very similar intervention was conducted by Crimmins, Bradlyn, St. Lawrence, and Kelly (1984) with a parent who was both abusive and neglectful toward her 4-year-old son with comparable results.

Group Comparison Studies of Parent-Training Interventions

In an extension of their earlier work with individual clinical cases, Wolfe, Sandler, and Kaufman (1981) offered child-management training to a group of eight abusive parents referred by a child welfare agency. Most of the parents were of low income, all had engaged in physical abuse, and their children ranged in age from 2 to 10 years. A demographically-comparable set of eight other abusive parents served as a no-treatment control group and completed assessment measures but received no parent training.

All parents in the study completed the Eyberg Child Behavior Inventory (ECBI) (Eyberg & Ross, 1978) and were evaluated on global measures of family functioning by social service caseworkers uninvolved in the parent-training program. In addition, all families in the study were observed in their homes during free (unstructured) interaction periods, during tasks in which the parent taught the child a new puzzle, and during tasks in which the parent was asked to elicit the child's compliance in picking up toys. All observed interactions were coded for the frequency of parent positive reinforcement techniques, appropriate commands and prompts, and appropriate punishment.

Following these baseline assessments, parents in the experimental condition attended a series of group sessions that provided instruction in child development and management, behavioral principles applied to parenting (such as positive reinforcement, time out, shaping, and appropriate punishment), problem-solving of child-management difficulties, and relaxation and self-management skills. In addition to the weekly groups, each family received individual in-home child-management training tailored to specific problems of that family. At the conclusion of the experimental group's intervention, all families were reassessed on the same set of measures that had been used during baseline. Significant improvement was found for experimental group parents relative to the control group parents on skill behaviors during the observed parent–child interaction tasks, and changes were well maintained at a 10-week followup of five of the parents. Differential change was not found between the child-management training and control groups for ECBI scores or caseworker ratings, perhaps because of the relatively small sample sizes in the study. Based on a 1-year follow-up inspection of welfare department records, none of the families that received treatment was suspected of further abuse.

The Wolfe et al. (1981) project, like most others reported in the literature on child-management training for abusive parents, taught parenting skills based largely on operant principles. Brunk, Henggeler, and Whelan (1987) compared the relative efficacy of operant-behavioral child-management training with a multisystemic family therapy intervention approach in a sample of 33 families with a history of child abuse or neglect Parents in the child-management training intervention attended an 8-session series of groups, modeled after the group treatment used by Wolfe et al. (1981), which taught general behavioral parenting skills and skills for handling specific child problems experienced by each family. In-the-home training was not conducted with individual families. Subjects in the multisystemic therapy condition received eight sessions of family therapy, conducted with individual family units rather than in groups; the intervention was based on family restructuring principles (cf. Haley, 1976; Minuchin, 1974) rather than behavioral training. Before and after intervention, all parents were assessed using symptom and child behavior problem checklists, family environment and social system self-report measures, and treatment satisfaction questionnaires. In addition, observations were made of parent–child interactions during a 10-minute, in-home talk in which the parent was asked to teach his or her child block designs of increasing difficulty level. These interactions were rated for verbal and nonverbal measures of parental control style using the Schaffer and Crook (1979) coding system.

Brunk et al. (1987) found that the child-management training and the multisystemic family therapy produced significant and comparable reductions in symptoms of parents' emotional distress, reduced overall family stress, and reduced severity of identified problems. The multi-systemic family therapy intervention produced greater improvement than did the child-management training on observational measures of effectiveness during the parent–child interaction task. Parents who received this treatment showed increased effectiveness in child control skills and were more appropriately responsive to child behavior. Also, some collateral improvements in child behavior were observed. However, these results must be viewed as preliminary because child-management training was conducted in groups, whereas the family therapy intervention was provided to individual family units, no follow-up was conducted, and a no-treatment control was not employed. Nonetheless, the results of Brunk et al. (1987) suggest that attention to factors beyond child-management skill alone may produce additional improvement in family functioning.

INTERVENTIONS THAT ADDRESS PARENT COPING

The treatment programs described in the previous section, with the exception of the Brunk et al. (1987) examination of family therapy and the Wolfe, Kelly, and Drabman (1981) inclusion of a relaxation training intervention component, entailed relatively direct and straightforward applications of behavioral child-management training. Although most empirical studies on child abuser treatment include such parent training, a number of researchers have incorporated other coping training elements in their interventions.

Denicola and Sandler (1980) combined child-management training with training in self-control, anger, and stress management skills for two physically abusive mothers. The child-management treatment compo-

nent was conducted in standard fashion and included reading assignments, verbal instruction, modeling, behavior rehearsal, and therapist
feedback concerning appropriate means to handle child behavior problems interactions with children. The self-control treatment element entailed deep muscle relaxation training, self-instructional training to control arousal and anger, stress inoculation procedures, and problem-
solving practice in citations that would typically produce aggressive
behavior. The child-management and self-control elements were introduced separately in a withdrawal experimental design, and each parent
received 12 treatment sessions. The introduction of intervention,
whether child management or self-control skills, produced reductions in
total aversive behavior for both the parent and the child during routine
interactions observed and coded in the home. Thus, both intervention
elements resulted in improved parent–child interaction patterns; in addition, each parent reported greater skill in handling child-related problems
and reduced anger and emotional upset.

In similar fashion, Scott, Baer, Christoff, and Kelly (1984) described
the treatment of a mother who physically abused her 11-year-old son
primarily at times when she was already angry and when the child then
misbehaved. Assessment revealed a recurrent pattern in which the parent (1) became frustrated following interpersonal conflicts with other
adults which she usually handled passively and unsatisfactorily, (2) experienced increased feelings of anger and stress as a result of these
problems, and (3) was then confronted by noncompliant, tantrum, or
"talking back" problems exhibited by her child. Because episodes of
violence appeared to be triggered by these multiple antecedents, Scott
et al. (1984) intervened with a combined therapy of assertiveness training (targeted toward the mother's relationship frustrations), child-
management skills training (to teach alternative means of handling child
behavior problems), and problem-solving training (to address life situations that were reported by the parent to create stress and generalized
anger). These three treatment elements were introduced sequentially in
a multiple-baseline design, and effects of training were examined with
measures of role-played assertiveness skill, subjective anger ratings,
problem-solving skill, and skill behavior during observed interactions
between parent and child in the clinic and home settings. Over the
course of a 20-session intervention, improvements were found on all
measures. In general, change in the various skill areas occurred at predicted points during the intervention (e.g., improved assertiveness followed assertiveness training and improved parent–child interaction behavior was found contingent upon training specific to child-

management skills). A 4-month follow-up revealed maintenance of change in all areas and no evidence of continued abuse or extreme punishment.

Most of the interventions described to this point were conducted with parents who were physically abusive or were both abusive and neglectful. In contrast, Dawson, de Armas, McGrath, and Kelly (1986) have reported on the treatment of three parents who endangered their children because of neglect rather than violent behavior. Each parent had a history of failing to meet child care needs properly, inadequately supervising the children, and otherwise exhibiting poor judgment in child-care responsibilities. All were referred by a child protective services agency. Following clinical interviews, Dawson et al. (1986) chose to focus treatment on parent cognitive problem-solving skills in areas related to child care.

Assessment measures in this study consisted of a set of 15 problem-solving vignettes. The situations described in the vignettes involved themes of leaving one's child in a potentially dangerous situation; handling conflicts between one's own leisure, social, or work needs and child-care responsibilities; establishing spending priorities; and handling child health emergencies. Prior to intervention, each parent responded verbally when asked how she would handle the situation. All responses were tape recorded and later rated for elements of effective problem-solving skill (D'Zurilla & Goldfried, 1971; Shure & Spivak, 1972). In addition, each family's caseworker completed more global measures evaluating perceived parent skill, judgment, and quality of family functioning.

Treatment in the Dawson et al. (1986) project consisted of problem-solving training introduced in a multiple-baseline design across parents. Each parent received seven to nine individual treatment sessions that focused on developing skills for effective problem solving in situations related to child care. Training was accomplished using modeling, shaping, problem-solving practice, feedback, and homework assignments. The examples practiced in sessions involved genuine problems that each parent had encountered in the past and had not handled successfully. In addition, parents received instruction in child-development principles. Analyses of parent performance on problem-solving assessment vignettes completed at the end of each training session revealed substantial increases in skill following the introduction of treatment. These changes were well-maintained throughout the intervention and through a 15-month follow-up. In addition, there was evidence of skill generalization to problems presented in novel vignettes, improvements in global caseworker ratings of family functioning, and no further reports of child maltreatment.

In the Dawson *et al.* (1986) study, cognitive problem-solving skills were taught in order to improve parents' judgment in child-care situations. A more direct environment modification approach to improve home safety condition has also been used by several investigators. Noting that poor home safety is frequently cited by investigators of child neglect and abuse cases, Tertinger, Greene, and Lutzker (1984) and Barone, Greene, and Lutzker (1986) have employed in-the-home interventions to train parents in ways to protect children from health and accidental injury hazards. In the Tertinger *et al.* (1984) project, an observational inventory was used to rate the homes of abusive and neglectful parents for hazards, accessible to children, that could produce child injury by poisoning, suffocation, electrical, fire, and other means. In-home counseling, which included instruction, modeling of hazard reduction steps, homework assignments, and feedback, was provided to each parent by community therapists. Subsequent observational checks revealed substantial reductions in the number of safety hazards in each family's home through a 7-month follow-up period. Barone *et al.* (1986) addressed the same problem with three abusive/neglectful families but employed audio-slide show instructional materials, a home safety review manual, and safety accessories rather than individual counseling in order to make the intervention more cost-efficient. Positive changes in home safety, again based on in-home observations of potential risks, were found for all three families.

In most of the studies reviewed thus far, relatively focused treatments have been used and evaluated with relatively small numbers of abusive parents. A different and larger scale treatment program has been described by Lutzker and his colleagues (Lutzker, Frame, & Rice, 1982; Lutzker & Rice, 1987; Lutzker & Rice, in press; Lutzker, Wesch, & Rice, 1984). Termed "Project 12-Ways," the program provides intervention services to child abusive and neglectful parents in a number of areas, including child-management training, stress management, assertiveness training, self-control therapy, job-finding skills assistance, alcoholism treatment, social support development, home safety improvement, and money management. Between 50 and 100 families receive in-the-home services in this program each year, and the intervention components offered to a given family are based on a clinical assessment of the family's needs and circumstances. Child-management training is the service most often provided, although the majority of parents receive intervention in other areas as well (Lutzker *et al.*, 1982). Global evaluation of this multiple component treatment approach has relied primarily on comparisons made between families that participate in the project with families from the same catchment area that do not, using welfare agency records of substantiated incidents of child abuse. These data indicate that program participation results in less frequent child abuse or neglect incidents during the year in which intervention is offered and less frequent reports of multiple abuse or neglect incidents in subsequent years, although some of the recidivism data are less clearcut (Lutzker & Rice, 1984, in press; Lutzker et al., 1982). Outcome analyses are considered preliminary by the investigators given nonrandom assignment of families to the project and control groups and unknown demographic equivalence of the groups. Nonetheless, the provision of multiple kinds of intervention to child abusive parents depending upon individual family needs is a logical and promising approach to abuser treatment.

RESEARCH CRITIQUE

Research on the effects of treatment for child abusive parents is difficult for a variety of reasons. Acts of parental violence typically occur in private. Although the physical consequences of abuse—child injury—can be detected in some cases, the vast majority of instances of parental violence are neither detected nor directly observable. Parent reports of violent behavior are susceptible to bias, inaccuracy, and distortion. Lack of candor is especially possible when a parent is under investigation or is involved in judicial processes related to child maltreatment. For these and other reasons, research on treatment outcome with abusive parents has relied on "probe" assessments of skill or behavioral competence in situations which are presumed to have a functional relationship to abuse. As we have seen, the most common paradigm employed in recent studies involves "sampling" parent and child behavior in naturalistic or staged interaction tasks, either in the home or in a clinic setting. To the extent that these parent–child interaction tasks approximate the real situations that give rise to family conflict and abuse, they constitute a valid assessment mode. To the extent that improvements in parent skill observed in these interactions following treatment then generalize to *in vivo* (and unobserved) interactions in the home that could actually trigger violence, the impact of therapy is also substantiated.

It now seems clear that training parents in child-management skills does produce positive change in parent–child interactional style during observational assessments and that change maintains over time when the same assessments are repeated. How adequately the effects of this training generalize outside formal interaction assessment observation tasks is largely unknown because data collection has relied primarily on performance in these tasks. Documentation that no further known abuse was reported to authorities over a follow-up period is a positive but, at best, imprecise indicator of intervention outcome because individual acts of maltreatment are unlikely to be reported to authorities. Increased attention to multimodal outcome assessment is needed in the child abuser treatment literature. Confidence that the effects of child-management training for abusers lessen violence and improve family functioning would be increased if changes in parent–child interaction skill were systematically corroborated with (1) ongoing self-monitoring of behavior and child-related problems made by the parent and perhaps also by the child; (2) evaluations made by significant others who regularly see family members such as teachers or relatives; (3) physical, emotional, and behavioral characteristics of the child; (4) measures sensitive to family stress and functioning; or (5) parent performance during novel, challenging parent–child interaction tasks different from those repeatedly practiced in training. Establishing change across several such measures following treatment could serve to validate more efficiently and corroborate the clinical impact of an intervention.

The issue of generality versus specificity in parent training focus may also play a role in clinical outcomes when treating child abusers. Some abusive parents appear to exhibit generalized skill deficiencies when interacting with their children in everyday, routine situations (Burgess, 1979; Burgess & Conger, 1978). However, there may also be specific and idiosyncratic child-problem situations that carry a high probability for violence or inappropriate handling within a given family. For example, Wolfe, Kelly, and Drabman (1981) described a case in which spankings and beatings were administered by a parent when her children "dawdled" excessively in the morning and at bedtime. Treatment in the case entailed an analysis of this particular child-management problem and the development of a parent-training intervention specifically tailored to it. The impact of child-management approaches would appear to be greatest when intervention is relevant to those specific conflict areas, child problems, and parent skill deficits known to affect the family being treated (Kelly, 1983). On the other hand, an overly narrow focus in child-management training may equip a parent to handle only a few isolated problem situations, but fail to grasp underlying principles needed to appropriately deal with other problems that were not specifically covered in training.

RESEARCH NEEDS ON MULTIFACTORIAL
TREATMENTS

Noted earlier was the observation that multifactorial conceptual models of child abuse imply the need for multifaceted treatment interventions targeted toward parent, child, social, and environmental variables functionally related to abuse in a given family. It is clear that child-management/parent training has received the bulk of attention in the empirical child abuser treatment literature. This is warranted given the now substantial evidence that abusers often lack the skills necessary to interact appropriately with their children and handle nonviolently child behavior problems, and also given the promising results of interventions that directly train abusive parents to use new child-management methods.

On the other hand, and as several investigators have noted (Kelly, 1983; Lutzker & Rice, 1987; Lutzker et al., 1982), ecological models of abuse suggest that abusing parents often have problems in areas outside child-management knowledge and skill alone. If this is the case, and if these other problems are also salient functional contributors to abusive behavior, attention to them may be needed to produce the most potent changes in family functioning. As one example, Wahler and his colleagues have found that parental "insularity," or isolation from positive interactions with friends in a parent's social network, predicts outcome and benefit following participation in general child-management training (Wahler, 1980; Wahler, Leske, & Rogers, 1979). Because abusive parents tend to be socially isolated (Helfer, 1973; Parke & Collmer, 1975), attention to this factor may well bear on therapy outcome. However, research in the child abuser treatment area has not directly examined this question to date. In similar fashion, some of the studies reviewed in this chapter incorporated stress management, anger control, or problem-solving techniques together with child-management training in their intervention packages (cf. Denicola & Sandler, 1980; Scott et al., 1984; Wolfe et al., 1981). Although these combination treatments yielded promising results, they are for the most part single-subject or small-sample demonstrations. Larger-scale research is needed to evaluate how (and perhaps for which abusive parents) the incorporation of anger–arousal control, problem-solving training, and skills training to handle other life stressors can amplify the effects of child-management intervention alone or promote more successful implementation of new child control methods. To date, there has been little or no research on these questions. If multifactorial conceptual models of abuse are advanced and prove useful, but if treatment focuses solely on child-management training, the impact of treatment interventions may be lessened.

TREATMENT FOR SPECIAL ABUSER POPULATIONS

As noted earlier, the populations most widely studied in the child-abuser treatment literature are parents who behave violently toward their children and who injure their youngsters as a result of inappropriate corporal discipline. In the majority of cases, research has focused on abuse toward young children. Very little treatment attention has been directed to parents who physically abuse their infants or, at the other end of the age range, their older children or adolescent children even though surveys indicate that these forms of family violence are both common and, often, severe (Gelles, 1978). Many studies have also found abuse to be disproportionately prevalent among parents of children with developmental disabilities and physical handicaps (see reviews by Ammerman, Van Hasselt, & Hersen, 1988; Kirkham, Schinke, Schilling, Meltzer, & Norelius, 1986), although reports of treatment for these families are rare. The development and evaluation of treatment programs for parents who abuse their infants, older children, or handicapped children are needed. Although many of the principles from the general child abuse treatment literature are no doubt relevant to these populations as well, families with infants, older children, and handicapped children may face different problems and experience stressors that require specialized attention in therapy. Finally, there is a striking paucity of empirical research on treatment for sexually abusive parents (see Kolko, 1987). Over the past several years, clinical researchers have started to evaluate methods to treat the problems experienced by child victims of sexual exploitation (Alter-Reid, Gibbs, Lachnmeyer, Sigal, & Massoth, 1986; Browne & Finkelhor, 1986; Kolko, 1987). However, research on methods to intervene with parents who perpetrate sexual abuse is very limited. Clinical research in the area of pedophilia treatment may prove relevant for some sexually abusive parents.

SUMMARY

Significant strides have recently been made in the development of treatment approaches for child abusive parents. A number of outcome studies now demonstrate the utility of child-management, parent-training, and other family intervention approaches in altering parents' reliance on excessively corporal, aversive, and violent child-control strategies. The effects of parent-training interventions have been confirmed by objective change in observed parent–child interactional patterns in clinic and, more importantly, in home settings.

Multifactorial models of child abuse stress the functional interplay between multiple parent, child, and environmental factors, and the reciprocal influences between them. Some case studies and group interventions have incorporated attention to such factors by training abusive parents in skills for anger and stress coping, problem-solving with respect to child-related and other life problem situations, and handling social and economic stressors as well as child-management skills. These approaches have produced positive outcomes and highlight the importance of addressing what may be multiple needs, skill deficits, pressures, and behavioral-social problems that affect some abusive parents. Research on the differential effectiveness of various therapy approaches for child abusers is rare in the literature but needed. Furthermore, because the antecedents of violent behavior may vary across families, it will be important to develop means to tailor treatment interventions more efficiently to specific problems that affect parent–child interactions and the family unit as a whole.

REFERENCES

Alter-Reid, K., Gibbs, M. S., Lachnmeyer, J. R., Sigal, J., & Massoth, N. A. (1986). Sexual abuse of children: A review of the empirical findings. *Clinical Psychology Review, 6,* 249–266.

Ammerman, R. T., Van Hasselt, V. B., & Hersen, M. (1988). Maltreatment of handicapped children: A critical review. *Journal of Family Violence, 3,* 53–72.

Azar, S. T., Robinson, D. R., Hekinans, E., & Twentyman, G. T. (1984). Unrealistic expectations and problems-solving ability in maltreating and comparison mothers. *Journal of Consulting and Clinical Psychology, 52,* 687–691.

Azrin, N. H., Holz, W. C., & Hake, D. F. (1963). Fixed ratio punishment. *Journal of the Experimental Analysis of Behavior, 6,* 141–148.

Barone, V. J., Greene, B. F., & Lutzker, J. R. (1986). Home safety with families being treated for child abuse and neglect. *Behavior Modification, 10,* 93–114.

Bell, G. (1973). Parents who abuse their children. *Canadian Psychiatric Association Journal, 18,* 223–228.

Belsky, J. (1980). Child maltreatment: An ecological integration. *American Psychologist, 35,* 320–335.

Bousha, D. M., & Twentyman, C. T. (1984). Mother-child interactional style in abuse, neglect, and control groups: Naturalistic observations in the home. *Journal of Abnormal Psychology, 93,* 106–114.

Browne, A., & Finkelhor, D. (1986). Impact of child sexual abuse: A review of the research. *Psychological Bulletin, 99,* 66–77.

Brunk, M., Henggeler, S. W., & Whelan, J. P. (1987). Comparison of multisystemic therapy and parent training in the brief treatment of child abuse and neglect. *Journal of Consulting and Clinical Psychology, 55*, 171–178.

Burgess, R. L. (1979). Child abuse: A social interactional analysis. In B. B. Lahey & A. E. Kazdin (Eds.), *Advances in clinical child psychology* (Vol. 2, pp. 142–172). New York: Plenum Press.

Burgess, R. L., & Conger, R. (1978). Family interactions in abusive, neglectful, and normal families. *Child Development, 49*, 1163–1173.

Burgess, R. L., & Richardson, R. A. (1984). Coercive interpersonal contingencies as determinants of child abuse: Implications for treatment and prevention. In R. F. Dangel & R. A. Polster (Eds.), *Behavioral parent training: Issues in research and practice* (pp. 239–259). New York: Guilford Press.

Crimmins, D. B., Bradlyn, A. S., St. Lawrence, J. S., & Kelly, J. A. (1984). In-clinic training to improve the parent-child interaction skills of a neglectful mother. *Child Abuse and Neglect, 8*, 533–539.

Dawson, B., de Armas, A., McGrath, M. L., & Kelly, J. A. (1986). Cognitive problem-solving training to improve the child-care judgment of child neglectful parents. *Journal of Family Violence, 1*, 209–221.

Denicola, J., & Sandler, J. (1980). Training abusive parents in child management and self-control skills. *Behavior Therapy, 11*, 263–270.

Disbrow, M. A., Doerr, H., & Caulfield, C. (1977). Measuring the components of parents' potential for child abuse and neglect. *Child Abuse and Neglect, 1*, 279–296.

D'Zurilla, T. J., & Goldfried, M. R. (1971). Problem solving and behavior modification. *Journal of Abnormal Psychology, 78*, 107–126.

Eyberg, S. M., & Ross, A. W. (1978). Assessment of child behavior problems: The validation of a new inventory. *Journal of Clinical Child Psychology, 7*, 113–116.

Finkelhor, D., & Hotaling, G. T. (1984). Sexual abuse in the national incidence study of child abuse and neglect: An appraisal. *Child Abuse Neglect, 8*, 23–33.

Frodi, A., & Lamb, M. E. (1980). Child abusers' responses to infant smiles and cries. *Child Development, 51*, 238–241.

Garbarino, J. (1976). A preliminary study of some ecological correlates of child abuse: The impact of socioeconomic stress on mothers. *Child Development, 47*, 178–185.

Garbarino, J., & Sherman, D. (1980). High risk neighborhoods and high risk families: The human ecology of child maltreatment. *Child Development, 51*, 188–198.

Gelles, R. J. (1978). Violence toward children in the United States. *American Journal of Orthopsychiatry, 48*, 580–592.

Giovannoni, J., & Billingsley, A. (1970). Child neglect among the poor: A study of parental inadequacy in families of three ethnic groups. *Child Welfare, 49*, 196–204.

Haley, J. (1976). *Problem solving therapy.* San Francisco: Jossey-Bass.

Helfer, R. E. (1973). The etiology of child abuse. *Pediatrics, 51*, 777.

Kelly, J. A. (1983). *Treating child-abusive families: Intervention based on skills-training principles.* New York: Plenum Press.

Kempe, C. H. (1973). A practical approach to protection of the abused child and rehabilitation of the abusing parent. *Pediatrics, 51*, 804–812.

Kempe, R. S., & Kempe, C. H. (1978). *Child abuse.* Cambridge: Harvard University Press.

Kirkham, M. A., Schinke, S. P., Schilling II, R. F., Meltzer, N. J., & Norelius, K. L. (1986). Cognitive-behavioral skills, social supports, and child abuse potential among mothers of handicapped children. *Journal of Family Violence, 1*, 235–245.

Kolko, D. J. (1987). Treatment of child sexual abuse: Programs, progress, and prospects. *Journal of Family Violence, 2*, 303–318.

Lahey, B. B., Conger, R. D., Atkeson, B. M., & Treiber, F. A. (1984). Parenting behavior and emotional status of physically abusive mothers. *Journal of Consulting and Clinical Psychology, 52,* 1062–1071.

Lutzker, J. R., & Rice, J. M. (1984). Project 12-ways: Measuring outcome of a large-scale in-home service for the treatment and prevention of child abuse and neglect. *Child Abuse and Neglect 8,* 519–524.

Lutzker, J. R., & Rice, J. M. (1987). Using recidivism data to evaluate project 12-ways: An ecobehavioral approach to the treatment and prevention of child abuse and neglect. *Journal of Family Violence, 2,* 283–290.

Lutzker, J. R., & Rice, J. M. (in press). Project 12-ways: Measuring outcome of a large in-home service program for the treatment and prevention of child abuse and neglect. *Child Abuse and Neglect.*

Lutzker, J. R., Frame, R. E., & Rice, J. M. (1982). Project 12-ways: An ecobehavioral approach to the treatment and prevention of child abuse and neglect. *Education and Treatment of Children, 5,* 141–155.

Lutzker, J. R., Wesch, D., & Rice, J. M. (1984). A review of project 12-ways: An eco-behavioral approach to the treatment and prevention of child abuse and neglect. *Advances in Behavior Research and Therapy, 6,* 63–73.

Mash, E. J., Johnston, C., & Kovitz, K. (1983). A comparison of the mother-child interactions of physically abused and non-abused children during play and task situations. *Journal of Clinical Child Psychology, 12,* 337–346.

Mastria, E. O., Mastria, M. A., & Harkins, J. C. (1979). Treatment of child abuse by behavioral intervention: A case report. *Child Welfare, 58,* 253–261.

Mayhall, P. D., & Norgard, K. E. (1983). *Child abuse and neglect: Sharing responsibility.* New York: Wiley.

Minuchin, S. (1974). *Families and family therapy.* Cambridge: Harvard University Press.

Mrazek, P. B. (1983). Sexual abuse of children. In Lahey, B. B. & Kazdin, A. E. (Eds.), *Advances in clinical child psychology* (Vol. 6, pp. 199–215). New York: Plenum Press.

Parke, R., & Collmer, M. (1975). Child abuse: An interdisciplinary analysis. In M. Hetherington (Ed.), *Review of child development research* (Vol. 5, pp. 509–590). Chicago: University of Chicago Press.

Patterson, G. R. (1977). A performance theory for coercive family interaction. In R. Cairns (Ed.), *Social interactions: Methods, analysis, and illustrations.* Society for Research in Child Development Monographs, University of Chicago, Chicago, IL.

Patterson, G. R., Ray, R., Shaw, D., & Cobb, T. (1969). *A manual for coding family interactions.* New York: Microfiche Publications.

Patterson, G. R., Reid, J. B., Jones, R. R., & Conger, R. E. (1975). *A social learning approach to family intervention* (Vol. 1). Eugene, OR: Castalia.

Reid, J. B., Taplin, P. S., & Lorber, R. (1981). A social interactional approach to the treatment of abusive families. In R. B. Stuart (Ed.), *Violent behavior: Social learning approaches to prediction, management, and treatment* (pp. 83–101). New York: Brunner/Mazel.

Reynolds, G. S. (1975). *A primer of operant conditioning* (rev. ed.). Glenview, IL: Scott, Foresman.

Rohrbeck, C. A., & Twentyman, C. T. (1986). Multimodal assessment of impulsiveness in abusing, neglecting, and nonmaltreating mothers and their preschool children. *Journal of Consulting and Clinical Psychology, 54,* 231–236.

Sandler, J., Van Dercar, C., & Milhoan, M. (1978). Training child abusers in the use of positive reinforcement practices. *Behaviour Research and Therapy, 16,* 169–175.

Schaffer, H. R., & Crook, C. K. (1979). Maternal control techniques in a directed play situation. *Child Development, 50,* 989–996.

Scott, W. O. N., Baer, G., Christoff, K. A., & Kelly, J. A. (1984). The use of skills training procedures in the treatment of a child abusive parent: A systematic case study. *Journal of Behavior Therapy and Experimental Psychiatry, 15,* 329–336.

Shure, M. B., & Spivak, G. (1972). Means-end thinking, adjustment, and social class among elementary school-aged children. *Journal of Consulting and Clinical Psychology, 38,* 348–353.

Tertinger, D. A., Greene, B. F., & Lutzker, J. R. (1984). Home safety: Development and validation of one component of an ecobehavioral treatment program for abused and neglected children. *Journal of Applied Behavior Analysis, 17,* 159–174.

Wahler, R. G. (1980). The insular mother: Her problem in parent child treatment. *Journal of Applied Behavior Analysis, 13,* 207–219.

Wahler, R. G., Leske, G., & Rogers, E. S. (1979). The insular family: A deviance support system for oppositional children. In L. A. Hamerlynch (Ed.), *Behavioral systems for the developmentally disabled: I. School and family environments.* New York: Brunner/Mazel.

Wolfe, D. A. (1985). Child-abusive parents: An empirical review and analysis. *Psychological Bulletin, 97,* 462–482.

Wolfe, D. A., Kelly, J. A., & Drabman, R. S. (1981). "Beat the buzzer": A method for training an abusive mother to decrease recurrent child conflicts. *Journal of Clinical Child Psychology, 10,* 114–116.

Wolfe, D. A., Fairbank, J. A., Kelly, J. A., & Bradlyn, A. S. (1983). Child abusive parents: Physiological responses to stressful and nonstressful behavior in children. *Behavioral Assessment, 5,* 363–371.

Wolfe, D. A., & Sandler, J. (1981). Training abusive parents in effective child management. *Behavior Modification, 5,* 320–335.

Wolfe, D. A., Sandler, J., & Kaufman, K. (1981). A competency-based parent training program for child abusers. *Journal of Consulting and Clinical Psychology, 49,* 633–640.

Wolfe, D. A., St. Lawrence, J. S., Graves, K., Brehony, K., Bradlyn, A. S., & Kelly, J. A. (1982). Intensive behavioral parent training for a child abusive mother. *Behavior Therapy, 13,* 438–451.

PART V

CONCLUSIONS

CHAPTER 12

FUTURE DIRECTIONS

JAMES GARBARINO

INTRODUCTION

In this chapter we will consider future directions in understanding factors contributing to child abuse and neglect. What does the future hold for this important field? We may examine five such directions: expanding definitions, increasing polarization of family experiences, proliferating linkage between child maltreatment and other dimensions of developmental risk, intensifying debate over the nature of community responsibility for children, and growing importance of psychological maltreatment as an integrating concept in the study of child abuse and neglect.

1. *Expanding definitions.* Child maltreatment is a social judgment. Thus, we create rather than discover categories of abuse and neglect.
2. *Polarization of family experiences.* Socioeconomic polarization, coupled with geographic segregation, predicts increasing concentration of risk for child maltreatment among low resource, high-stress families, who are increasingly estranged from affluent and socially connected families.
3. *Proliferating linkage.* As the definition of child abuse and neglect

---

JAMES GARBARINO • Erikson Institute for Advanced Study in Child Development, Chicago, Illinois 60610.

broadens, the link between child maltreatment and other developmental problems will increase. This includes linking physical abuse to subsequent criminal aggression, and sexual abuse to subsequent sexual assault. It also includes the linkage between prevention of child abuse and social reform.

4. *Community responsibility for children.* As definitions of child maltreatment expand and prevention initiatives increase, debate over the proper normal role of the community in the lives of children will intensify. Is child rearing presumed private until proven otherwise, or does the community have a vested right of access for purposes of preventing child maltreatment?

5. *Psychological maltreatment.* As research moves forward, there is growing recognition that psychological maltreatment is the common thread that binds together all forms of maltreatment and accounts predominantly for developmental outcomes.

EXPANDING DEFINITIONS

Child maltreatment is not a natural fact; it is a social judgment. In the future we must attend more to this basic principle. We do not "discover" child abuse and neglect; rather, we "create" it. Instead of being some set of objective categories of action (as is sometimes implied by standard definitions of "acts that harm the child"), child maltreatment is the product of child advocacy in raising the minimal standard of care for children. It is a social judgment that particular patterns of behavior are sufficiently inappropriate *and* dangerous as to warrant community action. Some parental treatment of children is judged to be inappropriate but not dangerous (e.g., letting children watch violently explicit television or permissively indulging children). Other potential treatment is dangerous but not thought inappropriate (e.g., playing football, or circumcision). To call something child maltreatment means that it meets both criteria (e.g., beating a child with board, taking sexually explicit pictures of the child, tying the child to a bed).

The key to this process is its historical dimension. It moves forward through a series of negotiated settlements between professional expertise and citizen values. We have seen this process at work actively in the last 25 years, as we see clearly in the case of vehicular neglect.

What proportion of injuries to children as occupants of automobiles were the result of child neglect in 1959? Virtually none: We did not have a minimal standard of care for children in automobiles then. We do now, and most injuries are now neglect related (because most injuries—and

90+% of deaths) are preventable if the minimal standard (car seats) is met. Through a process of advocacy based upon professional expertise a minimal standard was created. We now have a standard at a given time, in a specific political context.

Of course, one effect of this process is to increase the amount of child maltreatment (at least temporarily), as we raise the minimal standard and to create minimal standards in domains in which none existed before. This applies particularly to educational neglect, psychological maltreatment, and minimal physical abuse particularly (in the past two decades, at least).

The recent Straus and Gelles (1986) national survey of two-parent families may be seen as evidence of this phenomenon. From 1975 to 1985, Straus and Gelles found a 50% decrease in the (self-reported) physical abuse of children (at least 3-year-olds) among two-parent families. One interpretation of this evidence is to see in it the taking hold of the minimal standard of care with respect to physical assault. The field created physical child abuse in the period from 1962 to 1975 and then began to prevent it in the period from 1975 to 1985. We may envision this process continuing among families receptive to prevention messages and programs (i.e., normal families with sufficient resources to act responsively, and with sufficient prosocial relationships to motivate such responsible actions). The reciprocal of this hopeful prognostication is, however, a recognition of growing polarization of experience (the haves and the have nots) with concomitant bad news for the children of socioeconomic impoverishment.

POLARIZATION OF FAMILY EXPERIENCES

The mid-1960s were a time of socioeconomic optimism (and with good reason), because the peculiar workings of the post-1950s economy seemed to promise further extensions of affluence. Policy analysis suggested that poverty could be neutralized by institutional initiative. And indeed poverty was diminished dramatically for the elderly (who had traditionally been disproportionately poor). Poverty among families with children likewise declined.

But, the 1980s have been notable for growing poverty among families with children—now affecting about 25% of the young in America. This reflects public policy—a retreat from some key subsidy programs. But it also reflects an end to the peculiar economic conditions that gave rise to the spreading affluence of the 1960s and 1970s (Garbarino, 1988). The changed climate has exposed the underlying dynamics driving impoverishment in the fourth quarter of the twentieth century in the United States (including higher standards of minimal competence for participation in the affluent economy, public policies geared to enhancing the opportunities for the already affluent, and an individualistic ideology). All of the aforementioned facts portends growing polarization of family experiences, with a significant proportion (up to 25%) of families in even more deteriorated socioeconomic environments. Such an environment provides one feature of the future for studying and dealing with children at-risk for maltreatment.

We can see this insidious dynamic at work in many metropolitan and rural communities, where impoverishment is already dominant for a large segment of the population (a segment already often geographically concentrated in high-risk areas). Growing public discussion of the "underclass" serves to highlight this process of polarization. What is its relevance to child maltreatment?

In principle, nearly everyone is a potential child abuser. We know this from history and from Stanley Milgrim's laboratory studies of the "Eichmann Effect" (in which normal people perform acts of brutality under the impetus of situational stress and role pressure). Some few "saints" might be incapable of attacking or abandoning a child. Nevertheless, we must acknowledge significant *de facto* variations in risk. Child maltreatment becomes an ever more likely fact of life as we descend the socioeconomic ladder. Among the underclass it is so widespread that in most areas there is little or no attempt to employ the same standards of care that apply elsewhere in the community. Even with a triage system operating to screen in only the most immediately and indubitably threatening cases, protective service agencies are overwhelmed once they take the initiative in identifying child maltreatment in such environments.

But this matter of incidence is not the whole story. The polarization of family experience is occurring at a time when overall standards of social competence for full participation are rising. Thus, anything that diminishes academic success or employability becomes an ever more serious liability. Child maltreatment does this, and thereby participates in the various cycle of socioeconomic polarization. This leads to a third issue: proliferating linkage.

PROLIFERATING LINKAGE

Over the last twenty years child maltreatment has emerged as a central theme in efforts to understand the origins and consequences of developmental risks. Few psychological or social pathologies are unrelated (at least statistically) to child maltreatment. The reported consequences of child maltreatment include death, disability, delinquency, deviant personality, learning problems, and communication disorders, to list some of the more prominent.

Turning to the matter of causation, the origins of child maltreatment are found in a wide range of factors: psychological deficiency, sociological disability, social-psychological stress, and cultural impediments to caring for children. Thus, child maltreatment is linked to an extremely wide range of problems. Such linkage has proliferated as research has addressed a growing list of possible correlates *and* as the process of definition has created more and more categories of child maltreatment.

The future appears to hold more intense scrutiny of the links between child maltreatment and problems. For example, just how powerful is the role of child maltreatment in one generation in producing child maltreatment in the next? As this question is refined, attention focuses on the difficult task of specifying *under what conditions* intergenerational transmission takes place. Is child maltreatment an *independent* contributor to school failure or is it but another consequence of the same environmental and personality factors that produce school failure?

To the degree that improved research reaffirms the commonly perceived widespread linkage of child maltreatment to socioeconomic impoverishment then the public debate may come to focus on the issue of whether or not we can separate child abuse prevention from social reform. Will programs do the job, or must we have structural reform of a dramatic kind? Even to pose this question is to engage a fourth future concern: the nature of community responsibility for children.

COMMUNITY RESPONSIBILITY FOR CHILDREN

At its core, child maltreatment exists as a community judgment about the standards of care. Little wonder, then, that one of the key issues for the future is the nature of community responsibility for children. In the future, as in the past and present, the question is: What is the appropriate role for the community in the lives of children? Alternative models exist.

Soviet ideology casts parents as subsidiary to the state; parents rear citizens with *delegated* authority (delegated by the state to the parent). In the Puritan society of New England, parents acted as agents of God, with the Church as guarantor of God's interest in his children on earth.

Secular, individualistic American society recognizes parents as having natural authority over children by virtue of parenthood. The community's role is to intervene only when parents have abused or neglected their children.

Any other intrusion is generally unjustified (as the very word *intrusion* makes clear: the community is outside) unless it is voluntarily invited. All this has important implications for preventing child maltreatment and neutralizing or ameliorating risk.

Several years ago, I visited Sweden and Germany, and then returned to the United States. In Sweden, it was taken for granted that parents would produce their children regularly for community-sponsored evaluations (as part of a general preventive orientation to children). In Germany, such a model was thought to be an "intolerable intrusion." However, when families move, they routinely register with the local authorities (including children). Back home, *this* also was thought to be an intolerable intrusion. What, then, is the point? Different models (and perhaps levels) of community responsibility for children are possible, and in fact exist. However, communities take for granted as normal what they have, and consider weird, impossible, or immoral what they do not.

Child abuse prevention efforts hinge upon the community's conception of its relationship to children and their parents. Various models exist. One can define children as the property of parents and trusts that this proprietary relationship will ensure a minimal standard of care; but this model is largely discredited. Another defines the parent–child relationship as one of custody: parents have custody of children, with the community's responsibility being that of guardian of last resort (in cases of parental failure or voluntary request for services). This is the dominant American model. A third approach asserts the community's vested interest in children, and proposes some sort of shared custody of children between parents and community.

I believe that the latter approach is the best context in which to operate child abuse prevention efforts. It provides the basis for a supportive relationship that begins prenatally and that defines community connections as one element of the minimal standard of care for children. As such, it is the very foundation for child abuse prevention initiatives that go beyond enhancement and offer realistic prospects for dealing with the difficult dynamics posed by the concentrations of risks. It provides the philosophic and political foundation for such measures as comprehensive home health visiting that begins during pregnancy and continues as appropriate over the first 2 years of a child's life (cf. Olds,

Henderson, Chamberlin, & Tatelbaum, 1986). It is also what is needed to prevent psychological maltreatment.

PSYCHOLOGICAL MALTREATMENT

As the study of children at-risk matures, I believe it will turn increasingly to the concept of psychological maltreatment as its unifying theme. If we can set minimal standards of care that address directly emotional and intellectual development, identity, and self-esteem, we as a society will have arrived at a mature conception of the social dimension of normality. Armed with this conception, we will be able to formulate better policy and practice for preventing developmental risk.

A national survey revealed that roughly three quarters of American adults believe that repeated yelling or swearing at a child leads to long-term emotional problems for the child much of the time (National Committee for Prevention of Child Abuse, 1987). This is the cornerstone for community action to prevent one form of psychological maltreatment. The future could provide increasing specificity in research and programming around the component concepts of psychological maltreatment: rejection, terrorization, ignoring, isolation, and corruption (Brassard, Germain, & Hart, 1987; Garbarino, Guttmann, & Seeley, 1986). Such a development would advance our understanding of developmental risk and child maltreatment.

SUMMARY

Child maltreatment has emerged as a core issue for those of us concerned with the quality of life for children. Virtually nonexistent as a topic of study by students of child development until the 1970s, it has come to center stage. The future promises to continue this trend, with growing attention to issues of social context (definitions, polarizations of family experience and concentration of risk, and community responsibility) and the psychological processes linking maltreatment to development.

REFERENCES

Brassard, M., Germain, R., & Hart, S. (Eds.). (1986). *Psychological maltreatment of children and youth.* New York: Pergamon Press.

Garbarino, J. (1988). *The future as if it really mattered*. Longmont, CO: Bookmakers Guild.

Garbarino, J., Guttman, E., & Seeley, J. (1986). *The psychologically battered child: Strategies for identification, assessment, and intervention*. San Francisco: Josey-Bass.

National Committee for Prevention of Child Abuse (1987). *Public attitudes and actions regarding child abuse and its prevention*. Chicago, IL: Louis Harris Public Opinion Poll.

Olds, D., Henderson, C., Chamberlin, R., & Tatelbaum, R. (1986). Preventing child abuse and neglect: A randomized trial of nurse home visitation. *Pediatrics, 78,* 65–78.

Straus, M., & Gelles, R. (1986). Societal change and change in family violence from 1975 to 1985 as revealed by two national surveys. *Journal of Marriage and the Family, 48,* 465–479.

AUTHOR INDEX

Cohn, A.H., 61, 79, 99,
105, 232, 245, 253, 266
Cohn, J.F., 187, 195
Colbus, D., 8, 18
Colletta, N.,D., 154, 157,
160, 166
Collins, D., 127, 145
Collmer, C. W., 4, 5, 19,
89, 107, 109, 137, 144,
192, 197, 200, 201, 219
Collmer, M., 269, 270, 282,
286
Commonwealth v. Adams,
73, 79
Conerly, S., 87, 105, 199,
200, 219
Conger, R.D., 95, 105,
121, 130, 131, 141, 159,
165, 170, 190, 196, 270,
271, 272, 281, 285, 286
Conger, R.E., 272, 286
Connecticut v. Jarzbek, 73,
79
Connell, D.B., 116, 118,
124, 144, 158, 169
Conte, J.R., 241, 245, 251,
266
Cook, T.D., 99, 103, 105
Cooper, S.F., 178, 195
Cornelius, D., 251, 267
Cornely, P.J., 157, 165
Corson, J., 65, 81
Costa, J.J., 60, 79
Costello, A., 179, 198
Coster, W., 112, 142
Cotterell, J.L., 157, 166
Coulter, M.L., 71, 82
Cowen, E.L., 227, 245
Cox, W.R., 230, 244
Coy v. Iowa 59, 75, 79
Coyne, J.C., 181, 195
Craig, M.E., 68, 81
Crichton, L., 154, 165
Crimmins, D.B., 274, 285
Crittenden, P.M., 116, 118,
124, 141, 153, 156, 158–
160, 166, 206, 213, 217
Crnic, K.A., 157, 160, 166
Crockenberg, S., 137, 142,
157, 163, 166

Crook, C.K., 276, 286
Cross, A.H., 212, 218
Cross, C.E., 151, 162, 167
Crouter, A.C., 34, 51, 161,
165
Cumming, E., 226, 245
Cumming, J., 226, 245
Cummings, E.M., 157,
166, 188, 197
Curtis, G., 135, 142
Cytryn, L., 183, 198

D'Zurilla, T.J., 278, 285
Dachman, R.S., 8, 18, 239,
245, 246
Damon, L., 199, 200, 219,
260, 263, 266
Daniels, J.H., 153, 169
Dansky, L., 185, 196
Daro, D., 32, 51, 99, 105
Davenport, Y.B., 183, 198
Davidson, H.A., 59, 64–
66, 79, 80
Davis, G.E., 102, 107
Davis, H., 194, 196
Dawson, B., 278, 279, 285
de Armas, A., 278, 279,
285
DeConey, J.J., 62, 80
deLissovoy, V., 6, 17, 89,
105, 200, 207, 218
Denicola, J., 276, 282, 285
Diamond, L.J., 211, 214,
216, 218, 219
Dickens, B.M., 61, 62, 66,
80
Dietrich, K.N., 6, 12, 19,
158, 159, 166, 170, 214,
215, 220
DiLalla, D.L., 159, 166
Disbrow, M.A., 128, 142,
270, 271, 285
Dishion, T.J., 127, 143, 144
Doerr, H., 128, 142, 270,
271, 285
Donovan, W., 204, 205,
218
Dooley, D., 162, 170
Doran, L.D., 128, 129, 144
Dorr, D., 227, 245

Dowdney, L., 136, 142
Downey, G., 151, 155, 166
Drabman, R.S., 276, 281,
287
Draper, P., 202, 208, 217
Drapier, P., 13, 17
Droegemueller, W., 4, 5,
7, 18, 55, 63, 81, 109,
135, 143, 199, 219, 230,
246
Drotar, D., 211, 218
Dublin, C.C., 135, 145
Dubow, E.F., 155, 166
Dubowitz, H., 23, 26, 27,
51
Dumas, J.E., 127, 142, 145,
194, 198
Duncan, D.F., 203, 213,
219
Durfee, M., 199, 200, 219
Durlak, J.A., 255, 267

Easterbrooks, M.A., 157,
168
Eatman, R., 70, 80
Eddelman, J., 240, 246
Edelsohn, G., 71, 82
Edwards, B., 238, 248
Egeland, B., 8–12, 17, 89,
93, 105, 106, 110–113,
115, 116, 124, 134, 136,
137, 142, 145, 154–161,
163, 165–167, 169, 201,
204, 206, 212, 214, 216,
218
Egolf, B., 88–90, 97, 106,
107
Einbender, A.J., 5, 18, 199,
218, 257, 266
Elder, G.H., Jr., 151, 155,
162, 166, 169
Eldredge, R., 125, 126, 143
Elmer, E., 4, 8, 17, 89, 91,
93, 106, 110, 112, 114,
138, 142, 203, 218, 230,
245
Emde, R.N., 211, 218
Emery, R., 177, 196
Engfer, A., 151, 153, 157,
158, 161, 166, 167

308 AUTHOR INDEX

Straker, G., 128, 131–133, 145
Straus, M.A., 28, 37, 39–42, 48, 49, 51, 53, 86, 88, 89, 91, 108, 134, 145, 156, 162, 170, 212, 220, 234, 247, 293, 298
Stringer, S.A., 209, 220
Strock, B.D., 184, 198
Sturkie, K., 260, 263, 267
Sudia, C.E., 96, 108
Sugal, D.P., 255, 267
Sugarman, D., 97, 107
Sussman, E.J., 128, 145, 159, 170, 190, 197
Sylvester, C.E., 179, 197

Talbot, N.E., 162, 170
Taplin, P.S., 113, 128, 130, 145, 210, 22, 252, 254, 267, 270, 286
Tatelbaum, R., 297, 298
Taylor, D., 115, 140
Templin, K., 253, 267
Terrell, D., 227, 245
Tertinger, D.A., 239, 247, 279, 287
Thibaut, J., 71, 82
Thompson, R.,118, 142
Thompson, R.A., 56, 58, 64, 65, 82, 115, 118, 142, 143
Toedter, L., 89, 95, 97, 106
Tong, L., 94, 108
Tonge, W.L., 178, 195
Tooman, P., 29, 50
Toro, P.A., 93, 108
Trainor, C.M., 28, 30, 32, 38, 39, 53
Traylor, J., 194, 196
Treiber, F.A., 190, 196, 270, 286
Trickett, P.K., 128, 130, 131, 145, 159, 170, 190, 197, 209, 220
Tronick, E.Z., 154, 170, 187, 195
Trowell, J., 251, 267
Trudell, B., 236, 237, 243, 247

Tufts New England Medical Center, 257, 267
Turbett, P., 29, 38, 52
Turner, S.M., 179, 198
Twentyman, C.T., 8, 11, 17–19, 89, 90, 108, 128, 130, 132, 141, 143, 156, 168, 208, 217, 233, 234, 244, 245, 270, 272, 284, 286
Tyler, C.W., Jr., 41, 52

United States v. Iron Shell, 74, 83
Urquiza, A.J., 251, 257, 266
Urzi, T., 59, 60, 82

Valentine, D.P., 25, 53
Van Dercar, C., 272, 273, 286
Van Hasselt, V.B., 5, 6, 9, 12, 13, 17, 199, 207, 211–217, 220, 283, 284
Vaughn, B., 204, 214, 218
Vietze, P.M., 153, 154, 158, 164, 170, 203, 220
Von Eye, A., 115, 143
Vondra, J., 7, 18, 149, 154, 162, 163, 165, 167, 170

Wagner, N.N., 43–46, 51
Wahler, R.G., 127, 142, 145, 194, 198, 282, 287
Waisbren, S.E., 211, 221
Wald, M.S., 57, 58, 61, 83, 98, 108
Walker, A., 135, 142
Walker, C.E., 15, 19, 250, 252, 255, 256, 268
Walker, L., 71, 82
Wall, S., 114, 115, 140, 151, 164, 205, 217
Walsh-Allis, G., 184, 197
Walters, G.C., 209, 219
Warner, V., 184, 187, 198
Warren, D.A., 212, 221
Wasserman, G.A., 211, 212, 221

Waterman, J., 94, 107, 130, 133, 140, 159, 165, 199, 200, 219, 260, 263, 266
Waters, E., 112, 114, 115, 140, 141, 146, 151, 164, 205, 217, 220
Waters, G., 128, 130, 131, 144
Watson, D., 155, 170
Watson-Perczel, M., 15, 18, 239, 246
Webb, M.E., 8, 18, 239, 246
Weber, R.A., 157, 160, 168
Webster-Stratton, C., 189, 198
Weeks, D.G., 184, 198
Weinraub, M., 157, 160, 170
Weissman, M.M., 180, 184, 186, 187, 197, 198
Wells, E.A., 128, 129, 144
Wells, S., 66, 68, 81
Welsh, R.J., 214, 219
Werner, E.E., 172, 198
Wesch, D., 239, 246, 279, 286
West, M.O., 193, 198, 211, 219
Whatley, M.H., 236, 237, 243, 247
Wheeler, J.R., 265, 266
Whelan, J.P., 275, 276, 285
Whitcomb, D., 70, 72, 74, 78, 83
White, K.M., 234, 239, 243, 247
White, R., 211, 221
Whitnig, L., 27, 53
Whittaker, J.K., 160, 170
Wieder, S., 152, 161, 168
Williams, D.P., 26, 53, 86, 87, 93, 94, 96, 107
Williams, G.J., 252, 268
Wilson, A., 227, 245
Wilson, H.B., 230, 247
Wilson, S.K., 186, 194, 198
Wimberley, R.C., 91, 107
Wisconsin v. Yoder, 56, 83
Wittig, B., 113, 114, 140

SUBJECT INDEX

/